Neuroanatomy for Medical Students

Second edition

J. L. Wilkinson OBE, MD, FRCS

*Formerly Senior Lecturer, Anatomy Department,
University of Wales College of Cardiff, UK*

with a Foreword by Lord Walton of Detchant

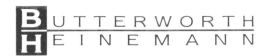
BUTTERWORTH
HEINEMANN

Butterworth–Heinemann Ltd
Linacre House, Jordan Hill, Oxford OX2 8DP

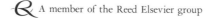 A member of the Reed Elsevier group

OXFORD   LONDON   BOSTON
MUNICH   NEW DELHI   SINGAPORE   SYDNEY
TOKYO   TORONTO   WELLINGTON

First published 1986
Second edition 1992, 1993

British Library Cataloguing in Publication Data
Wilkinson, J.L.
   Neuroanatomy for medical students. — 2nd ed.
   I. Title
   616.8

ISBN 0 7506 1447 1

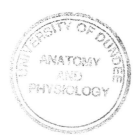

Typeset by Cambridge Composing (UK) Ltd
Printed and bound in Great Britain by
Bath Press Ltd, Bath, Avon

Contents

Foreword

In my Foreword to the first edition of this excellent book, I pointed out that for many years descriptive and topographical anatomy had been under attack by medical educationalists, with the implication that much of the detail taught to medical students of a generation ago was no longer relevant to modern medical practice. However, I went on to say that I firmly believe that medical students should be taught basic neurobiology. This means that they must achieve a thorough grounding in those principles which are relevant to understanding the structure and function of the nervous system. Inevitably this requires them to acquire a core of fundamental knowledge of neuroanatomy, without which it is in my opinion impossible for any doctor to be able to interpret the symptoms and signs of dysfunction of the nervous system in such a way as to construct a differential diagnosis which leads in turn to a planned programme of investigation and treatment.

The first edition, clearly and succinctly written by Dr Wilkinson and beautifully illustrated, presented, as I indicated, that basic core of essential knowledge which provided the infrastructure upon which a stable edifice of neurological pathophysiology could be established by those also possessing the essential physiological and biochemical knowledge. As Dr Wilkinson's Preface makes clear, the second edition is somewhat longer than the first, including more neurophysiology, neuropharmacology and applied anatomy. There are also many new illustrations, a comprehensive glossary has been added and the bibliography has been substantially expanded. Hence, this is not simply a text on neuroanatomy but neuroanatomical principles, clearly outlined and illustrated, are integrated throughout with other essential neurobiological information. In other words, it is an admirable primer of neuroscience which I believe that medical students will find extremely useful. This book provides that fundamental knowledge base which in my view is essential to a proper understanding of the clinical neurosciences. I am happy to commend it most warmly.

Lord Walton of Detchant
Oxford, 1991

Preface

Rapid developments in neuroscience make this second edition necessary: an expanded bibliography, with references throughout the text, includes literature consulted during its preparation. More neurophysiology, neuropharmacology and applied anatomy have been incorporated. Revision of artwork is considerable: 47 new illustrations have been produced, of which 14 are additional, the rest, including the entire brainstem series have been redrawn or photographed. A comprehensive glossary has been added.

Present advances in investigation and understanding will probably accelerate, producing new forms of therapy: it is very desirable that today's students should realize that knowledge is expanding, and exciting progress is taking place. To this end some chapters present a brief account of recent research. Included here are subjects such as nerve growth factor, neural transplantation, dorsal column transection, cerebellar memory, perivascular spaces, neurotransmitters and neuromodulators, nuclear magnetic resonance and position emission tomography. Other topics updated or expanded are: cell membrane structure and function, motor control, muscle spindles, spinocerebellar tracts, reticular formation, striatal transmitters, retinal neurons, pineal gland, pituitary tumours, split brain effect, visual cortex, neural plasticity and barrel fields. A revision section on topography of ventricles and a summary table of cranial nerve are added.

Because the term 'extrapyramidal' is still widely used clinically in describing disorders of basal ganglia, it has been retained in relation to these structures, and collectively to related cortical efferents, corticostriate, -rubral, -olivary, -nigral and -reticular fibres. It is not used in classification of spinal motor pathways.

I am most grateful to Lord Walton for his foreword to this book and his continued interest. My thanks are due to Professor J.Z. Young for Figure 2.6 and to Sir Sydney Sunderland for Figure 3.2; Dr Gordon Armstrong of the Bristol MRI Unit, and Dr J.R. Bradshaw of Bristol Frenchay Hospital Radiology Department kindly provided the new magnetic resonance and computerized tomography scans; Professor D.M. Armstrong of the Physiology Department, Bristol University advised on current cerebellar research; Professor R.O. Weller of the Neuropathology Department, Southampton University on his investigations into perivascular spaces of the brain. In addition to recent research papers and reviews, revision of Chapter 15 owes much to Profesor R. Nieuwenhuys' classical monograph '*Chemoarchitecture of the Brain*'. Glaxo Laboratories and Parke Davis supplied information on Sumatriptan and Tacrin respectively.

My thanks go to many colleagues for their advice, particularly to Dr Robert Santer and Dr Alan Watson for helping me to keep up to date with recent publications. As with the first edition, I am greatly indebted to Catherine Hemington for her excellent line drawings and to Mr Peter Hire for the photography. Finally I wish to acknowledge the support and cooperation of Sue Deeley, Christine Hamer, Michael Maddalena and other staff at Butterworth-Heinemann.

JLW

Chapter 1

Development and topography of the nervous system

The purpose of this chapter is to present a preliminary overall view of the central nervous system. Those who have not yet studied embryology may prefer to start with general topography on page 12. Initially there may seem to be much new terminology, but this unfamiliarity resolves as studies progress: the glossary at the end of the book provides an explanation of all the neuroanatomical and clinical terms used. Many of the features briefly mentioned here can only be fully understood after further description and dissection. Commonly used descriptive terms are *rostral* (towards the beak, or nose); *caudal* (towards the tail); *ventral* (towards the belly) and *dorsal* (towards the back). These terms are equally applicable throughout the animal kingdom.

Development

An understanding of development helps to explain the nervous system's organization (*Fig.* 1.1). In the early embryonic disc, ectoderm overlying the newly-formed notochord thickens to form a midline *neural plate*. The edges of the neural plate become elevated as folds, creating a *neural groove*. Fusion of these folds extends caudally from the cervical region, creating a *neural tube*, with small openings, the *neuropores*, at its rostral and caudal ends, which close by the end of the fourth intrauterine week. Vertebral bodies develop around the notochord, which persists as the nucleus pulposus of intervertebral discs. (Incomplete closure of the caudal neuropore and defective development of associated vertebral arches produce *spina bifida*). The lateral margins of the neural plate comprise specialized *neural crest* cells; neural tube formation segregates these, and in the process of embryonic segmentation they become dorsal root ganglia. (Other neural crest cells provide neurolemmal sheath cells for spinal nerve fibres or migrate to become sympathetic ganglion cells and chromaffin cells of suprarenal medulla.) The rostral part of the neural tube enlarges into forebrain, midbrain and hindbrain vesicles; the remainder remains cylindrical as the spinal cord; neural proliferation in its walls eventually narrows the lumen to a minute central canal.

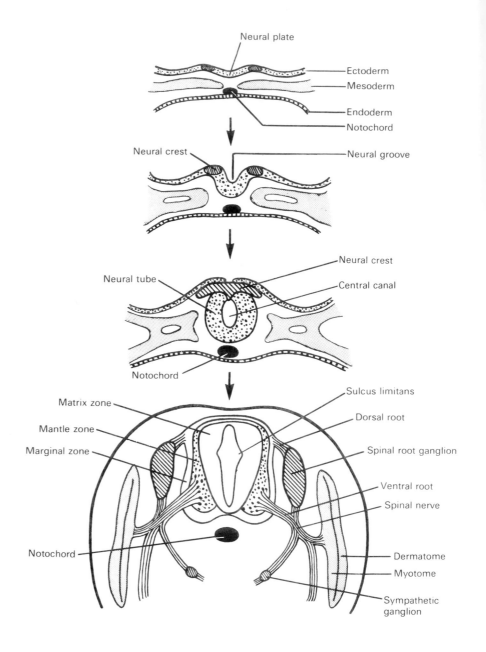

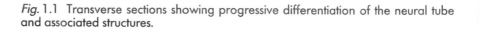

Fig. 1.1 Transverse sections showing progressive differentiation of the neural tube and associated structures.

The spinal cord

Details of histogenesis are beyond this brief account. Transverse sections of the neural tube reveal three layers (*Fig.* 1.1). The inner *matrix zone* is a wide germinal layer, its numerous cells undergoing mitosis; it produces neuroblasts and spongioblasts, the former developing into neurons, the latter into neuroglial cells (astrocytes and oligodendrocytes). The neuroblast cell bodies migrate outwards and form a surrounding *mantle zone*, the future spinal grey matter; their axons pass out further into a *marginal zone*, the future white matter. Central processes from the dorsal root ganglia grow into the neural tube; some ascend in the marginal zone, while others synapse with neurons in the mantle zone. When cell differentiation is complete, the residual cells of the matrix zone form the ependymal lining of the central canal.

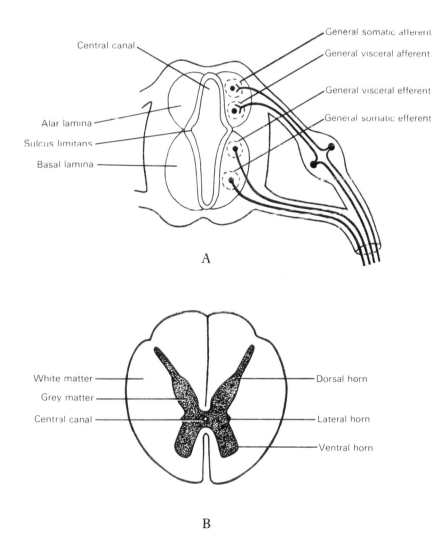

Fig. 1.2 Transverse sections of developing spinal cord showing (A) four cell columns in grey matter; (B) mature (thoracic) spinal cord.

The dorsal and ventral walls of the neural tube remain thin as *roof and floor plates*. On each side the wide mantle zone is demarcated into dorsal (alar) and ventral (basal) regions by an inner longitudinal *sulcus limitans*. Neurons of the *alar lamina* are functionally sensory (afferent). Neurons of the *basal lamina* are motor (efferent), their axons leaving the spinal cord as ventral roots which, with peripheral processes of the dorsal root ganglia, form spinal nerves (*Fig.* 1.2).

Alar and basal laminae are subdivided into four longitudinal *cell columns* with specific functions. These grey columns are seen as 'horns' in cross-sections of a mature cord. The two afferent columns of each alar lamina receive axons from the dorsal root ganglia. Axons from the efferent columns form ventral nerve roots.

The *general somatic afferent* column ('ordinary' sensation) extends throughout the spinal cord and occupies most of the dorsal horn. It receives impulses from superficial (cutaneous) and deep (proprioceptive) receptors.

The *general visceral afferent* column (visceral sensation) at the base of the dorsal horn of cord segments T1–L2 and S2–4, receives impulses from viscera and blood vessels.

The *general visceral efferent* column (to smooth muscle) provides autonomic innervation for viscera, glands and blood vessels. Sympathetic outflow is from a lateral horn (T1–L2). Parasympathetic outflow is via certain cranial nerves and from S2–4 spinal segments. These fibres are termed 'preganglionic' because they all synapse in ganglia before reaching their targets.

The *general somatic efferent* column (to skeletal muscle) extends throughout the spinal cord in the ventral horn.

These four columns are termed 'general' because additional 'special' components are required in the brainstem for faculties such as taste and hearing. Aggregations of nerve cell bodies (somata), visible in transverse sections of grey matter, are often referred to as *'nuclei';* each nucleus has particular functions and its neurons share common pathways.

Developmentally one cord segment (neuromere) serves one myotome and one dermatome on each side. In contrast to the very obvious segmentation of mesodermal somites, embryonic cord segments are not distinctly separated from one another because the developing cord must have internal structural continuity. Functional segmentation is marked externally by the attachments of pairs of spinal nerves.

Initially the spinal cord and vertebral canal are of equal length, but the former grows less rapidly; at birth its caudal end is level with the third lumbar vertebra and in adults reaches only to the disc between the first and second lumbar vertebrae. The more caudal spinal nerve roots are therefore elongated and pass obliquely within the canal before emerging via intervertebral foramina; beyond the spinal cord's tip the vertebral canal contains a bundle of lumbar, sacral and coccygeal roots descending to their respective foramina.

Three membranes, derived from mesenchyme, surround the brain and spinal cord; these *meninges* are termed, from within outwards, pia mater, arachnoid mater and dura mater, and will be described later.

The brain

Three brain vesicles in the rostral part of the neural tube indicate the early division of the latter into *forebrain* (prosencephalon), *midbrain* (mesencephalon) and *hindbrain* (rhombencephalon) (*Fig.* 1.3); their cavities become ventricles in the mature brain. Three flexures appear in this region (*Fig.* 1.4); two are convex dorsally, a *cephalic flexure* (at midbrain level) and a *cervical flexure* (at the junction of hindbrain and spinal cord). A *pontine flexure*, concave dorsally, produced by unequal growth at future pontine level, has a buckling effect, everting the lateral walls and attenuating the roof of the neural tube here (*Fig.* 1.5 and *see Fig.* 5.4). The sensory alar laminae thus become lateral to the motor basal laminae in the floor of a rhomboid-shaped fossa (hence the name rhombencephalon). The part of the hindbrain caudal to the pontine flexure is the *myelencephalon* (future medulla oblongata); the rostral part, from which the pons and cerebellum develop, is the *metencephalon;* the hindbrain cavity becomes the *fourth ventricle*. In contrast, the mesencephalic cavity remains narrow as the *cerebral aqueduct*. The forebrain vesicle develops bilateral outgrowths which together constitute the *telencephalon* (= 'end-brain'); these overgrow and cover the original

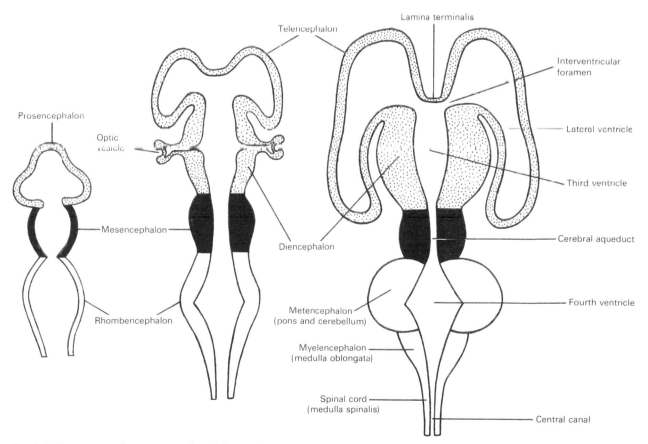

Fig. 1.3 Diagrams of stages in the differentiation of cerebral vesicles and the ventricular system.

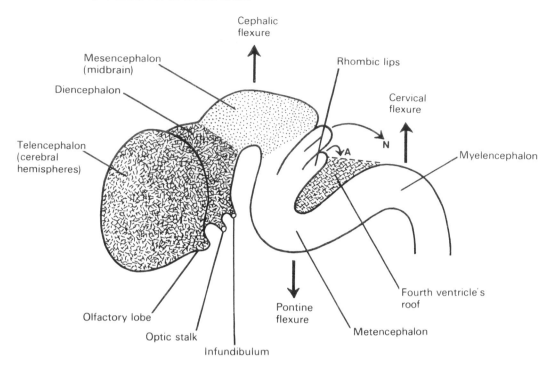

Fig. 1.4 Diagram of the external form of a developing brain and its flexures. Arrows from the rhombic lips indicate the direction of growth of the cerebellum: the neocerebellum (**N**) comes to overhang the fourth ventricle's thin roof, dorsal to the archecerebellum (**A**).

forebrain, which becomes the diencephalon (= 'between-brain'). The twin cavities of telencephalon develop into two *lateral ventricles;* the midline cavity of diencephalon is the *third ventricle.*

The hindbrain (rhombencephalon)

The caudal myelencephalon has a central canal and becomes the closed part of the medulla. Rostrally this canal widens into the fourth ventricle: its floor, derived from myelencephalon (medulla) and metencephalon (pons), has a longitudinal sulcus limitans on each side, separating the alar and basal laminae. Cranial nerves with nuclear origins in these laminae differ from spinal nerves in the number and type of their components. In addition to four general components, there are special sensory nuclei concerned with taste (gustatory), hearing (cochlear) and equilibration (vestibular), and special motor nuclei innervating muscle of branchial origin. Some cranial nerves have only one component, either sensory or motor, while others have more, for example the vagus nerve has five. Concerned with input to the developing cerebellum, numerous *pontine nuclei* and the medullary *inferior olivary nucleus* migrate ventrally from the alar laminae. Long ascending and descending fibres ultimately traverse the ventral region.

The attenuated roof of the developing fourth ventricle is a single layer of ependymal cells with a thin covering of pia mater; this is a *tela choroidea*, a vascularized membrane in which a *choroid plexus* of blood vessels forms (*Fig. 1.5*). Cerebrospinal fluid formed within the ventricular system leaves the fourth ventricle through three apertures, one median and two lateral (*see* p. 88).

The *cerebellum* grows from *rhombic lips*, which are bilateral dorsal extensions of the alar plates of the metencephalon (*Fig. 1.5*). These meet and fuse over the fourth ventricle's roof, developing there and folding the tela choroidea and its plexuses inwards towards the ventricular cavity. The neocerebellum, phylogenetically recent and forming much of the cerebellar hemispheres, grows rapidly to overlie the more primitive archecerebellum (*Fig. 1.4*).

The *otocyst*, from which the membranous labyrinth of the internal ear develops, is an invagination of a small area of thickened surface ectoderm (otic placode) on each side of the hindbrain; it becomes isolated from the surface.

The midbrain (mesencephalon)

The mesencephalon retains a generally cylindrical form; its lumen becomes the narrow cerebral aqueduct (*Fig. 1.3*, and *see Fig. 1.13*). The nuclei of two

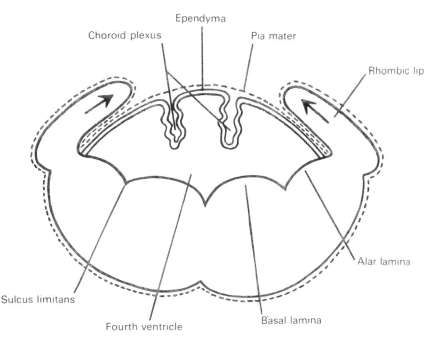

Fig. 1.5 Developing fourth ventricle and cerebellum. Pia mater vascularizes ependyma to form a choroid plexus in the roof. Alar laminae lie lateral to basal laminae. Rhombic lips, derived from alar laminae, grow together to form the cerebellum, dorsal to the ventricular roof.

motor cranial nerves (oculomotor and trochlear) develop in its basal laminae. Cells of the alar laminae invade the roof plate, forming bilateral longitudinal ridges which later become subdivided by a transverse groove. Thus four small elevations, the *corpora quadrigemina*, develop in the tectum (roof) dorsal to the aqueduct. The developmental origins of the red nuclei and substantia nigra are less certain.

The forebrain (prosencephalon)

At an early stage, before closure of the anterior neuropore, paired, hollow, lateral *optic vesicles* diverge forwards from the forebrain. On reaching the surface ectoderm, these invaginate to form retinae, from which nerve fibres grow proximally through the hollow optic stalks to form optic nerves.

The *diencephalon* develops from the original forebrain vesicle. The two *thalami* form on each side in the dorsal part of the third ventricle's walls, the *hypothalamus* in their lower regions and floor. A downgrowth from the floor, the *neurohypophysis*, joins an upgrowth from the stomodeum which becomes the *adenohypophysis;* together these constitute the *hypophysis cerebri* (pituitary gland). The roof is thin, comprising ependyma and pia mater; as in the fourth ventricle, this forms a *tela choroidea* with *choroid plexuses*. The *epithalamus*, consisting of the pineal gland and habenular nuclei, develops posteriorly in the roof. The closed rostral end of the neural tube persists as a thin *lamina terminalis*.

The *telencephalon* comprises paired cerebral vesicles, their developing lateral ventricles each communicating with the third ventricle through an interventricular foramen (*Fig.* 1.6). The developing cerebral hemispheres enlarge upwards and forwards, then backwards and inferiorly in a C-shaped manner, their caudal growth flanking the diencephalon, then fusing with it on each side (*Fig.* 1.7). The lowest part of the medial walls of the ventricles remains thin, only ependyma. Pia vascularizes this ependyma to form a tela choroidea, edged with choroid plexuses, invaginating the lateral ventricles through a linear *choroid fissure* which extends posteriorly on each side from the interventricular foramen (*Fig.* 1.8). Early in development, the phylogenetically ancient *hippocampus* (archecortex) forms a thickening of the medial wall above the interventricular foramen and choroid fissure on each side. The two hippocampi are connected by a bundle of fibres, the *fornix;* the choroid fissure develops between fornix and thalamus. Subsequent massive development of the cerebral hemispheres (neocortex) displaces the hippocampi posteroinferiorly, the fornix being drawn out as an efferent tract on the medial side of each hippocampus. The choroid fissure also becomes curved, bounded peripherally throughout by the fornix.

Commissural fibres interconnect the growing hemispheres and initially the only median structure which can be bridged is the lamina terminalis (*Fig.* 1.8). The *anterior commissure* develops in, and remains connected to, the lamina terminalis, passing from the olfactory bulbs and temporal lobes of one hemisphere to those of the other. The *corpus callosum*, the major interhemispheric commissure, also starts in the upper lamina terminalis but it grows massively as the hemispheres develop, expanding posteriorly above

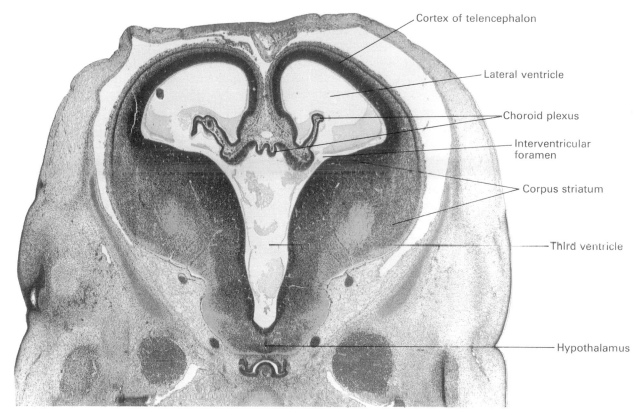

Cortex of telencephalon

Lateral ventricle

Choroid plexus

Interventricular foramen

Corpus striatum

Third ventricle

Hypothalamus

Fig. 1.6 Coronal section through the forebrain of a 20-mm pig embryo, × 23.

the fornix and connected to it by a thin midline *septum pellucidum*. Thus the corpus callosum invades the areas formerly occupied by the hippocampi; vestigial hippocampal remnants remain on its superior surface as a very thin mantle of grey matter, the *indusium griseum*, embedded in which are white *longitudinal striae*. The pia mater roofing the third ventricle is continuous anteriorly with that under the corpus callosum; as the latter grows posteriorly, the two pial layers fuse in the tela choroidea, whose plexuses project into the third and lateral ventricles. Between the caudal edge of the developing corpus callosum and the epithalamus (pineal gland), the two pial layers separate at the *transverse cerebral fissure*, through which choroidal arteries enter and internal cerebral veins leave (*Fig.* 1.10).

The *corpus striatum* develops on each side in the floor of the telencephalon, alongside the thalami (*Fig.* 1.7) (primitively these deep areas of grey matter were motor and sensory 'control centres'). Development of the cerebral hemispheres requires a major pathway for descending fibres from the cortex and ascending fibres from thalamus to cortex; the only route is through this region. Thus, on each side, an aggregation of fibres, the *internal capsule*, divides the corpus striatum into a dorsomedial *caudate nucleus* which bulges

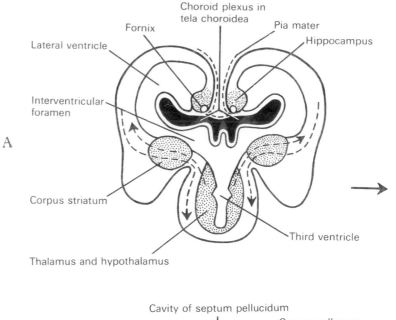

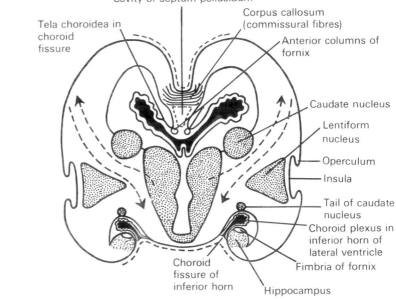

Fig. 1.7 Coronal sections through the forebrain to show development of the internal capsule: arrows indicate the path taken by its descending and ascending fibres. In (A) the telencephalon is a bilateral outgrowth, its cortex thin, the corpus striatum in its floor, the interventricular foramina are wide, choroid plexuses project into the lateral and third ventricles. In (B) the telencephalon has enlarged down around the diencephalon, fusing with its lateral surfaces; the internal capsule has divided corpus striatum into caudate and lentiform nuclei; the corpus callosum has separated tela choroidea from dorsal surface; ependyma and residual pia mater form a septum pellucidum with small central cavity; the hippocampus has been displaced into the floor of inferior horn of lateral ventricle.

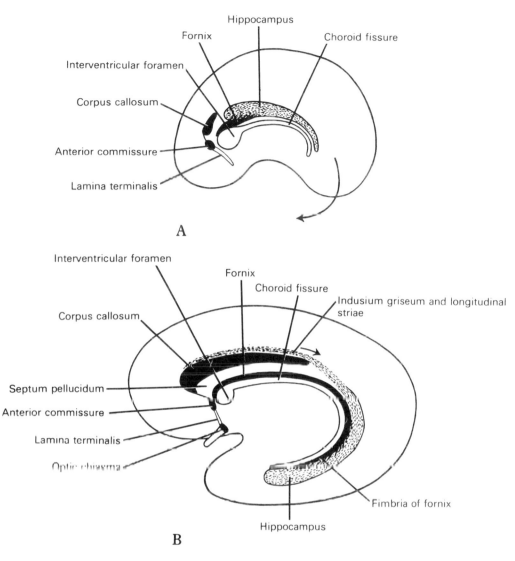

Fig. 1.8 Medial aspects of right foetal cerebral hemispheres to show development of commissures and choroid fissure. In (A) the corpus callosum is rudimentary and the hippocampus overlies the interventricular foramen. In (B) the corpus callosum is much larger and the hippocampus is being displaced into the developing temporal lobe; its fornix bounds the choroid fissure peripherally.

into the lateral ventricle, and a ventrolateral *lentiform nucleus* which is deep to the cortex (here known as the *insula*).

The *cerebral hemispheres* grow rapidly forwards (frontal region), posteriorly (occipital region), then anteroinferiorly (forming the temporal lobe). This curved pattern of expansion from the interventricular foramina round the diencephalon explains the C-shaped formation of related structures such as the lateral ventricles, choroid fissures and fornix (*Fig.* 1.8). The caudate nucleus is so-called because it has a tail (= cauda) which curves round into the temporal lobe. Initially the cortical surface is smooth. At the end of the third intrauterine month a lateral depression appears over each lentiform nucleus; rapid growth in adjoining areas causes a *lateral cerebral fissure* to develop here, the submerged cortex forming the insula. With continued development the cortical surface becomes furrowed by *sulci*, the intervening convolutions forming *gyri*. Neuroblasts, developed in the deep (matrix) zone have here migrated superficially to form the cortex, the intervening zone becoming white matter.

General Topography in the Adult

The *central nervous system* comprises the brain and spinal cord; the *peripheral nervous system* comprises the cranial and spinal nerves and their ramifications.

Peripheral nervous system

There are 12 paired cranial and 31 paired spinal nerves. The constituent nerve fibres innervate somatic or visceral structures and convey afferent (sensory) or efferent (motor) impulses. *Somatic efferent fibres* pass directly from their cells of origin in the central nervous system to skeletal muscle. *Autonomic (visceral) efferent fibres* from the central nervous system are pre-ganglionic, synapsing in peripheral ganglia with neurons that innervate smooth muscle and glands. *Somatic* and *visceral afferent fibres* pass from peripheral receptors to their cells of origin in spinal dorsal root ganglia, or in equivalent ganglia of certain cranial nerves.

The autonomic nervous system has *sympathetic* and *parasympathetic* divisions. Sympathetic outflow is from the spinal *thoracolumbar* region (T1–L2). Parasympathetic outflow is *craniosacral* in origin, occurring from two widely separated sources, via the oculomotor, facial, glossopharyngeal, and vagus cranial nerves and S2–4 spinal nerves. Sympathetic and parasympathetic systems generally have opposing actions. Sympathetic activity accompanies expenditure of energy, as in an emergency situation ('fright, fight, flight') producing such symptoms as pupillary dilatation, cardio-acceleration, cutaneous vasoconstriction, increased blood pressure, reduced peristalsis and contraction of sphincters. Parasympathetic activity conserves and restores energy ('repose and repair'), slowing the heart rate and increasing peristalsis and glandular activity.

Central nervous system

The brain and spinal cord may be described (in a simplified way) as consisting of grey matter (nerve cell bodies and mostly non-myelinated fibres) and white matter (chiefly myelinated fibres) with neuroglial cells and blood capillaries occurring throughout. Topographically the central nervous system may be divided into forebrain (cerebral hemispheres and diencephalon), midbrain, hindbrain (pons, medulla oblongata and cerebellum) and spinal cord. The midbrain, pons and medulla oblongata collectively form the *brainstem*.

The forebrain

The paired *cerebral hemispheres* have an external grey *cortex* and a white centre; in the latter there are deep grey masses, the *basal ganglia*. The two hemispheres are separated by a median longitudinal fissure, and joined by a massive bridge or commissure, the *corpus callosum*, whose fibres interconnect corresponding cortical areas. The cerebral cortex is convoluted by *gyri* and furrowed by *sulci*. The *insular cortex* is submerged in the *lateral fissure* (of Sylvius). The *central sulcus* extends from the superomedial border of the hemisphere, slightly posterior to its mid-point, down and forwards towards the lateral fissure. Sulci partially divide the hemispheres into lobes named after the cranial bones adjacent to them (*Fig. 1.9*). The *frontal lobe* is anterior

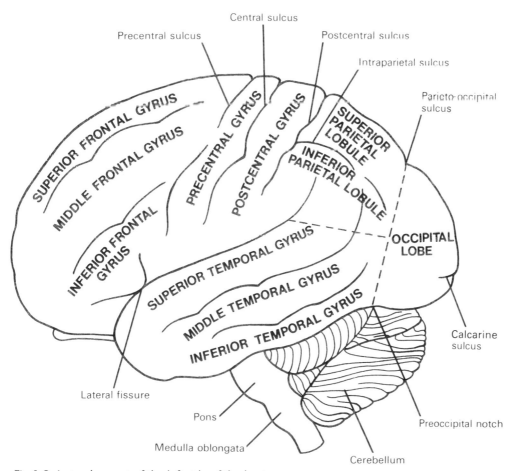

Fig. 1.9 Lateral aspect of the left side of the brain.

to the central sulcus and above the lateral fissure; the *parietal lobe* is posterior to the central sulcus and above the lateral fissure; the *occipital lobe* is behind a line from the parieto-occipital sulcus to the pre-occipital notch; the *temporal lobe* is below the lateral fissure and in front of the pre-occipital notch. The so-called limbic lobe is a composite bordering zone (limbus) between the telencephalon and diencephalon, extending through the septal area (anterior to the lamina terminalis) and the cingulate gyrus (above the corpus callosum) to the parahippocampal gyrus (on the inferior surface of the temporal lobe, adjacent to the brainstem and continuous with the hippocampus).

Sensory tracts to the cerebral cortex comprise three neurons: the cell bodies of primary sensory neurons are in dorsal root ganglia, secondary neurons are in spinal cord or medulla, tertiary neurons in the thalamus. Input from one side of the body projects to the opposite (contralateral) cerebral hemisphere. Cortical motor control of the limbs is also contralateral.

The *diencephalon*, lying between the cerebral hemispheres and brainstem, consists of thalami, hypothalamus and epithalamus. Each *thalamus*, an egg-shaped grey mass lateral to the third ventricle, is a major relay and integration centre for ascending fibres, receiving axons of secondary sensory neurons; thalamic tertiary sensory neurons project to the cerebral cortex. The thalami also integrate motor functions, relaying impulses from the cerebellum and

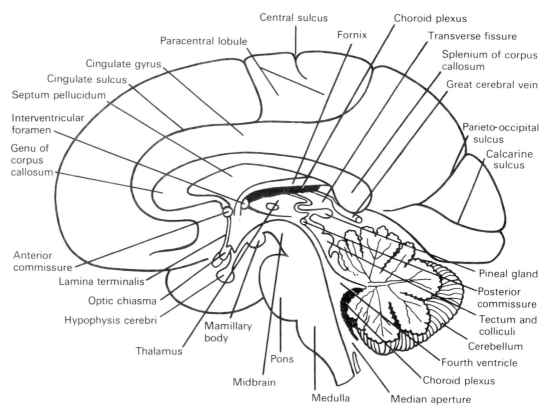

Fig. 1.10 Median sagittal section of the brain.

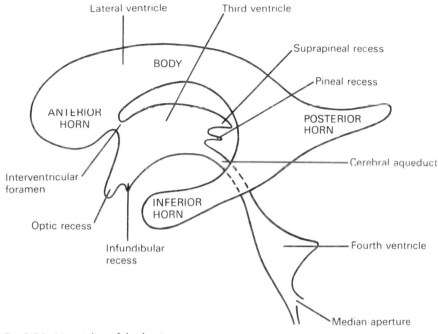

Fig. 1.11 Ventricles of the brain.

corpus striatum to the motor cortex. Connexions with the limbic system influence behaviour, mood and memory. The *hypothalamus* (= 'below thalamus') regulates visceral activity through the autonomic nervous system and hormonal activity through the hypophysis cerebri. The *epithalamus*, sited posteriorly in the diencephalic roof, includes the pineal gland and habenular nuclei. Reduction of pineal secretion precipitates puberty; the habenular nuclei have olfactory and limbic connexions. The subthalamus is between the diencephalon and midbrain.

The *basal ganglia* include the corpus striatum within each cerebral hemisphere and the substantia nigra and red nuclei in the midbrain: relaying through the thalamus to the cortex, they influence the quality of motor performance and are sometimes termed 'extrapyramidal nuclei'. The red nuclei also have caudal connexions. The compact mass of white fibres in the *internal capsule* partially divides each corpus striatum into a medial caudate and a lateral lentiform nucleus (*see Figs* 9.2 and 9.4). Between the internal capsule and the cortex, nerve fibres diverge as the *corona radiata*.

Within each cerebral hemisphere the *lateral ventricle* has a central body, anterior horn (in the frontal lobe), posterior horn (in the occipital lobe) and inferior horn (in the temporal lobe) (*Fig.* 1.11). It connects via an *interventricular foramen* (of Monro) with the third ventricle, which continues via the cerebral aqueduct to the fourth ventricle. Cerebrospinal fluid, formed by ventricular *choroid plexuses*, passes through apertures in the fourth ventricle into the subarachnoid space around the brain and spinal cord. The two lateral ventricles are separated anteriorly by the midline *septum pellucidum* (between corpus callosum and fornix) (*Fig.* 1.10); posteriorly the lateral ventricles diverge from one another. Each interventricular foramen is bounded in front by the fornix, behind by the thalamus.

The brain and spinal cord are surrounded by three meninges, the pia mater, arachnoid mater and dura mater. The *pia mater* is adherent to the brain and spinal cord. The subarachnoid space (between pia mater and arachnoid mater) contains cerebrospinal fluid and the major arteries; the latter may rupture and produce a subarachnoid haemorrhage. The *dura mater* adheres to the internal cranial surface, and is infolded vertically between the cerebral hemispheres as a sickle-shaped *falx cerebri* (*see Fig.* 13.1). The *tentorium cerebelli* is a horizontal dural partition over the posterior cranial fossa, between the cerebrum and the cerebellum, its free edge at midbrain level. The dura mater encloses *venous sinuses* which receive all the venous drainage of the brain.

The midbrain

The *mesencephalon* (*Figs* 1.10 and 1.13) is traversed by the *cerebral aqueduct;* dorsal to this the roof, or *tectum*, has four little hillocks (colliculi) which comprise the *corpora quadrigemina*. Ventral to the aqueduct a central *tegmentum* is separated ventrally from two *crura cerebri* by pigmented grey matter, the *substantia nigra*. Each crus is in continuity with the internal capsule of the same side and contains fibres descending to the spinal cord (corticospinal fibres), pontine nuclei (corticopontine fibres) and brainstem (corticobulbar fibres). Between the crura is an *interpeduncular fossa*. In the tegmentum are two large, oval, pinkish, nuclear masses, the red nuclei. Two *superior cerebellar peduncles* enter the lower midbrain and their fibres decussate (cross over), some entering red nuclei, most ascending to the thalamus. The oculomotor and trochlear cranial nerves have midbrain origins.

The hindbrain

The *rhombencephalon* consists of pons, medulla oblongata and cerebellum. The pons is continuous above with the midbrain and below with the medulla oblongata, which blends into the spinal cord just below the foramen magnum (*Fig.* 1.12). The hindbrain cavity is the fourth ventricle.

The *pons*, as the name suggests, is a broad, bridge-like structure on its ventral aspect, its transverse fibres forming the *middle cerebellar peduncles;* a ventral median sulcus adjoins the basilar artery. In transverse section (*Fig.* 1.13) it is seen to consist of a large ventral and a smaller dorsal region. In the ventral region, numerous *pontine nuclei* give rise to transverse fibres which cross the midline into the opposite middle cerebellar peduncle; bundles of fibres descend from the crura of the midbrain to the pyramids of the medulla. In the dorsal part, or *tegmentum*, there is a diffuse *reticular formation* of small cells and fibres (which extend throughout the brainstem) and nuclei of the trigeminal, abducent, facial and vestibulocochlear cranial nerves.

The *medulla oblongata* (*Fig.* 1.10, 1.12 and 1.13) is somewhat conical, its caudal closed part and central canal continuous with the spinal cord; rostrally the canal opens into the fourth ventricle. Bilateral ventral surface elevations,

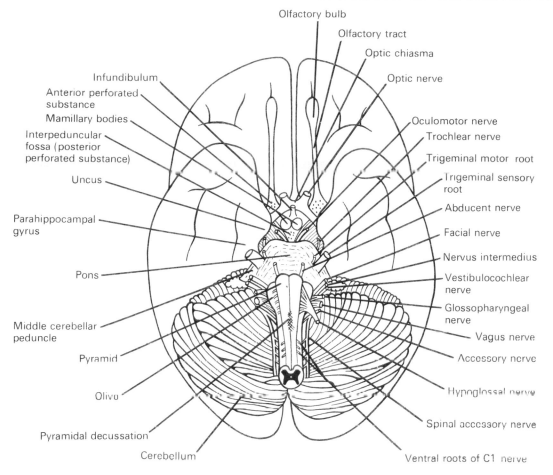

Fig. 1.12 Inferior aspect of the brain and origins of the cranial nerves.

the *pyramids*, contain corticospinal (pyramidal) fibres, most of which cross in a *pyramidal decussation* to descend contralaterally in the spinal cord. Alongside each pyramid an oval surface swelling, the olive, contains the *inferior olivary nucleus*, where various cerebellar afferents converge. Dorsal to each olive is an *inferior cerebellar peduncle*. On each side of the dorsal surface of the lower medulla there are *gracile and cuneate tubercles* produced by similarly named nuclei which receive ascending fibres from the dorsal columns of the spinal cord. The medulla contains nuclei of the glossopharyngeal, vagus, cranial accessory and hypoglossal cranial nerves. The trigeminal sensory nuclear complex extends throughout the brainstem and into the first two spinal cord segments.

The *cerebellum*, dorsal to the pons and medulla, has two lateral *hemispheres* and a midline *vermis*. It is connected to the midbrain, pons and medulla respectively by superior, middle and inferior *peduncles*. Its *cortex* has narrow transverse *folia* (leaf-like in sections), separated by deep fissures. The white

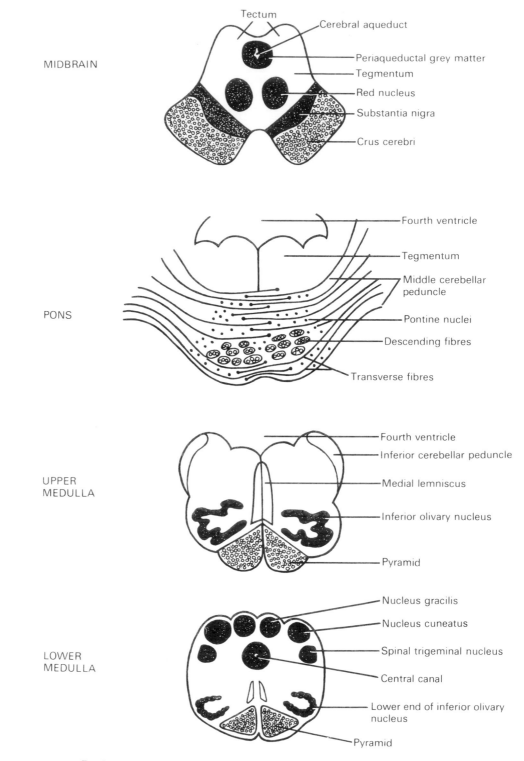

Fig. 1.13 Transverse sections of the brainstem.

medullary centre contains *intracerebellar nuclei*, the largest is termed the *dentate nucleus* because it has a tooth-like profile. The cerebellum is close to the fourth ventricle's roof, formed by *superior and inferior medullary vela*, the latter invaginated by a choroid plexus and perforated posteriorly by a median aperture. The ventricular floor (rhomboid fossa) has a recess on each side, leading to two lateral apertures.

Connexions between cerebellum and spinal cord are predominantly uncrossed (ipsilateral = 'to the same side'). Afferent tracts to the cerebellum comprise two neurons, their primary and secondary cell bodies located in dorsal root ganglia and spinal cord respectively.

The spinal cord

The spinal cord is continuous rostrally with the medulla oblongata and ends caudally as a tapered *conus medullaris*; in adults this reaches the level of the first lumbar intervertebral disc (between L1 and L2). The dura mater, arachnoid mater and the *subarachnoid space*, containing cerebrospinal fluid, extend to vertebral level S2. External to the dura mater an *epidural space* contains fat, blood vessels and lymphatics.

The cord is not of uniform diameter throughout: there are *cervical* and *lumbar enlargements*, associated with innervation of the limbs. The region of origin of a pair of spinal nerves marks a *cord segment*. The paired spinal nerves are: 8 cervical, 12 thoracic, 5 lumbar, 5 sacral and 1 coccygeal, each attached by a dorsal (sensory) and a ventral (motor) root. The spinal nerves pierce the dura mater, traverse the epidural space and leave the vertebral canal through intervertebral foramina. The lumbar, sacral and coccygeal nerve roots extend beyond the spinal cord as the *cauda equina*, so-named because it resembles a horse's tail.

The spinal cord has central grey and peripheral white matter. In transverse sections the grey matter has an irregular H-shape (*Fig. 1.2*) with two *ventral horns*, two *dorsal horns* and a *grey commissure* containing a minute *central canal*. In the thoracic there are also *lateral horns*. These horns, seen on section, represent columns of grey matter in the intact cord. White matter is demarcated bilaterally into *ventral*, *lateral* and *dorsal white columns* (*funiculi*) by the lines of attachment of spinal nerve roots.

Chapter 2

Neurons and neuroglia

The Neuron

Neurons are cells specialized for the reception, integration and transmission of information. Each has a cell body or *soma* and processes or *neurites*. Receptor neurites, known as *dendrites*, are usually numerous; each soma has only one efferent process, the *axon*. The cytoplasm or *perikaryon* of the soma contains perinuclear basophilic material in the form of granular *Nissl bodies*. These are absent close to axonal origin in the *axon hillock*, whose continuation is the *initial segment* of the axon. Axons have an external plasma membrane, the *axolemma*, enclosing their cytoplasm, known as *axoplasm;* they may have *collateral branches* and end by *synapses* either with other neurons or with effectors at neuromuscular or neuroglandular junctions.

Neuronal somata vary in size from 5 μm to 120 μm. According to their dendritic patterns they are classified as unipolar, bipolar and multipolar (*Fig. 2.1*). *Unipolar neurons* (e.g. in dorsal root spinal ganglia) have a spherical soma and a single process which bifurcates to pass centrally and peripherally; sometimes termed *pseudo-unipolar*, each develops from a bipolar cell whose processes fuse near the soma. *Bipolar neurons* have an elongated soma with a process at each pole; associated with some special senses, they exist in the retina, the olfactory mucosa, and the cochlear and vestibular ganglia. *Multipolar neurons*, afferent or efferent in function, are irregular in somal shape with many dendrites and are the most numerous neurons in the central nervous system; they are classified as Golgi Type I or II. *Golgi Type I* neurons have a large soma and a long axon, for example pyramidal cells of the cerebral cortex, Purkinje cells of the cerebellar cortex and spinal ventral horn cells; they transfer information from one region to another. *Golgi Type II* are interneurons with a small, often stellate, soma and a short axon which terminates locally.

Neurocytological investigation

For light microscopy, neural tissue may be stained in various ways. *Nucleic acid dyes*, including cresyl violet and toluidine blue, stain nuclei and Nissl bodies, demonstrating somata but not axons. *Silver stains* (e.g. *Cajal* and *Golgi* methods) depend on the affinity of neural tissue for silver; nerve cells and their processes stain darkly while myelin is unstained. *Myelin stains:*

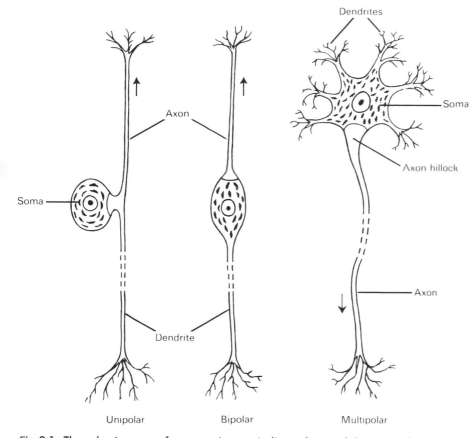

Fig. 2.1 Three basic types of neuron. Arrows indicate the usual direction of impulse transmission.

(a) in the *Weigert* method, potassium dichromate makes myelin sheaths stainable by haematoxylin and they become dark blue; (b) the *Marchi* technique demonstrates degenerating fibres, potassium dichromate rendering normal myelin yellow-brown, osmic acid staining fatty acids of degenerating myelin black.

In recent years, *histochemical* and *immunocytochemical techniques* have made possible the identification of individual neurotransmitters and associated enzymes in neurons. For example, using formaldehyde-induced fluorescence, noradrenaline (norepinephrine) appears pale green and serotonin (5–HT) yellow when exposed to ultraviolet light. Neurotransmitter pathways have been classified, and these are described in Chapter 15.

Axon-tracing in the past depended on degeneration techniques. If central connexions are destroyed, the axons degenerate; following axonal damage the soma undergoes *chromatolysis*, it swells, the nucleus becomes eccentric in position, and the Nissl bodies disintegrate and are dispersed as fine granules (*Fig.* 2.2). This is the *acute reaction;* after 14 days the cells may show signs of recovery or may die if the axon is damaged near its origin. By removing individual ocular muscles, thereby severing their nerves, Warwick (1953)

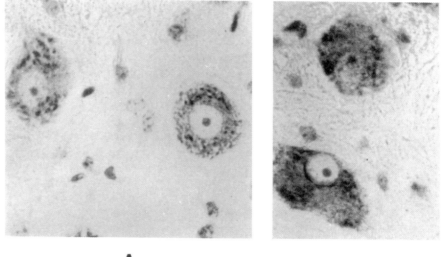

A   B

Fig. 2.2 Chromatolysis in the oculomotor nuclear complex. (A) Normal somatic motor neurons with uniformly distributed large discrete chromatin granules and central nuclei. (B) Following resection of one extra-ocular muscle, somata of affected neurons show disintegration and dispersal of granules and eccentricity of nuclei. (Cresyl violet stain, × 580.) (From an illustration by Warwick R. (1953) *J. Comp. Neurol.* **98**, 499, reproduced by kind permission of author and publisher.)

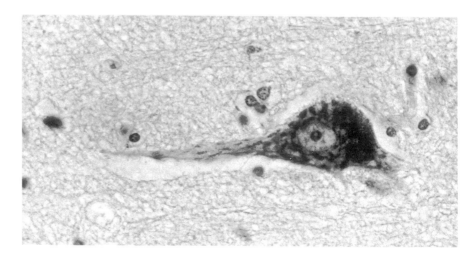

Fig. 2.3 Giant pyramidal (Betz) cell of cerebral motor cortex. (Cresyl violet stain, × 520.)

was able to define their central representation by mapping the resultant chromatolytic neurons. More recent methods utilize orthograde or retrograde axonal transport (Cowan & Cuénod, 1975). Uptake by somata of injected radioactive-labelled amino acids and their subsequent distal (orthograde) axonal transport may be traced by autoradiography. An injection of the enzyme horseradish peroxidase (HRP) is taken up by axon terminals or damaged axons and transferred to somata, where it can be identified histochemically.

Electron microscopy has greatly increased detailed knowledge of cell membranes, organelles, synapses and myelin sheath structure. In combination with other techniques, synaptic relationships between identified neurons are now being elucidated at the ultrastructural level.

Cytology (*Fig.* 2.4)

The *cell membrane* is a bilaminar phospholipid structure with an external layer of glycoprotein. A mosaic of specialized protein molecules within the membrane provides *channels* which are individually selective for the passage of sodium (Na^+), potassium (K^+) or chloride (Cl^-) ions. Some of these channels are *open*, others are *gated*. There are two types of gating. Channels associated with synapses are opened when a neurotransmitter binds to a receptor on the soma or dendrite: this is *ligand gating* (the substance that binds is the ligand). Other channels, mostly on the axon, are *voltage-gated*, being actively opened or closed by changes in the electrical potential of the membrane; the soma has relatively few of these. In the resting state, the concentration of intracellular K^+ is high and that of Na^+ low, relative to extracellular fluid and this is maintained by an adenosine triphosphate (ATP)-driven *sodium–potassium pump*. Potassium ions tend to diffuse out through ungated channels. Unequal distribution of ions across the membrane creates a negative *resting potential* of about -70 mV. Synaptic excitation produces *depolarization*, a reduction of membrane potential, brought about by a neurotransmitter-mediated opening of sodium channels, allowing a sudden influx of Na^+. When a critical threshold is reached, an all or none response, the *action potential*, begins in the initial segment of the axon. The presence of voltage-gated sodium channels here and throughout the axon allows the action potential to develop in the initial segment and then, as a wave of depolarization, to become a self-propagating nerve impulse. Multiple sub-threshold synaptic stimuli can summate to trigger an action potential. The impulse, lasting about 5 ms, is followed by a return to the resting potential and then by a *refractory period* during which the cell is unresponsive to stimuli. Inhibitory synaptic stimuli cause *hyperpolarization* or increased potential in the cell membrane, for example by opening ligand-gated chloride channels.

The *nucleus* has a double membrane with pores. Its *chromatin* consists of large molecules of deoxyribonucleic acid (DNA), which regulates ribonucleic acid (RNA) synthesis; RNA probably leaves via the *nuclear pores* and controls cell protein synthesis in the ribosomes. There is usually a single *nucleolus*. In

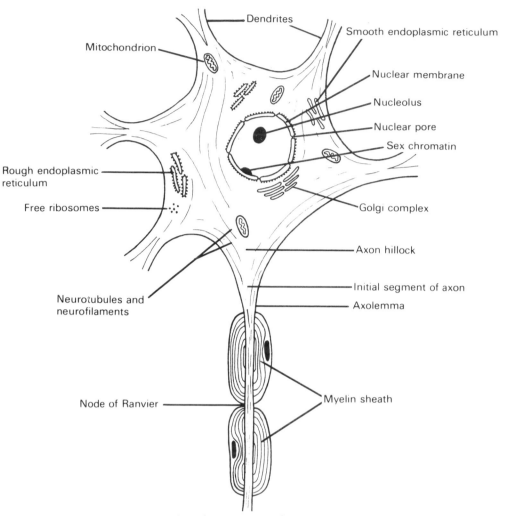

Fig. 2.4 Diagram of the fine structure of a neuron.

females there is a *nucleolar satellite* (Barr body) of sex chromatin. Some binucleate somata appear in sympathetic ganglia.

Cytoplasmic organelles

Nissl bodies (chromatin granules), intensely basophilic and stained by cresyl violet and similar dyes, occupy the perikaryon and dendrites but not the axon hillock (*Figs* 2.1 and 2.3). They are more prominent in motor than in sensory neurons, amounts varying with cell activity. With electron microscopy they are seen to consist of *granular (rough) endoplasmic reticulum*, groups of cisternae with attached and free ribosomes containing RNA and concerned in production of proteins necessary for cell metabolism and structural maintenance; some neurons synthesize peptide neurotransmitters or hormones.

Golgi complexes, which are clusters of flattened cisternae near the nucleus and similar in appearance to agranular (smooth) endoplasmic reticulum, enclose glycoprotein in membrane-bound vesicles for axonal transport. They also produce *lysosomes*, which are membrane-bound enzymes, able to destroy intracellular bacteria or other foreign material and to dispose of effete intracellular organelles.

Mitochondria, numerous throughout the soma, dendrites and axon, are spherical, ovoid or filamentous, with a double membrane folded internally into cristae. Regarded as the 'powerhouse' of cells, they store energy in ATP. They are particularly evident at sites of metabolic activity, for example near synapses, motor and sensory endings.

Electron microscopy reveals prominent microtubules, *neurotubules*, 20–30 nm in diameter and composed of the protein tubulin, running through the perikaryon into the neurites; these are concerned with the transport of large molecules along the neurites in either direction. In addition there are *neurofilaments*, about 10 nm thick. Neurofilaments aggregate in silver-stained preparations to form the 'neurofibrils' which are visible in light microscopy.

Centrosomes (centrioles), usually a feature of dividing cells, have been observed in mature neurons incapable of division; they may be associated with the formation or maintenance of neurotubules.

In addition to organelles, *cytoplasmic inclusions* may appear in neurons. *Melanin*, most evident in the substantia nigra, increases in amount up to puberty, then remains constant; it is chemically related to the neurotransmitter dopamine which is utilized by neurons located there. The pontine nucleus ceruleus (caeruleus = dark blue) contains melanin and copper. With increasing age, most neurons develop yellowish-brown *lipofuscin* ('age pigment') granules.

Dendrites and axons

Dendrites are slender extensions from the soma which greatly increase its receptive field and contain the same organelles. They commonly have numerous branches whose configurations characterize neuron types (*see Fig. 12.1*), for example the Purkinje cells of the cerebellar cortex have a dendritic field arranged in one plane (*see Fig. 7.6*). Frequently their surface area is extended by synaptic *dendritic spines*.

A single *axon*, generally the longest neurite, usually arises from an *axon hillock*; this narrows into an *initial segment*, beyond which the diameter remains uniform. Axons thicker than 1 μm generally have a *myelin sheath* which commences after the initial segment and is interrupted at intervals by the nodes of Ranvier (*see* p. 35). In the central nervous system myelin sheaths are formed by neuroglia (oligodendrocytes), in peripheral nerves by neurolemmal cells of Schwann. At the nodes, the bare axolemma is exposed to ionic exchange, while the myelinated segments (internodes) are insulated; this arrangement is the structural basis for '*saltatory conduction*', by which action potentials 'jump' from node to node. The speed of conduction is proportional to the thickness of the axon and its sheath. Slender axons are non-myelinated. *Collateral branches* arise at nodes, a recurrent collateral recurving towards the parent soma and synapsing with nearby neurons. The *axon terminals* have presynaptic expansions (*boutons terminaux*), or a row of many such swellings (*boutons de passage*). The *axoplasm* contains neurotubules, neurofilaments, agranular (smooth) endoplasmic reticulum and mitochondria; RNA and ribosomes, concerned with protein synthesis, are usually absent from the axoplasm.

Axoplasmic transport

Products synthesized in the soma travel along the axon in the *orthograde* direction in two modes. Bulk flow of axoplasm undergoes *slow transport* at about 1–3 mm/day, the mechanism for which is unknown. *Rapid transport* of membrane-bound vesicles, including neurotransmitters, has a velocity of about 400 mm/day (2800 mm/day in the hypothalamo-hypophyseal tract); this transport probably occurs on the external surfaces of the neurotubules. *Retrograde transport* provides a feedback whereby information on peripheral activity is relayed to the soma. It is used experimentally in axon-tracing, as with HRP, and has clinical implications in centripetal invasion by neurotoxic and infective agents (e.g. tetanus toxin and rabies).

Synapses (Fig. 2.5)

Each neuron is an anatomical unit; this was proposed by Ramón y Cajal (1900, 1908), but was finally proven only by electron microscopy. Unidirec-

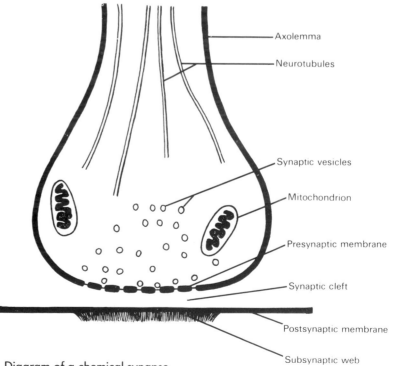

Fig. 2.5 Diagram of a chemical synapse.

tional communication occurs between neurons at foci of specialized contact, the *synapses*, generally sited between the axon of one neuron and the cell surface of another. Myelinated axons lose their sheaths near their terminals. Each axon may have thousands of boutons; similarly each neuron may be contacted by a few terminals or by thousands, some excitatory, some inhibitory (*Fig. 2.6*). This general pattern provides for discrete, convergent or divergent transmission of information. Commonly the synapses are between an axon and the soma or dendrites of another neuron (*axosomatic*, *axodendritic*); synapses from one axon to another (*axoaxonic*) are inhibitory. Synapses also occur between dendrites in areas of complex activity. There is continuous turnover and remodelling of synapses, for example, in the cerebral cortex (Jones, 1988). Neurons also synapse with *effectors* at neuromuscular and neuroglandular junctions.

In the central nervous system most synapses are of the type called *chemical synapses*, in which the *presynaptic* and *postsynaptic membranes* are separated by a *synaptic cleft* about 20 nm wide. The presynaptic membrane may have local thickenings, the postsynaptic membrane a dense *subsynaptic web;* these, together with other variable factors, such as width of cleft or type and shape of vesicles, are used in classifying synapses. A presynaptic terminal, has *synaptic vesicles* which contain a chemical *neurotransmitter*. Neurotransmitters, released from the presynaptic terminal, have a transient action of a few milliseconds because specific mechanisms exist to remove them from the synaptic cleft. Many peptides are neuroactive, but have a longer action, sometimes because there is no mechanism for rapidly terminating this. They may co-exist with, and modulate the effects of neurotransmitters, and are termed *neuromodulators* (*see* Chapter 15). Low molecular weight neurotransmitters may be synthesized at terminals but peptide production is dependent upon the mechanisms of protein synthesis located in ribosomes of the cell body.

Arrival of nerve impulses at a terminal creates an influx of calcium ions, which causes release of neurotransmitter by exocytosis into the synaptic cleft, where it binds to *receptors* of the postsynaptic membrane. Each receptor comprises a binding component which protrudes into the cleft and a neurotransmitter-activated ionic channel through the cell membrane. In excitatory synapses, Na^+ channels open and depolarization follows; in inhibitory synapses, K^+ or Cl^- channels open and hyperpolarization of the postsynaptic membrane occurs. The neurotransmitter acetylcholine is inactivated in the cleft by acetylcholinesterase. Catecholamines such as noradrenaline are located in dense-cored vesicles, and the duration of their postsynaptic effect is limited by their re-uptake to the presynaptic terminal as well as by enzymatic means and diffusion. Monoamine oxidase, an intraneuronal enzyme produced by mitochondria, degrades catecholamines. Monoamine oxidase inhibitors may be used clinically in treating depressive illness. Other transmitters include: monoamines such as noradrenaline, dopamine and 5–HT; amino acids such as gamma-aminobutyric acid (GABA), glycine and glutamate; and many peptides, including enkephalin and substance P.

Electrical synapses, common in invertebrates, also occur in the sensory

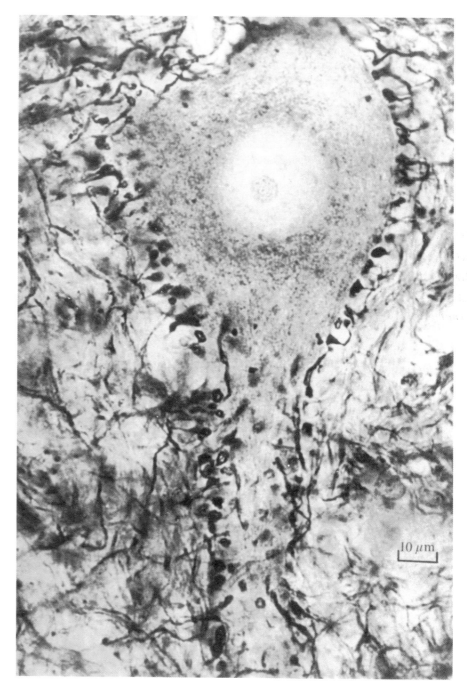

Fig. 2.6 Section through a ventral horn neuron showing numerous nerve endings on its cell body and on one of its dendrites, from a cat spinal cord. (Cajal silver stain.) (From Young, J.Z. (1978) *Programs of the Brain*, Oxford University Press, Oxford, by kind permission of the author and publisher.)

nervous system of lower vertebrates. A narrow *gap junction*, 2 nm wide, contains small channels between apposed membranes, which effect rapid direct transmission of impulses by ionic flow; this can be bi-directional. Gap junctions are like those in cardiac and non-striated muscle.

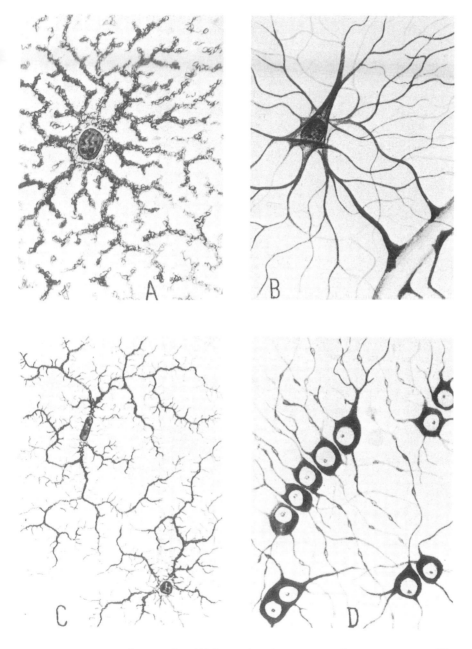

Fig. 2.7 Four types of neuroglia. (A) Protoplasmic astrocytes from grey matter. (B) Fibrous astrocytes from white matter. (C) Microglia. (D) Interfascicular oligodendrocytes. (From del Río-Hortega, P. (1920) *Trab. Lab. Invest. Biol., Madrid* **18**, 37–82.)

Neuroglia (*Fig.* 2.7)

Neurons are surrounded by more numerous, non-excitable glial cells, comprising about half the volume of the central nervous system. Unlike neurons, they are able to divide. There are several varieties.

Astrocytes, the most numerous, are star-shaped (Greek *astron* = star), with many processes which contact non-synaptic neuronal surfaces, and have 'perivascular feet' which cover 85% of the surface of capillaries within the central nervous system. These processes form an external glial membrane under the pia mater and an internal membrane under the ventricular ependyma. Their cytoplasm contains bundles of filaments. There are two main subtypes: *fibrous astrocytes*, in white matter, have long slender processes and many filaments; *protoplasmic astrocytes*, in grey matter, have shorter, flattened, branched processes with few filaments. They support neurons, structurally and functionally. When damaged, they hypertrophy and proliferate to form a 'glial scar'. A so-called 'blood–brain barrier' is primarily due to tight junctions between capillary endothelial cells, but astrocytes also

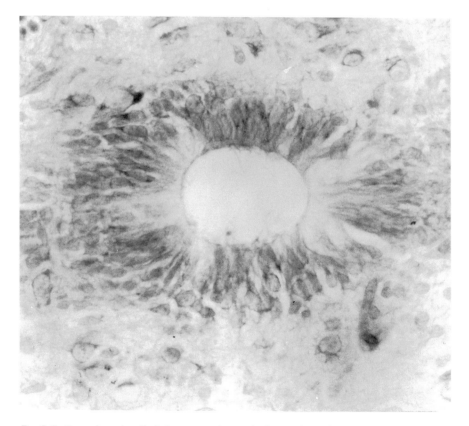

Fig. 2.8 Ependymal cells lining central canal of spinal cord in a chick embryo. The canal's dark outline represents tight junctions between adjacent cells. At this stage of development the ependymal surface is ciliated. Pale-staining neuroblasts are visible in the surrounding mantle zone. (Toluidine blue stain, × 570.)

contribute a selective nutritive path between blood vessels and neurons. They also occur in the retina (cells of Müller). Astrocytes are the commonest source of primary malignant tumours in the central nervous system.

Oligodendrocytes differ in having a smaller, denser nucleus, fewer processes (Greek *oligos* = few) and no cytoplasmic filaments. *Interfascicular oligodendrocytes* are arranged along myelinated axons and have processes which form myelin internodes on several adjoining axons. This contrasts with myelinated axons in peripheral nerves where there is one neurolemmal Schwann cell to each internode. *Perineuronal satellite cells* surround somata. Both types of oligodendrocyte may have nutritive functions, possibly related to high oxygen need.

Microglia, small, irregular cells with a few branched processes, are normally inactive but, like connective tissue macrophages, can become phagocytic.

Ependyma lines the cerebral ventricles and the central canal of the spinal cord; comprising a single layer of cuboidal cells, its surface generally has microvilli and cilia. Subjacent to it is an internal limiting membrane of astrocytes. Embryonic ependyma (*Fig.* 2.8) has more than one cell layer, with processes extending through the width of the neural tube to an external limiting membrane. *Choroidal epithelium* (*see Fig.* 13.8) modified for active and selective secretion of cerebrospinal fluid (CSF), is convoluted, its surface further extended by microvilli. Tight intercellular junctions form a 'blood–CSF barrier'; the cell cytoplasm has numerous mitochondria, Golgi complexes and endoplasmic reticulum. Specialized astrocytes, termed *tanycytes*, located between ependymal cells of the third ventricle's floor, extend from the hypothalamic median eminence to the hypophyseal portal system and provide a pathway whereby hormones may enter or leave cerebrospinal fluid.

Chapter 3

Peripheral nervous system

Impulses enter and leave the central nervous system via the cranial and spinal nerves. Cranial nerves may be motor, sensory or mixed; they may be purely somatic or mostly visceral in distribution. The spinal nerves, formed by dorsal (sensory) and ventral (motor) roots, are segmentally arranged; the intercostal nerves, in their cutaneous and muscular supply to the *dermatomes* and *myotomes*, retain the primitive pattern. The dermatomes are prolonged into the limbs but still retain a general numerical sequence except at axial lines (*Fig.* 3.1). The division and redistribution of the embryonic myotomes into individual muscles and their segmental innervation is much more complicated, as the following generalizations indicate. Most muscles are supplied from two segments (although the intrinsic muscles of the hand are unisegmental). Muscles sharing a common primary action are supplied by the same segments, opposing muscles by segments in sequence with the former. Thus in elbow movements, spinal cord segments C5 and 6 supply flexors and C7 and 8 supply extensors. The emergence of motor skills and the evolution of functionally specialized muscles in mammalian limbs required an interchange of fibres from segmental spinal nerves in the brachial, lumbar and sacral *plexuses*, from which plurisegmental nerves enter the limbs. Moreover there is a correlation between the supplies to joints, muscle and skin: *Hilton's law* states that those 'nerves whose branches supply the groups of muscles moving a joint furnish also a distribution of nerves to the skin over the insertions of the same muscles and the interior of the joint'. In addition to primary segmental interchange in large plexuses, there are secondary *intraneural plexuses* of fibres in plurisegmental nerves within which appropriate branches are formed (*Fig.* 3.2). This has implications in nerve injuries, since even the loss of a few millimetres renders accurate reapposition impossible.

Structure of Peripheral Nerves

Peripheral nerves comprise fasciculi of nerve fibres, myelinated and non-myelinated, enclosed in three sheaths of connective tissue. The nerve trunks are surrounded by *epineurium*, fasciculi by *perineurium* and individual nerve fibres by *endoneurium* (*Fig.* 3.3). Capillaries and lymphatics ramify in this connective tissue. Major arterial occlusion in the limbs may cause severe pain due to ischaemic neuritis.

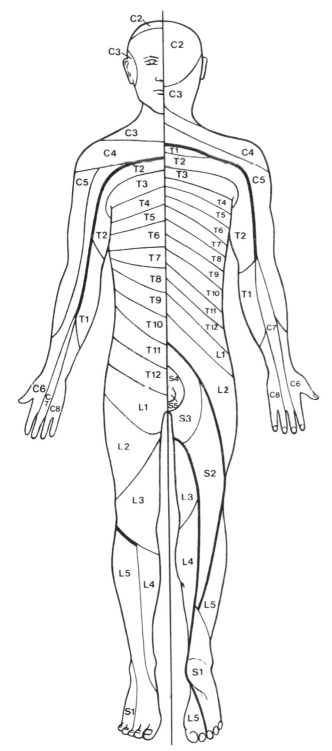

Fig. 3.1 Dermatomes on the anterior and posterior surfaces of the body. Axial lines, where there is numerical discontinuity, are drawn thickly.

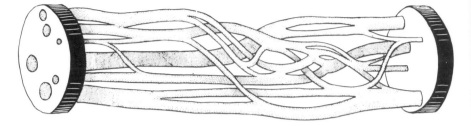

Fig. 3.2 Funicular plexus formation in a 3 cm segment of a musculocutaneous nerve of the arm. (From Sunderland S. (1978) *Nerves and Nerve Injuries*, London, Churchill Livingstone, reproduced by kind permission of the author and publisher.)

Classification of nerve fibres

According to axonal diameter (including the myelin sheath if present) and to the speed of conduction, nerve fibres may be divided into three main groups, A, B and C; group A, large and myelinated, are further classified into somatic sensory (I, II, III) (alternative nomenclature Aα, Aβ, Aδ) and motor (α, β, γ) sub-groups. In the following list only *maximum* diameters and conduction rates are given.

Afferent A fibres

Group I (Aα): from annulospiral endings of muscle spindles (Ia) and tendon organs (Ib) (20 μm, 120 m/s).
Group II (Aβ): from 'flower-spray' endings in muscle spindles, touch and pressure receptors (15 μm, 70 m/s).
Group III (Aδ): from pain and temperature receptors (5 μm, 30 m/s).

Efferent A fibres

α *fibres:* supply skeletal (extrafusal) muscle (17 μm, 120 m/s).
β *fibres:* few in number, probably the same as Aα.
γ *fibres:* supply intrafusal muscle (of muscle spindles) (8 μm, 30 m/s).

B fibres

Myelinated, preganglionic autonomic (3 μm, 15 m/s).

C fibres

Non-myelinated, postganglionic autonomic efferents; also visceral and somatic afferents for pain and temperature sensations (2 μm, 2 m/s).

Myelinated and non-myelinated nerve fibres (*Fig.* 3.4)

During development, axons leaving the spinal cord as ventral roots unite with peripheral processes of dorsal root ganglia to form segmental spinal nerves; they are accompanied at regular intervals by peri-axonal *Schwann cells*.

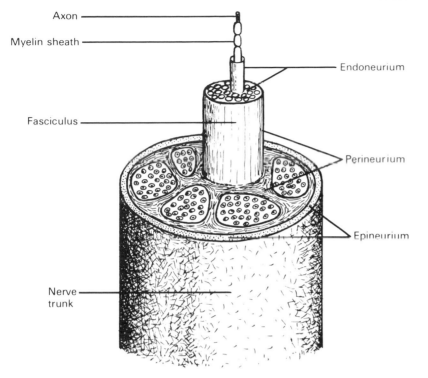

Axon

Myelin sheath

Endoneurium

Fasciculus

Perineurium

Epineurium

Nerve
trunk

Fig. 3.3 Diagram of the structure of a peripheral nerve.

Small fibres, usually 1 μm or less in diameter, remain *non-myelinated*, and several invaginate the plasma membrane of a single Schwann cell. Action potentials travel continuously along the axolemma, not by the more rapid saltatory conduction, in the absence of nodes of Ranvier.

Myelinated fibres have a regularly segmented *myelin sheath* interrupted by *nodes of Ranvier*, each myelinated *internode* being up to 1 mm long. Myelin sheaths begin to develop before birth but are not complete until a year or more later; a neurolemmal Schwann cell spirals round an axon, its plasma membrane forming concentric lamellae. On electron microscopy these lamellae show a major dense line, where two inner protein layers of plasma membrane are in apposition, and a less dense double thickness of lipid, in which a thin intraperiod line represents fused outer membrane surfaces (*Fig.* 3.4C). The cytoplasm and nucleus of the Schwann cell are peripheral in the *neurolemma;* only a very thin collar of cytoplasm remains next to the axon. The most external and internal infoldings of the plasma membrane form a *mesaxon. Myelin incisures* (of Schmidt-Lanterman) are regular spiral zones in the sheath where cytoplasm penetrates centrally between myelin layers towards the axon. Nodes of Ranvier separate consecutive sections of the myelin sheath, whose lamellae here form terminal loops (*Fig.* 3.4D). In peripheral nerves the neurolemma extends on to the node, while in the central nervous system the axolemma is more exposed. Action potentials

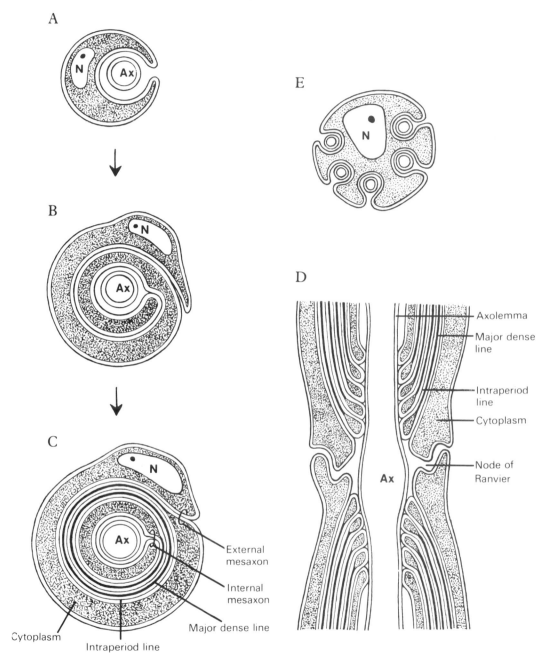

Fig. 3.4 (A,B,C) Diagrams of stages in development of a myelinated sheath. Schwann cell cytoplasm is stippled and its nucleus (**N**) shown; **Ax**, axon. (D) Longitudinal section of a myelinated nerve showing fine structure of node of Ranvier. (E) Several non-myelinated axons are related to one Schwann cell.

jump from node to node by the process called *saltatory conduction*, giving greater velocity (particularly in large axons with long internodes) than in non-myelinated fibres.

Ganglia

Sensory ganglia of spinal dorsal roots and in some cranial nerves have a connective tissue *capsule* continuous with the epineurium and perineurium. The somata of primary sensory neurons, 20–100 μm in size, are mostly peripheral, their processes lying centrally in the ganglion. They are *unipolar*, a single process bifurcating to pass to peripheral receptors and to the central nervous system. The peripheral process, conducting towards the soma, is functionally a dendrite but has the structural and physiological characteristics of an axon. Impulses pass directly from the peripheral to the central process, bypassing the soma. *Satellite cells* surround each soma, separating it from capillaries; they serve nutritive functions and are structurally like neurolemmal cells.

Autonomic ganglia are situated in the sympathetic paravertebral chains, prevertebral thoracic and abdominal plexuses (e.g. cardiac, pulmonary, coeliac, mesenteric) and in visceral walls (*see Fig.* 3.12). Structurally and functionally they differ from sensory ganglia, being visceromotor and containing synapses. The postsynaptic (principal) cells are multipolar, uniform in size, smaller than many cells in the sensory ganglia, sometimes binucleate and their axons are non-myelinated. There are also interneurons near synapses. Somata and nerve fibres are intermingled. Some myelinated preganglionic fibres pass through the paravertebral ganglia to synapse more peripherally; the afferents also are 'fibres of passage', their somata lying in dorsal root ganglia (*see also* p. 49). The distribution of parasympathetic ganglia is described on p. 114.

Degeneration and Regeneration After Injury

Damage affects nerves both proximally and distally. The soma, the trophic centre of the neuron, undergoes *chromatolysis* (p. 21). From the site of injury *retrograde degeneration* of each axon and its myelin sheath spreads proximally only to the first node and this is quickly followed by regeneration. Distally, *Wallerian degeneration* affects the whole nerve fibre; its axon disintegrates, its myelin sheath breaks into lipid droplets. Schwann cells then proliferate to fill the endoneurial tube, emerging from its cut end.

The soma begins to recover after about 3 weeks, swelling subsides, Nissl bodies reappear, and the nucleus returns to a central position. Much earlier, within 24 four hours after injury, axons in the proximal stump start to regenerate. Successful restoration is greatly influenced by the nature of the injury; if the nerve is crushed, the endoneurial tubes may remain intact, and axons may then reach their original territories; when a nerve is severed this is much less likely.

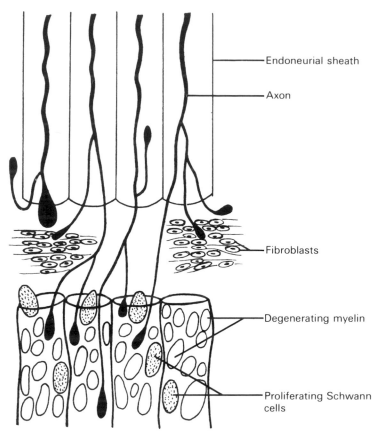

Fig. 3.5 Diagram showing axonal regeneration following nerve severance.

Following section, totally accurate reapposition of cut ends is most unlikely; destruction of only a few millimetres of nerve renders this impossible because constituent fibres change orientation in a plexiform fashion throughout its length; proliferating axons are unable to cross a major gap and become entangled in a 'stump neuroma'. Local events such as haemorrhage, infection and fibroblastic proliferation may inhibit successful repair. In mixed nerves, somatic, autonomic, motor and sensory fibres may travel to inappropriate endings. Proximal axons develop multiple sprouts and are guided along Schwann cells into the distal, severed parts of endoneurial tubes. Several sprouts from different axons may enter one tube (*Fig.* 3.5), but only one will establish effective contact with the peripheral receptor or effector organ, thicken and remyelinate. In a mixed nerve, regeneration of non-myelinated fibres may be poor and vasomotor control imperfect.

Axons may grow as much as 5 mm/day but functional recovery is generally estimated at 1.5 mm/day; crossing the site of injury entails delay, as does establishing effective peripheral contact, thickening and remyelinating. Functional recovery is often incomplete; apart from the factors mentioned, it is affected by the length of fibre to be restored and by the ability of atrophied muscle, sense organs and stiff joints to recover. If, for example, the sciatic nerve is severed, the recovered power in the calf muscles may be only 50%; 'foot drop', due to weakness of extensors, persists in most cases and sensory recovery in the foot is usually limited to pain and deep sensation.

If a nerve is only partly divided, some recovery is due to development of *collateral sprouts* from intact fibres, a marked feature in autonomic nerves. If intentional section (e.g. sympathectomy, vagotomy) is incomplete, the long-term results may hence be disappointing. (For further reading, *see* Sunderland, 1978).

Peripheral Receptors and Effectors

Receptors

Receptors are transducers, converting mechanical and other stimuli into electrical impulses. They are classified as superficial *exteroceptors* responding to external stimuli, deeper *proprioceptors* stimulated by movement, pressure and change of body position and *interoceptors* from viscera and blood vessels. They may be either *encapsulated* by connective tissue or *unencapsulated* (free or expanded).

Cutaneous receptors (Figs. 3.6 and 3.7)

These are grouped functionally into mechanoreceptors, thermoreceptors and nociceptors, respectively serving mechanical deformation, thermal change and potentially damaging stimuli. This subdivision indicates preferential selectivity rather than absolute specificity; for example, an intense thermal stimulus can ultimately activate nociceptors.

Free nerve endings.   Finely myelinated group Aδ (III) and non-myelinated C fibres form subcutaneous and intradermal plexuses, whose rami terminate as naked axons between cells. They are the only type of nerve ending present in the cornea or in dental pulp. Often regarded as nociceptors, they are the most widely distributed receptors and also serve more general functions, including thermal sensation and light touch. *Peritrichial* expanded endings occur in the outer root sheath of hair follicles and are stimulated by light touch causing movement of hairs. One nerve fibre supplies many follicles; each follicle is supplied by several myelinated fibres, which lose their sheaths and form a peritrichial plexus. *Tactile discs* (of Merkel) are expanded nerve endings in the germinative epidermal layer of hairless skin. They contact *Merkel cells*, which are specialized epithelial cells with a lobulated nucleus and cytoplasmic secretory granules near the nerve terminal.

Encapsulated nerve endings.   Lamellated (Pacinian) corpuscles (*Fig.* 3.7) are the largest and most numerous encapsulated receptors. Ovoid, up to 4 mm long, each has an outer multilaminated capsule of flat cells, and is

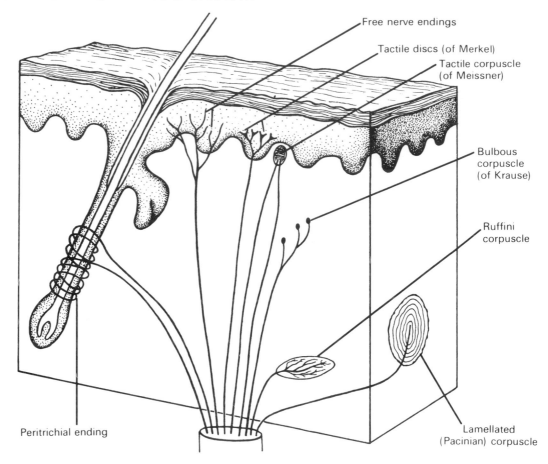

Free nerve endings

Tactile discs (of Merkel)

Tactile corpuscle (of Meissner)

Bulbous corpuscle (of Krause)

Ruffini corpuscle

Lamellated (Pacinian) corpuscle

Peritrichial ending

Fig. 3.6 Sensory nerve endings and receptors present in hairy skin.

innervated by a thick myelinated group I (Aα) nerve fibre, which loses its sheath to enter the central core. They respond to deformation, resulting from pressure or vibration. *Tactile (Meissner's) corpuscles* are ovoid, about 100 μm long, sited in the dermal papillae and most numerous in the fingertips. They contain transversely arranged epithelioid cells; each corpuscle is supplied by up to four myelinated nerve fibres. Sensitive to tactile stimuli, they probably serve close spatial ('two point') discrimination. *End bulbs* of various types consist of multiple branched nerve terminals, encapsulated: the *bulbous corpuscles* (of Krause), found mainly at mucocutaneous junctions, are spherical and up to 50 μm in diameter; slightly different *genital corpuscles* (of Golgi-Mazzoni) occur in the genital skin. The afferent branches of a sensory neuron serve a group of nerve endings of the same type and the receptive fields of neurons overlap.

The primary sensations (modalities) of touch, pain, cold and warmth are represented in the skin by a pattern of spots, each specific to one of these; for example a 'cold spot'. This is not explicable simply by an equivalent local distribution of particular receptors. Other factors include intensity and

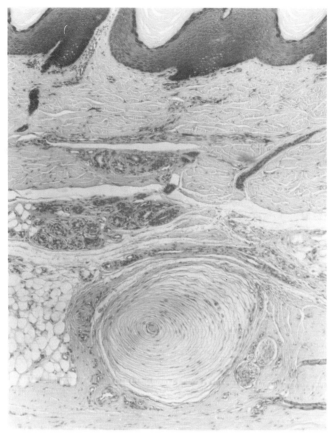

Fig. 3.7 Lamellated (Pacinian) corpuscle in the skin. (Haematoxylin and eosin stain, × 8.)

duration of stimulus, size of receptive field, type of neuronal innervation and its central nervous system connexions. Some free endings are polymodal: polymodal nociceptors respond to a variety of noxious stimuli. Free endings in dentine, cornea and periosteum appear to serve nociception only.

Classically there are said to be two types of pain: 'fast pain' is a sharp, well localized pricking sensation involving Aδ (III) fibres, while 'slow pain' is longer lasting, burning in quality, poorly localized and mediated by C fibres. Central processing of painful stimuli is discussed later (p. 66). Touch and pressure sensations are served by more heavily myelinated A fibres. Complex stimuli may involve several types of receptor; perception presumably requires abstraction, correlation and analysis of the resultant impulses, but the nature of this is largely speculative.

Muscle receptors

The receptors of *neuromuscular spindles* (*Fig.* 3.8) respond to stretch and have motor functions. Up to 8 mm long, the spindles consist of specialized

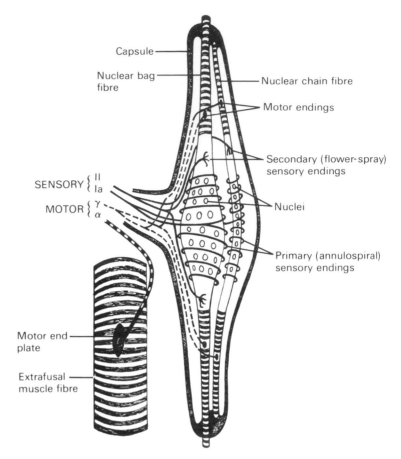

Fig. 3.8 A neuromuscular spindle. Note the innervation of nuclear bag and nuclear chain intrafusal fibres. Motor nerves are shown as interrupted lines.

intrafusal muscle fibres, motor and sensory endings, in a fluid-filled fusiform capsule, oriented parallel to the surrounding (extrafusal) muscle. They are attached at each pole to intramuscular connective tissue; thus when a muscle lengthens, the spindles are stretched. The intrafusal muscle fibres are slender, with cross-striations only at each end; centrally many nuclei are arranged in sarcoplasm, either in a chain formation (*nuclear chain fibres*) or in an expanded equatorial zone (*nuclear bag fibres*). Nuclear bag fibres are thicker and longer than chain fibres, projecting beyond the capsule at each end and attached to extrafusal connective tissue.

There are two types of sensory ending, termed annulospiral and flower-spray. *Annulospiral (primary) endings* surround the equator of intrafusal fibres and come from thickly myelinated (type Ia) nerves; they respond rapidly, transmitting information on velocity of change as well as length (dynamic response). *Flower-spray (secondary) endings* are located some distance from the equator, mostly on nuclear chain fibres; they are terminal varicosities of more thinly myelinated (type II) nerves and respond more slowly, signalling information only on length (static response). Small muscles involved in precise movements such as the interossei and lumbricals of the hand are richly endowed with spindles; in muscles of mastication they ensure accurate dental occlusion. (For detailed distribution of spindles *see* von Voss, 1971.)

Extrafusal muscle is innervated by α motor neurons. Axons of smaller, γ motor neurons terminate at the striated poles of intrafusal fibres. Neuromuscular spindle receptors are stimulated in the stretch reflex (*see Fig.* 4.7), their sensitivity adjusted by contraction of intrafusal muscle. As in the familiar knee-jerk response, stretching of a muscle stimulates its spindle receptors and, via a spinal reflex arc, α motor neurons are activated, and the extrafusal muscle contracts, this in turn reducing intrafusal tension. Under supraspinal control this mechanism regulates muscle tone; by opposing passive length changes it is essential to the maintenance of a set posture.

In the γ *reflex loop hypothesis*, upper motor neurons at cranial level are said to activate γ neurons, intrafusal muscle contracts, spindle receptors respond and, through spinal reflex connexions to α motor neurons, extrafusal muscle contracts. It has been shown however that spindles begin to fire **after** extrafusal muscle contraction has started, an observation inconsistent with a follow-up length servo system of control. In voluntary movement, α *and* γ *motor neurons are usually activated synchronously*, thereby enabling spindles to continue transmitting information about muscle length. The γ loop may sometimes reinforce α activity in response to load. Motor control mechanisms which involve spindles are described on p. 61.

Tendon and ligament receptors

Neurotendinous fusiform receptors (of Golgi), up to 500 μm long, are most numerous near musculotendinous junctions. A fusiform capsule contains slender and cellular intrafusal tendon fibres, innervated by group Ib nerves with bulbous terminals. Excitation requires a tension greater than that to which muscle spindles respond. Through spinal interneurons tendon receptors are inhibitory to α motor neurons, thus preventing excessive tension, and balancing excitatory input from neuromuscular receptors. Tendons and ligaments also have free (nociceptor) nerve endings.

Joint receptors

Free nerve endings, profuse in synovial membrane and articular capsules, react to painful stimuli. *Ruffini corpuscles* and *lamellated (Pacinian) corpuscles* in capsules respond to movement and pressure. *Neurotendinous spindle receptors* prevent excessive stretch of the capsular ligaments. Awareness of joint position depends on neuromuscular spindle afferents, aided by capsular and cutaneous pressure receptors.

Receptors in muscles, tendons, joints and ligaments participate in spinal reflexes; they also provide information to the cerebellum (subconscious proprioception) and cerebrum (conscious proprioception or *kinaesthesia*).

Effectors

Somatic effectors are the terminals of myelinated axons of motor neurons that pass without interruption from spinal cord to striated muscle. Visceral effectors are supplied by non-myelinated axons from cells in the autonomic ganglia.

Somatic effectors

A single motor neuron and the muscle fibres innervated by it constitute a *motor unit*, which may include up to 200 muscle fibres in large muscles such as gastrocnemius. Where movements are very precise, as in intrinsic hand muscles, the motor units are small; extra-ocular muscles have only 6 muscle fibres per unit (Basmajian, 1978). Having branched a few or many times, an axon ends the central region of each muscle fibre at a *neuromuscular junction* or motor end plate (*Fig.* 3.9). The myelin sheath is lost from the final branches, which are covered by neurolemmal Schwann cells and endoneurium; the former are superficially placed, the latter blends with the endomysium. The expanded, naked, axonal terminal is apposed to the *sole plate* of a muscle fibre; here the sarcolemma forms a 'synaptic gutter', many junctional folds increasing the surface area of this *subneural apparatus*. The axolemma and sarcolemma are separated by a synaptic cleft of 20–50 nm. The terminal axoplasm has mitochondria and synaptic vesicles containing acetylcholine; the subneural apparatus has acetylcholine receptors on the apices of the

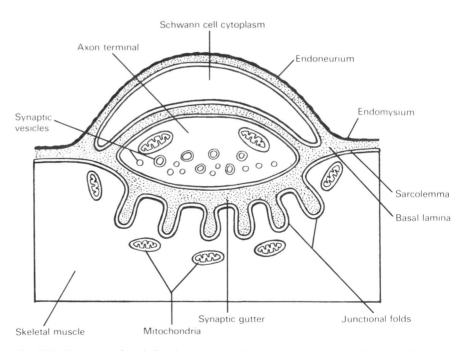

Fig. 3.9 Diagram of a skeletal neuromuscular junction (motor end plate). Between Schwann cell, axon and muscle there is a basal lamina (stippled).

junctional folds, its sarcoplasm containing many nuclei, mitochondria and the enzyme acetylcholinesterase, which inactivates acetylcholine. Nerve impulses cause exocytosis of the presynaptic vesicles into the synaptic cleft and acetylcholine then binds to postsynaptic receptors and depolarizes the sarcolemma, creating an action potential. Muscle contraction ensues, limited in duration by the action of acetylcholinesterase.

Visceral effectors

Postganglionic fibres are non-myelinated. Where precision and speed are required, as in the iris, innervation is discrete; in enteric muscle, where peristalsis is slow and diffuse, the fibres form plexuses with much branching, each neuron supplying many muscle fibres. There are no specialized endings as in striated muscle; a naked varicose axon terminal, its neurolemmal cytoplasm retracted, occupies a shallow groove in the plasma membrane of cardiac or visceral muscle, and these endings are more widely separated than in skeletal muscle. The terminals are similar in glands. By electron microscopy axoplasmic membrane-bound vesicles of cholinergic terminals (containing acetylcholine) are clear, while adrenergic terminals (containing noradrenaline) are dense.

Autonomic Nervous System

The general functions of sympathetic and parasympathetic nerves have been briefly described in Chapter 1; their distribution is shown in *Figs* 3.10 and 3.11. Details of the parasympathetic components in cranial nerves are provided in Chapter 6.

Visceral afferents

Physiological impulses travel mainly in parasympathetic fibres, while nociceptor impulses travel via sympathetic pathways.

Baroreceptors in the carotid sinus signal fluctuations in the arterial blood pressure via the glossopharyngeal nerve. Similar receptors in the right atrium respond via the vagus nerve to central venous pressure changes. *Chemoreceptors* in the carotid bodies respond to reduced arterial oxygen, stimulating a brainstem inspiratory centre. Vagal bronchial afferents, activated progressively by stretch during inspiration, eventually inhibit this centre. Vagal afferents from the upper gastrointestinal tract mediate visceromotor, vasomotor and secretory reflexes. Sacral parasympathetic afferents convey awareness of vesical and lower colonic distension.

The gastrointestinal tract is insensitive to cutting and burning; pain results from the distension of hollow viscera, tension on mesenteries and compression of solid viscera. Impulses pass centrally via sympathetic afferents, but are often interpreted as 'referred pain', diffusely localized to the body surface with the same segmental innervation. Thus the early pain of appendicitis is

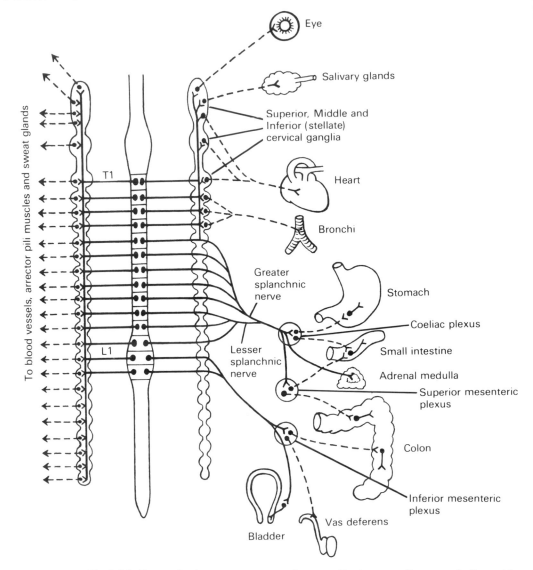

Fig. 3.10 Sympathetic nervous system. Postganglionic nerve fibres are indicated by interrupted lines.

referred to the periumbilical skin, since the midgut is median during development; if inflammation progresses, the parietal peritoneum (which has somatic innervation) is irritated and local pain occurs in the right iliac fossa. The heart is supplied by cervical and thoracic sympathetic branches, connecting with spinal segments T1–5; pain from coronary ischaemia (angina) is referred to the left side of the chest and lower neck and inner surface of the left arm. Whereas the somatic muscle spasm which frequently accompanies visceral pain is a spinal reflex, referred pain is probably due to the central (thalamic) proximity of equivalent somatic and visceral connexions.

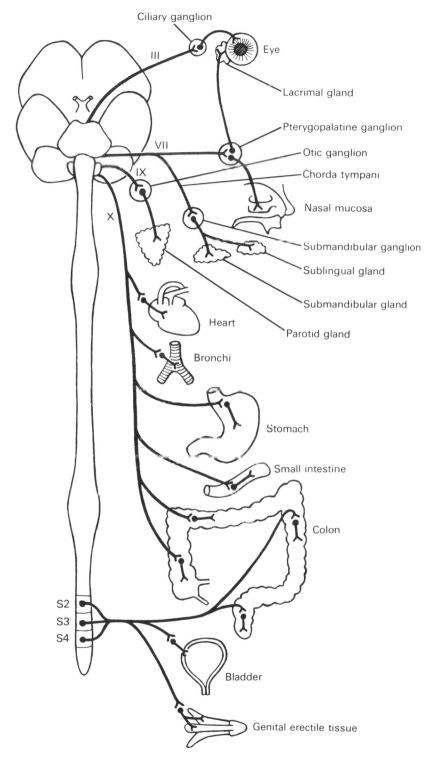

Fig. 3.11 Parasympathetic nervous system.

Visceral efferents

All *preganglionic fibres* (sympathetic and parasympathetic) are cholinergic. *Postganglionic* parasympathetic fibres are cholinergic; postganglionic sympathetic fibres are adrenergic except for sudomotor fibres, which are cholinergic. Enteric innervation involves additional neurotransmitters and requires separate consideration (*see below*).

Neurotransmitters bind to *receptors* sited on postsynaptic membranes or effector organ cells. Their chemical specificity is of crucial importance pharmacologically. There are two main groups of adrenergic receptors. *Alpha* receptors respond to noradrenaline (e.g. for cutaneous vasoconstriction and pupillary dilatation). *Beta* receptors respond more to adrenaline than noradrenaline; there are sub-groups β_1 (e.g. increasing cardiac muscle contractility and atrio-ventricular conduction velocity) and β_2 (e.g. relaxing bronchial muscle). There are two groups of cholinergic receptors, termed 'nicotinic' and 'muscarinic', because they can be activated either by nicotine or muscarine. *Nicotinic receptors* are present at the neuromuscular junctions of skeletal muscle, also at synapses between pre and postganglionic neurons in autonomic ganglia. *Muscarinic receptors* are located in all effector cells which are stimulated by parasympathetic postganglionic neurons (e.g. for pupillary constriction, salivary secretion, and increased intestinal motility), and also in the postganglionic cholinergic endings of sympathetic nerves (sweating).

Sympathetic efferents leave via ventral roots (T1–L2), enter the spinal nerves, then form *white rami communicantes* (myelinated) to the ganglia of the sympathetic trunks which are paravertebral (*Fig.* 3.12). Having synapsed, some rejoin the spinal nerves by *grey rami communicantes* (non-myelinated) as vasomotor, sudomotor and pilomotor fibres. Some rostral efferents ascend in the sympathetic trunks and synapse in cervical ganglia, passing on to cervical nerves and, via carotid plexuses, to cranial structures; similarly some caudal efferents descend to lumbar and sacral ganglia. Alternatively, efferents may pass through paravertebral ganglia to synapse in *prevertebral ganglia* (coeliac, superior and inferior mesenteric plexuses); a few terminate in the *suprarenal medulla*.

Parasympathetic outflow is via *cranial nerves* (oculomotor, facial, glossopharyngeal, vagus) and via the second to fourth sacral nerves, whose visceral efferents separate as *pelvic splanchnic nerves*. At cranial level preganglionic fibres synapse in the ciliary, pterygopalatine, submandibular and otic ganglia to supply intrinsic ocular muscles, lacrimal and salivary glands. Sympathetic efferents from the carotid plexus traverse but do not synapse in these ganglia. The vagus has a diffuse distribution to thoracic and abdominal viscera, but the pelvic organs and terminal third of the colon are supplied by pelvic splanchnic nerves (*nervi erigentes*, being also vasomotor to erectile tissue). Parasympathetic ganglia are close to the viscera, or in their walls; they form *cardiac* and *pulmonary plexuses*, an *intermuscular myenteric plexus* (*of Auerbach*) and *submucosal plexus* (*of Meissner*). Pelvic splanchnic nerves join the pelvic sympathetic plexuses and synapse in minute ganglia; some ascend (in the sympathetic hypogastric plexus) to the descending and sigmoid colon.

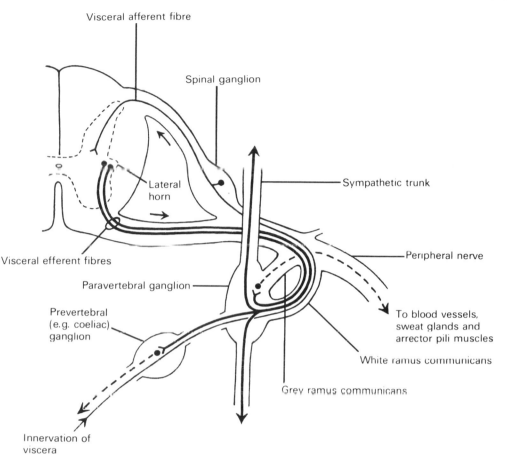

Fig. 3.12 Sympathetic efferent and afferent fibres. Postganglionic efferents are indicated by interrupted lines.

Fibres leaving *autonomic ganglia* are more numerous than those entering, thus providing a dissemination of effect. Integration and processing also occur by connexions between the principal cells and via interneurons (containing dopamine or noradrenaline) which form circuits between the afferent fibres and the principal cells. Parasympathetic effects are more discrete than sympathetic effects; there is less divergence and the action of the main parasympathetic neurotransmitter, acetylcholine, is quickly reversed by acetylcholinesterase.

Enteric innervation

This has considerable anatomical and physiological independence from the central nervous system. Peristalsis is locally coordinated and is maintained even when central connexions are severed. The enteric ganglia are unusual; the submucosal plexus contains unipolar and bipolar primary afferent neurons. The myenteric plexus (between circular and longitudinal muscle layers) has features resembling the central nervous system: supporting cells like astrocytes surround all the neuronal elements; it is avascular; paraneuronal capillaries with tight intercellular junctions outside 'glia' resemble those in the brain. Postganglionic parasympathetic terminals are cholinergic; sympathetic terminals do not affect smooth muscle directly, but act by inhibiting parasympathetic fibres in ganglia. Numerous intrinsic neurons may contain acetylcholine, serotonin or substance P. Other neurotransmitters have been identified. Langley (1921) considered the 'enteric nervous system' unique and a third component of the autonomic system (in addition to sympathetic and parasympathetic). This subject attracts much research.

Research: nerve growth factor

In 1951 Levi-Montalcini and Hamburger observed that implantation of a piece of mouse sarcoma into a 3-day chick embryo caused a remarkable increase in sympathetic ganglion cell numbers. This was attributed to a diffusable substance they termed 'nerve growth factor' (NGF). Subsequently this chemical was isolated and purified. Its structure is now known and it has been studied extensively in vivo and in vitro (cell culture). Its presence is critical for the development of sensory and sympathetic neurons in the peripheral nervous system, and their survival. Thus, if an antiserum to NGF is given to newborn mice, the sympathetic ganglia atrophy. Since deprivation causes death of these neurons and excess produces proliferation, it appears that NGF regulates the number of neurons that normally survive to maturity.

During development, 20–80% of neurons in dorsal root ganglia die shortly after innervating their target areas, being surplus to the particular peripheral requirements. This innervation density is regulated by the amount of NGF which is present in developing skin, taken up by endocytosis into peripheral processes of sensory neurons and transported to the somata (Davies and Lumsden, 1990).

NGF does not affect growth of motor neurons towards muscle. It has no effect on sensory regeneration following a crush injury to a mature nerve. Its effect on cholinergic neurons in the central nervous system will be described later; other central effects are partially understood. Investigations indicate that NGF is only one member (albeit the best known) of a family of growth factors that orchestrate normal neuronal development, maturation and survival in the peripheral and central nervous systems. It is hoped that current and future research will lead to potential therapy for degenerative diseases, at present incurable. For further reading see Zaimis and Knight (1972), Berg (1984), Purves and Lichtman (1985) and Cheney (1990).

APPLIED ANATOMY

There are three main kinds of peripheral nerve injury. *Compression* results in *neurapraxia*, that is dysfunction without structural damage; temporary paralysis ensues, but there is rapid and total recovery. *Crushing* (axonotmesis) damages axons and myelin sheaths but endoneurial tubes are relatively intact, so full functional recovery is possible; after *severance* (neurotmesis) recovery is slower and usually incomplete, for reasons discussed above. Individual fasciculi can be reapposed by microsurgery. Sensory recovery follows a pattern: first there is the return of awareness of deep pressure, then of superficial pain poorly localized, followed by thermal sensation and, much later, light touch. Recovery of the most discriminative aspects of sensation is often imperfect, more so in proximal than in distal lesions. Amputation may be followed by continued, and sometimes painful, awareness of a '*phantom limb*'. Rarely, nerve injury is followed by continuous, intractable, disabling, burning pain (*causalgia*) and intense hyperaesthesia; it is imperfectly understood. One theory was that efferent sympathetic fibres artificially synapse with fine afferent (pain) fibres. It is now known that severed sensory fibres may develop α adrenergic receptors, responsive to locally released and circulating noradrenaline. Sympathetic denervation, or destruction of sympathetic terminals in a limb by perfusion with the drug guanethidine, is often curative. Alternatively, 'pathological pain' may be of central origin.

A variety of conditions, nutritional (e.g. vitamin B deficiency), metabolic (e.g. diabetes mellitus), infective and toxic may cause *peripheral neuropathy*, resulting in negative phenomena due to loss of conduction and positive symptoms such as paraesthesiae ('pins and needles') due to spontaneous discharge.

The clinical relevance of retrograde axonal transport in rabies and tetanus is mentioned in Chapter 2. *Herpes zoster* ('shingles'), a viral infection of a spinal dorsal root ganglion or cranial sensory ganglion, causes pain in the corresponding dermatome, followed 24–48 hours later by a cutaneous blistering in the area, due to orthograde transport.

Occasionally clinical disorders directly affect neuromuscular transmission. *Botulism*, a potentially fatal form of food poisoning, inhibits acetylcholine release at neuromuscular junctions. *Myasthenia gravis*, a rare state of weakness and fatigue in skeletal muscles, is due to an auto-immune reduction of acetylcholine receptors at neuromuscular junctions; it is alleviated by the anti-cholinesterase drug, neostigmine.

Curarine, used in relaxant anaesthesia, produces muscle paralysis by blocking acetylcholine uptake at the postsynaptic receptors of motor end plates. Postoperatively this action is reversed by neostigmine, which inhibits cholinesterase, thereby causing acetylcholine to accumulate and competitively to displace curarine from the blocked receptors.

Stimulation or blockage of receptors is used therapeutically. Asthmatic bronchospasm is relieved by a β_2 stimulant such as salbutamol; a cardioselective β_1 blocker decreases the heart rate by an action at the sinoatrial and atrioventricular nodes. Atropine blocks acetylcholine at muscarinic receptors: an injection reduces salivation and bronchial secretion during anaesthesia, atropine eye drops dilate the pupil, oral belladonna reduces gastrointestinal motility.

Local anaesthetics block axolemmal ionic exchange and affect non-myelinated and thinly myelinated (e.g. pain) fibres more rapidly and longer than thickly myelinated fibres.

Chapter 4

Spinal cord

Gross Anatomy

The spinal cord lies within the vertebral canal. In foetuses up to the age of 3 months, cord and canal are of equal length. Thereafter, the vertebral column grows more rapidly, so that at birth the caudal end of the cord is level with vertebra L3; in adults its caudal end is usually at the level of the first lumbar intervertebral disc (between L1 and L2). Cranially it continues into the medulla, just below the foramen magnum, its total length approximately 45 cm.

The cord is not of uniform diameter. It has two enlargements associated

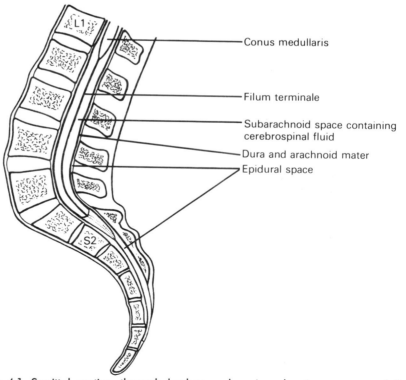

Fig. 4.1 Sagittal section through lumbosacral region showing conus medullaris, filum terminale and lower end of the subarachnoid space.

with the innervation of the limbs. The greatest diameter occurs at the *cervical enlargement* in cord segments from C4 to T1, and is associated with the brachial plexus. The *lumbar enlargement* extends from cord segments L1 to S3. The caudal end forms the conical *conus medullaris;* from its tip, a fine thread of connective tissue, the *filum terminale*, extends to the dorsal side of the first piece of the coccyx (*Fig.* 4.1).

The spinal cord is enclosed in three layers, or *meninges*. The innermost *pia mater* adheres to the cord's surface. The *dura mater*, outermost, is lined by the *arachnoid mater*, both these extending to the level of vertebra S2. The *subarachnoid space* between the pia and arachnoid is filled by cerebrospinal fluid. To sample this, lumbar puncture can be safely carried out using a needle inserted in the midline between the third and fourth lumbar spines. The pia mater extends out on each side as a *denticulate ligament*, attached to the dura by 21 'teeth' which serve to anchor the spinal cord. External to the dura mater an *epidural space* is occupied by adipose tissue and venous plexuses.

Each spinal cord segment gives origin to a pair of spinal nerves. There are 31 pairs of spinal nerves: 8 cervical, 12 thoracic, 5 lumbar, 5 sacral and 1 coccygeal. Since there are only seven cervical vertebrae, the first seven nerves pass cranial to the numerically corresponding neural arches but the eighth passes between the pedicles of C7 and T1 vertebrae. Caudal to this, each nerve occupies an intervertebral foramen below the vertebra of the same number. Each dorsal and ventral root pierces the dura mater separately, the latter fusing with their epineurium. Extradurally the roots traverse the epidural space and unite immediately distal to the dorsal root ganglion, within an intervertebral foramen.

An adult spinal cord is considerably shorter than its vertebral column and spinal cord segments are generally situated rostral to the numerically corresponding vertebrae. Thus segment T1 is opposite vertebra C7, L1 is opposite T11, sacral and coccygeal segments are behind the body of L1 vertebra. Hence some nerve roots pass obliquely from the cord, this obliquity increasing caudally. The lumbar, sacral and coccygeal roots together form a leash, the *cauda equina*, around the filum terminale (*Fig.* 4.2).

A *ventral median fissure* throughout the whole ventral aspect is partly filled superficially by a thickening of the pia, the glistening *linea splendens*, and contains the anterior spinal artery. Immediately deep to the fissure is the white commissure. From a shallow *dorsal median sulcus*, a midline neuroglial septum extends to the grey commissure.

Grey Matter and Nuclei

The grey matter has a variable butterfly profile (*Fig.* 4.3). The grey commissure encloses a small central canal. On each side there are dorsal and ventral grey columns, referred to in sections as 'horns'. The intermediate area has a small lateral horn in segments T1–L2. The amount of grey matter is increased in the cervical and lumbar enlargements. The cord segments are

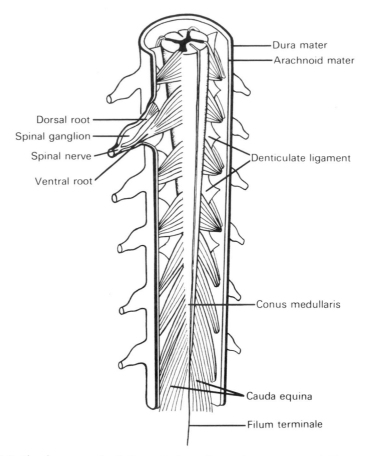

Fig. 4.2 The lower end of the spinal cord, cauda equina and filum terminale, exposed from the ventral side and viewed obliquely.

not of equal length: lumbar and sacral segments are relatively short, increasing the area of grey matter seen in sections at these levels.

'Nuclei' of grey matter are aggregations of nerve cell bodies, or somata, usually with common functions and on a common pathway. In the following description, these extend throughout the cord unless otherwise stated *Figs.* 4.4 and 4.5). Histological sections are usually stained either to show neuronal somata (e.g. cresyl violet stain) or myelin sheaths (silver stains).

Dorsal horn (somatic and visceral afferent)

Note: somata of primary sensory neurons are located in dorsal root ganglia.

1. *Substantia gelatinosa*. This caps the apex of the dorsal horn, and contains small Golgi Type II neurons and fine fibres. It modulates afferent patterns in respect of pain perception. At its tip is a small posterior marginal nucleus.

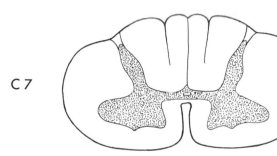

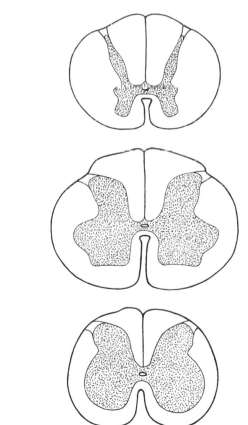

C2

C 7

T6

L 4

S 2

Fig. 4.3 Transverse sections of the spinal cord to indicate general profiles and relative amounts of white and grey matter at various levels.

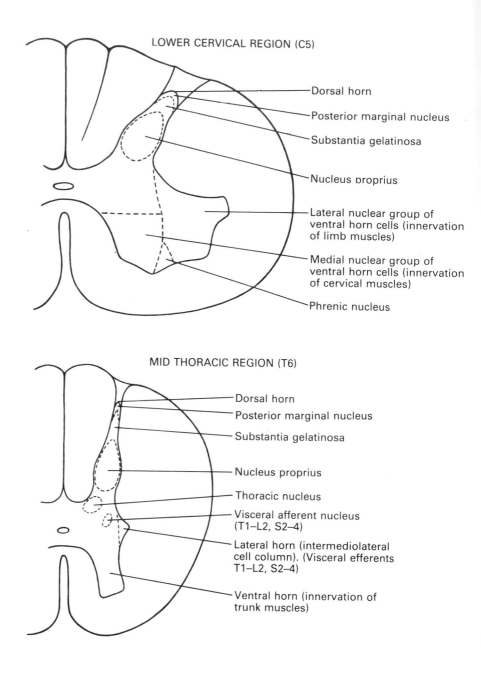

Fig. 4.4 Grey matter of the spinal cord.

2. *Nucleus proprius*. Forming most of the dorsal horn, this contains bodies of secondary sensory neurons subserving pain, temperature and touch.
3. *Thoracic nucleus* (nucleus dorsalis of Clarke). Extending through T1 to L2, this is the location of bodies of secondary sensory neurons carrying proprioceptive impulses to the cerebellum and is situated medial to the base of the dorsal horn. An ascending input enlarges the caudal end of Clarke's column, which also has, at its cranial end, a descending input from the lower cervical region. Proprioceptive afferents from the upper cervical spinal nerves ascend to the medulla (accessory cuneate nucleus). Cell bodies for other (rostral and ventral) spinocerebellar tracts are not aggregated into such clearly defined nuclei.
4. *Visceral afferent nucleus*. This extends from TI to L2 (sympathetic), and from S2 to S4 (parasympathetic), and is sited laterally in the base of the dorsal horn. It receives visceral afferents from nerve cells in the dorsal root ganglia.

Lateral horn (visceral efferent)

The cell bodies of preganglionic sympathetic efferent neurons occupy the intermediolateral cell column (T1–L2), a characteristic feature of thoracic sections. The cells of origin of the sacral parasympathetic outflow have a similar location in segments S2–4 but do not form a projecting lateral grey horn.

Ventral horn (somatic efferent)

Many descending pathways, often referred to as 'upper motor neurons', converge on individual ventral horn cells, the lower motor neurons which form the 'final common pathway' (*see Fig.* 2.6). There are two cell types: large α motor neurons innervating extrafusal muscle fibres and smaller γ motor neurons supplying intrafusal muscle fibres of the neuromuscular spindles.

A medial column of neuron somata, extending throughout all levels, supplies trunk and neck musculature. The cervical and lumbar enlargements are characterized by lateral extensions of the ventral horn; subgroups of neurons supply muscles with a common effect on a joint, such as flexion or extension.

A *phrenic nucleus* in cord segments C3–5 is the origin of the phrenic nerve. The spinal accessory nerve, unique in emerging by a row of rootlets from the lateral aspect of the cord, ascends via the foramen magnum. It originates from an *accessory nucleus*, located dorsolateral in the ventral horn of the upper five or six cervical segments and supplies muscles of branchial arch origin, hence its unusual features.

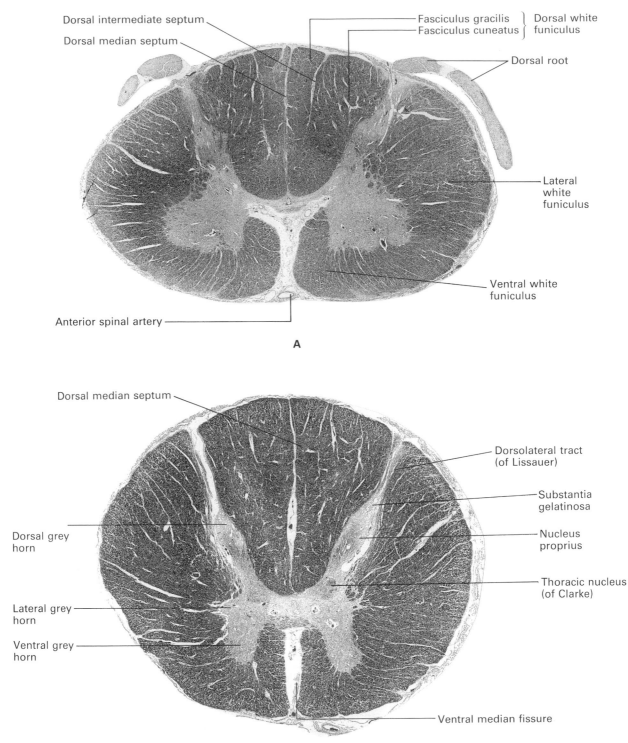

Dorsal intermediate septum

Dorsal median septum

Fasciculus gracilis ⎱ Dorsal white
Fasciculus cuneatus ⎰ funiculus

Dorsal root

Lateral white funiculus

Ventral white funiculus

Anterior spinal artery

A

Dorsal median septum

Dorsolateral tract (of Lissauer)

Substantia gelatinosa

Nucleus proprius

Dorsal grey horn

Thoracic nucleus (of Clarke)

Lateral grey horn

Ventral grey horn

Ventral median fissure

B

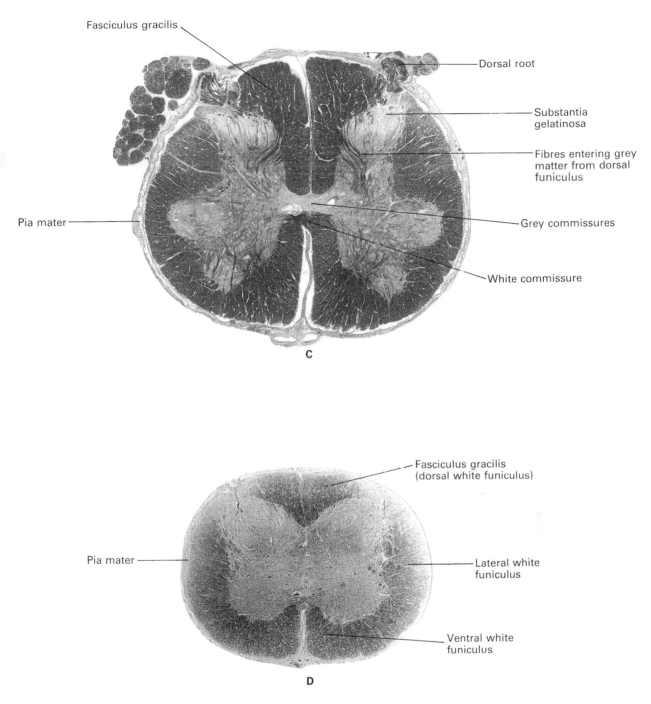

Fasciculus gracilis

Dorsal root

Substantia gelatinosa

Fibres entering grey matter from dorsal funiculus

Pia mater

Grey commissures

White commissure

C

Fasciculus gracilis (dorsal white funiculus)

Pia mater

Lateral white funiculus

Ventral white funiculus

D

Fig. 4.5 (A) Transverse section of lower cervical cord (Weigert stain × 8.2). (B) Transverse section of midthoracic cord (Weigert stain, × 10.7) (C). Transverse section of lumbar cord (Weigert stain, × 8.7). (D) Transverse section of sacral cord (Weigert stain, × 12).

The laminar architecture of Rexed

As might be expected, the organization of spinal grey matter is much more complex than is evident from the study of large nuclei at low magnification. Detailed investigation of cytoarchitecture, experimental examination of the effects of cutting dorsal nerve roots and supraspinal paths, and electrophysiological recordings have revealed a laminar functional pattern of cells: 10 laminae, as described by Rexed (1954) in cats, and shown in *Fig.* 4.6, are briefly described here.

Laminae I–IV, near the apex of the dorsal horn, are receptive zones for cutaneous afferents. Each layer has identifiable cell patterns and synaptic fields. Laminae V and VI are at the base of the dorsal horn. Lamina V receives input from superficial laminae in addition to primary afferents; efferent fibres form contralateral spinothalamic tracts. Lamina VI is only prominent in cord segments associated with the limbs and appears to receive proprioceptive impulses: microelectrode studies show that only these cells respond to movement. Lamina VII is the intermediate zone between the dorsal and ventral horns, including the thoracic nucleus, visceral afferent and efferent nuclei and many interneurons. Lamina IX largely consists of α and γ motor neurons whose dendritic fields extend into lamina VII. Lamina X is part of the grey commissure.

Corticospinal fibres from 'sensory' cortical areas terminate in laminae IV and V and, with descending fibres from the brainstem, influence sensory input. In cats, corticospinal fibres from the 'motor' cortex terminate on interneurons in laminae V–VII. In primates some corticospinal fibres synapse directly with α and γ motor neurons. Reticulospinal and vestibulospinal fibres synapse with interneurons in laminae VII and VIII.

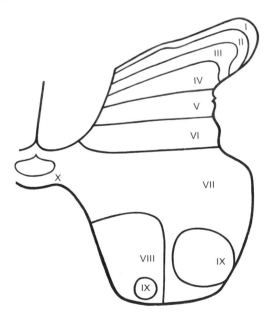

Fig. 4.6 Laminae of Rexed in the spinal grey matter of a lower lumbar segment.

Spinal cord nuclei and corresponding laminae

Nuclei	Laminae	Regions
Posterior marginal nucleus	I	Dorsal horn
Substantia gelatinosa	II, III	Dorsal horn
Nucleus proprius	IV, V	Dorsal horn
Thoracic nucleus (T1–L2)	VII	Intermediate zone
Visceral nuclei (T1–L2, S2–4)	VII	Intermediate zone
Somatomotor nuclei	IX	Ventral horn

Intrinsic Spinal Mechanisms and Motor Control

Between the dorsal and ventral horns there are many small cells with short axons known as *internuncial neurons*, or interneurons: they are commonly interposed between descending fibres and motor neurons or they may form part of a reflex arc. *Association neurons* are restricted to one side of the cord (ipsilateral); axons of *commissural neurons* cross the midline (contralateral connexion). Interneurons may be intersegmental or limited to one cord segment. Some are inhibitory, for example when a 'prime mover' is stimulated, its antagonist must synchronously be inhibited ('reciprocal inhibition').

Renshaw interneurons are sited between an axon collateral and the cell body of motor neurons (*Fig 4.7B*); being inhibitory they limit the duration of discharge. When directed towards adjacent neurons their 'surround inhibition' sharpens the signal and eliminates unwanted action, for example during precise digital movements which have very discrete (monosynaptic) corticospinal control.

A *reflex arc* comprises: a sensory receptor, a sensory neuron, a central synapse sometimes via interneurons, a motor neuron and an effector such as muscle fibres, glands etc. In the *flexor reflex* (*Fig. 4.7A*) a limb is withdrawn in reaction to a painful cutaneous stimulus. Its path is polysynaptic and its response clearly involves several cord segments. A *stretch reflex* (*Fig. 4.7C*) is monosynaptic and exemplified by tapping a patellar tendon. When a muscle is stretched, receptors in its neuromuscular spindles respond; afferent impulses then cause spinal α motor neurons to fire and the skeletal muscle contracts. By counteracting stretch this reflex is important in maintaining posture.

Neuromuscular spindle receptors can be stimulated either by passive stretch or by active contraction of intrafusal muscle. The postulated γ reflex loop (*Fig. 4.7D*) is no longer regarded as a commonly used length-servo system in supraspinal motor control because experiments in man have shown that γ motor neuron firing seldom precedes that of α motor neurons. Fusimotor activity usually occurs 10–50 ms after skeletomotor contraction: this observation is not inconsistent with simultaneous α and γ outflow from the spinal cord because their nerve conduction velocities and response times differ slightly (Vallbo, 1971).

The ways in which motor neurons are recruited can vary according to the task required. Thus, during muscle lengthening, γ activation is not required because the spindles are already being stimulated mechanically. Usually during muscle contraction there is synchronous *coactivation* of α and γ neurons in order that the spindles can continue to monitor muscle length. Coactivation appears to be supervised by an α–γ *linkage* control sited in the anterior lobe of the cerebellum: dysfunction of this contributes to the neuromuscular incoordination of cerebellar disease (e.g. ataxia, dysmetria, asynergia — *see* chapter 7).

Theoretically coactivation also provides a compensatory local mechanism whereby, within limits (potential mechanical gain is low), muscle contraction may be increased or decreased reflexly in response to load. Thus if unexpected resistance to movement stops extrafusal muscle shortening but intrafusal muscle contraction continues, spindle receptors might reflexly augment α motor neuron firing. This *servo-assist* theory is attractive; unfortunately the strength of reflexly augmented contraction is probably inadequate for major load compensation and its functional significance is uncertain (Brooks, 1986).

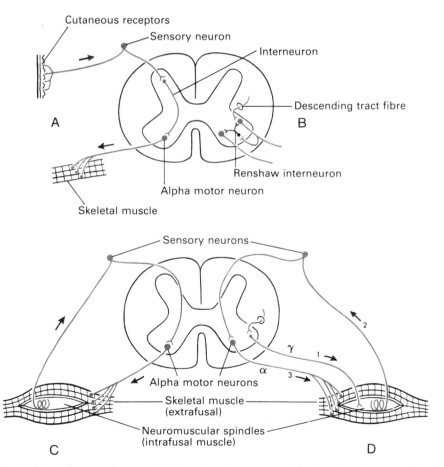

Fig. 4.7 (A) Flexor reflex arc. (B) Renshaw interneuron. (C) Stretch reflex arc. (D) γ reflex loop hypothesis.

Intrinsic spinal mechanisms include stereotyped simple motor programs such as stepping. The flexor reflex involves a complex and prolonged sequence of muscular activity, flexing one limb and sometimes extending another. Intrinsic spinal programs are an integral feature of motor control and of current research interest. One line of investigation seeks to discover whether, after cord injury it may be possible to reactivate such spinal 'motor pattern generators' through neuron transplantation, so restoring locomotion and other stereotyped movements.

White Matter and Tracts

The white matter of the cord (*Fig.* 4.8) is in three columns or *funiculi*. The *ventral funiculus* is between the ventral median fissure and the ventral spinal roots, the *lateral funiculus* between the dorsal and ventral roots, and *dorsal funiculus* between the dorsal spinal roots and dorsal median septum. The two dorsal funiculi are often termed *dorsal columns*. The absolute amount of spinal white matter increases cranially, ascending tracts enlarging upwards

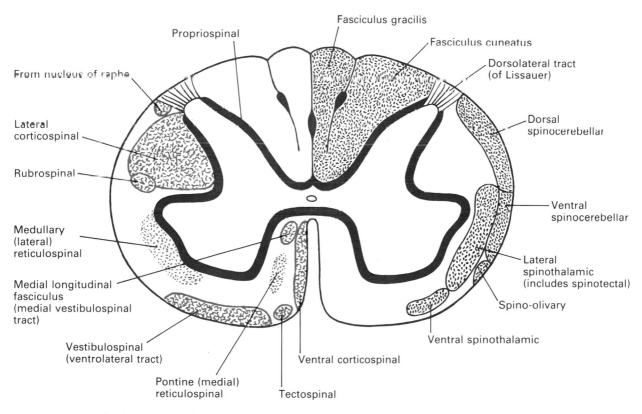

Fig. 4.8 A simplified diagram of the main tracts in the cervical spinal cord. Ascending tracts are on the right of the diagram, descending tracts (in red) on the left. Propriospinal tracts, containing ascending and descending intersegmental fibres, are shown in black. The reticulospinal tracts are not well localized.

with added input, descending tracts progressively reduced by output as they descend. The cord diameter is greatest in the lower cervical region.

Ascending tracts

Pathways to the cerebral cortex via the thalamus

Tracts ascending to the contralateral cerebral cortex are in three-neuron chains: all the primary neurons have their somata in dorsal root ganglia; the secondary are either in the spinal dorsal grey matter or the dorsal medulla; tertiary neurons are in the thalamus. Most of the ascending tracts in the dorsal half of the cord ascend uncrossed, but ventral tract fibres have crossed the midline.

Dorsal root fibres enter the cord as two groups. Heavily myelinated fibres form a *medial division*, entering the dorsal columns and conveying impulses concerned in proprioception, vibration, touch and pressure. Non-myelinated and thinly myelinated fibres form a *lateral division*, concerned in pain and temperature modalities. The following account is supplemented by a research review on p. 70.

PAIN AND TEMPERATURE PATHWAYS

Fine (Aδ and C) fibres enter the *dorsolateral tract* (of Lissauer), their branches ascend or descend one or two segments and terminate in the marginal zone and substantia gelatinosa (laminae I and II) of the dorsal horn. Their secondary neurons are in the *nucleus proprius*, with dendrites extending into the substantia gelatinosa to synapse with incoming fibres either directly or via interneurons. Axons from the nucleus proprius cross in the white commissure, ascending by one segment as they do so, to form the *lateral spinothalamic tract*. Of recent evolution, this tract contains only 1500–2000 fibres even in humans. If the tract is severed surgically there is loss of pain and temperature sensation contralaterally; the upper border of sensory loss is one or two dermatomes below the level of section. Pathological cord compression is often of gradual onset and tract destruction may be incomplete. Since input to the tract is from the mesial aspect, fibres from the opposite lower limb are most superficial and affected first. If untreated, the sensory 'level' then ascends as pressure increases but is arrested some dermatomes below the level of the lesion.

Alternative *spinoreticular* pain pathways involve the reticular formation, a diffuse, phylogenetically ancient bilateral network of polysynaptic fibres, ascending and descending throughout the cord and brainstem. Visceral pain is mediated by both pathways: hence surgical division of the lateral spinothalamic tract may only partly relieve intractable pain of visceral origin. Dorsal root autonomic afferents synapse with neurons of the visceral afferent nucleus at the base of the dorsal horn.

General sensory afferents from the face are in the trigeminal nerve, the primary sensory neurons in its ganglion, the secondary neurons in the

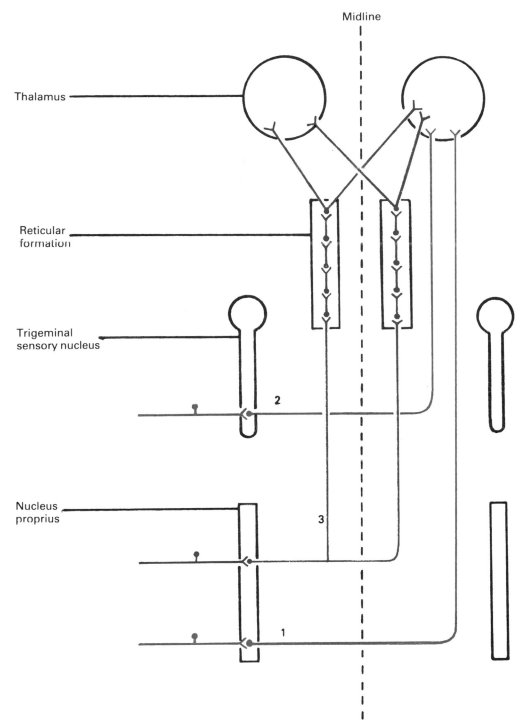

Fig. 4.9 Diagram of pain pathways. 1: Lateral spinothalamic tract. 2: Trigemino-thalamic tract. 3: Bilateral spinoreticular pathways. (Adapted from Sinclair D.C. (1967) *Cutaneous Sensation*. Oxford, Oxford University Press.)

trigeminal sensory nucleus of the brainstem and upper cervical cord. From this nucleus *trigeminothalamic tracts* arise. (Trigeminal nuclei and tracts are described in Chapter 6.) Pain pathways are illustrated in *Fig.* 4.9.

PAIN RESEARCH

Increased understanding of pain has accrued in recent years. In 1965 Melzack and Wall proposed the gate control theory of pain. In 1969 Reynolds showed that stimulation of mesencephalic central grey matter produces deep analgesia without loss of consciousness. In 1974 Pert et al. localized endogenous opiate-like substances, enkephalins and endorphins, in synaptic membranes and their release was later shown to be associated with pain relief.

PAIN PERCEPTION

All perception is complex and largely still under investigation. Individuals vary in their 'pain threshold'; anticipation and fear lower it and increase the perceived intensity of pain. A soldier may sustain a grievous wound but, in the heat of battle, be unaware of it. Modulation of incoming information from nociceptors occurs at several levels in the spinal cord, able to produce inhibition of its transmission (e.g. rubbing a bumped elbow appears to relieve the pain). An explanation of such inhibition was proposed in the 'gate theory' (*Fig.* 4.10). In simple terms, this transmission from spinal nerves to higher brain centres is dependent upon the relative activities in large and small diameter afferents. It is thought that the activity in the large diameter,

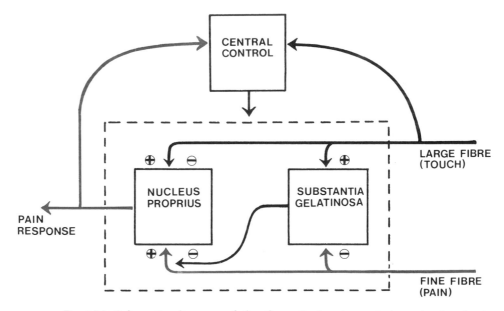

Fig. 4.10 Schematic diagram of the theoretical gate control mechanism in the perception of and response to painful stimuli. Note excitation (+) and inhibition (−). (Adapted from Melzack R. and Wall P. D. (1965) *Science*, **150**, 971.)

low threshold fibres (e.g. from touch corpuscles) inhibits nociceptive transmission via activation of inhibitory interneurons of the substantia gelatinosa: these 'close the gate'. Small (nociceptor) fibres de-activate these inhibitory interneurons and 'open the gate' to the nucleus proprius. Thus artificially increased activity in low threshold cutaneous receptors (e.g. those stimulated by rubbing the skin) can 'close the gate' and then less information from nociceptors is transmitted supraspinally. A major nociceptive barrage 'opens the gate'. This dorsal horn complex also receives corticospinal fibres (originating in sensory cortex), and reticulospinal fibres, providing paths to influence sensory input if required. The original form of the theory has now been reviewed (Wall, 1978): the general 'gate' concept is maintained but its mechanisms are imperfectly understood (particularly regarding pre- and post-synaptic inhibition, and the precise role of the substantia gelatinosa). The clinical implications are valuable: appropriate electrical transcutaneous stimulation of sensory nerves may relieve intractable pain.

A signal advance in concepts of pain mechanisms has been the identifica-

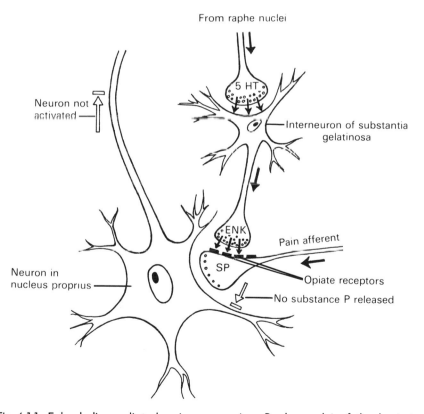

Fig. 4.11 Enkephalin-mediated pain suppression. Raphe nuclei of the brainstem (which produce the neurotransmitter serotonin, **5-HT**) synapse by descending fibres in the dorsolateral spinal tract with interneurons of the substantia gelatinosa (containing enkephalin, **ENK**). Enkephalin binds to opiate receptors of the afferent pain terminals, blocking the release of substance P (**SP**); neurons in the nucleus proprius are not activated. (Adapted from Ottoson D. (1983) *Physiology of the Nervous System.* London, Macmillan.)

tion of opiate receptors in several regions of the central grey matter. In the spinal cord, receptors and enkephalin occur in the substantia gelatinosa and act as pain suppressors (*Fig.* 4.11). Cells in the periaqueductal mesencephalic grey matter and medullary raphe nucleus can be activated by collaterals from ascending or descending pathways. Axons from raphe nuclei project via a small dorsolateral spinal tract (neurotransmitter, serotonin) to interneurons of substantia gelatinosa, some of which release enkephalin, and this, in turn, causes inhibition in the pain pathway. This *raphe-spinal* pathway forms part of a complex descending system that can profoundly affect the rostral transmission of nociceptive information.

A peptide, substance P, appears in the central terminals of pain fibres (Aδ and C), probably as one of the primary transmitters in the pathway. Substance P is not present in dorsal column nuclei.

SIMPLE TOUCH AND PRESSURE (*Fig.* 4.12)

Dorsal root fibres concerned in these modalities are large and myelinated; they enter the cord by the roots' medial divisions, bifurcate into short descending and longer ascending fibres in the dorsal columns, then enter and terminate in the dorsal grey horns of six to eight segments. There is thus a marked overlap of central input from adjacent dorsal roots. Secondary fibres, arising in the *nucleus proprius*, cross to form the contralateral *ventral spinothalamic tract*. Finer tactile and spatial discriminations are not served by this pathway.

DISCRIMINATIVE TOUCH, CONSCIOUS PROPRIOCEPTION, VIBRATION (*Fig.* 4.12)

The dorsal columns convey long (ipsilateral) projection fibres for the above modalities, extending from the dorsal root ganglia to the medulla, forming the *dorsal column–medial lemniscal pathway*. Fibres entering the cord below midthoracic level accumulate medially to form the *fasciculus gracilis;* the input above this is to the *fasciculus cuneatus*. Cell bodies of secondary neurons are in the *nuclei gracilis* and *cuneatus*, located dorsally in the lower medulla. The pathway then crosses in the *sensory decussation* to form the *medial lemniscus*, which ascends through the brainstem to the thalamus and en route receives a trigeminothalamic input ('lemniscus' means a ribbon or fillet).

The pathway is a highly discriminative one, both spatially and in the specificity of fibres for each modality, ensured by relatively discrete synapses, limited divergence, and by 'surround inhibition'. Dorsal column integrity may be tested clinically to illustrate these features. If a subject's finger or toe is moved by an examiner, the individual can state, with closed eyes, which digit is being moved, and in what direction (conscious proprioception or kinaesthesia). Spatial touch is tested by 'two-point discrimination'. Such analytical abilities become apparent in the recognition of familiar objects by manipulation. Vibration (rapidly repeated signals of short duration) is tested by applying a tuning fork to a bony prominence such as the medial malleolus.

Since fibres feed into the dorsal columns from the lateral aspect, the lower

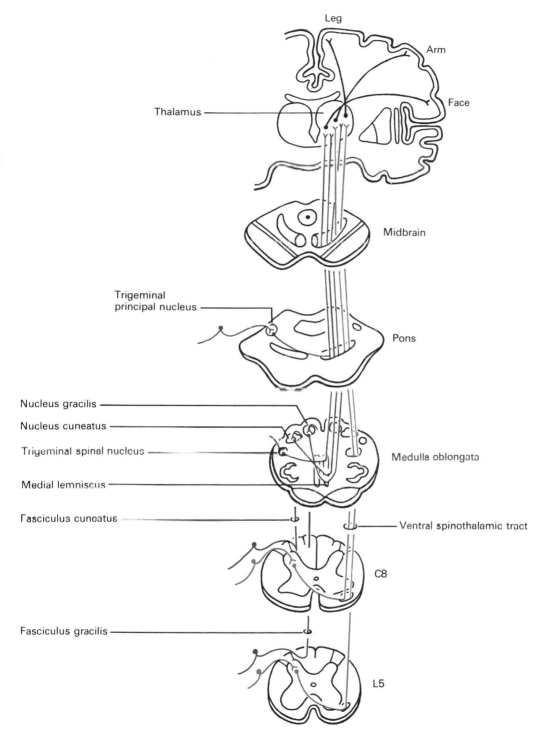

Fig. 4.12 Ascending pathways for tactile sensation. The dorsal column-medial lemniscal path is in blue, the ventral spinothalamic tract is in red.

half of the body is represented medially and the upper half laterally. In the crossed spinothalamic tracts, input accumulates from the mesial aspect and somatic representation is reversed. Since both paths project to the same thalamic region, somatic orientation must be aligned in the brainstem; this occurs in the medial lemniscal pathway. The sensory decussation involves one 90° rotation, and a further 90° rotation occurs as the medial lemniscus ascends (*Fig.* 4.12).

The dorsal columns also carry 'passenger fibres' which ascend or descend before entering dorsal grey horns, synapsing there with secondary sensory neurons of nucleus proprius or the thoracic nucleus. Intersegmental fibres are also necessary for some spinal reflexes, such as the flexor reflex, in which the response implicates motor neurons of several segments.

DORSAL COLUMN RESEARCH

This account of the functions of dorsal column and spinothalamic pathways accords with most clinical experience. There is, however, evidence of a more complex relationship and views on this are briefly summarized here.

Animals trained to discriminate cutaneous stimuli for weight, texture, vibration and two-point position can continue to do so after dorsal column section. Observed functional losses are primarily related to movement, such as failure of orientation, failure to handle objects, the adoption of immobile postures, particularly when deprived of vision. It is proposed that environmental stimuli are of two main types: those which are 'passively impressed on the animal or man' (carried by spinothalamic tracts) and 'those that must be actively explored by motor movement or sequential analysis before they can be successfully discriminated'. Dorsal columns are considered to be essential only for the latter (Wall, 1970). After dorsal column severance, cats have difficulty in **learning** discriminative tasks (Kitai and Weinberg, 1968) and monkeys cannot detect the direction of movement of a tactile stimulus (Vierck, 1974). Examination by Wall and Noordenbos (1977) of three human subjects with dorsal column lesions of known extent (severance extended ventrolaterally in two) showed that: 1) they were unable to carry out tasks requiring simultaneous analysis of spatial and temporal characteristics of a stimulus, e.g. detection of the direction of its movement on the skin; 2) kinaesthesia, tactile localization and vibration sense were impaired rather than lost.

The pathway for lower limb afferents mediating conscious proprioception is also under review: in cats these impulses ascend initially in the fasciculus gracilis of the lumbar cord but synapse in the thoracic nucleus; the pathway then joins the ipsilateral dorsal spinocerebellar tract as far as the medulla, leaving via collaterals to enter the *nucleus z* (of Brodal and Pompeiano, 1957). This lies immediately rostral to the nucleus gracilis and its axons enter the sensory decussation to join the opposite medial lemniscus. This atypical four-neuron pathway has been widely quoted in textbooks of human neuroanatomy as also applicable to humans; if so, then lower limb proprioception should be relatively unaffected by cervical dorsal column compression and that is not the usual clinical finding. Patients with dorsal column dysfunction due to pressure from buckled ligamenta flava in cervical spondylosis have been reviewed by MacFadyen (1984). Most of these complained of ataxia of gait and sensory changes (numbness, paraesthesia); on examination they had loss of joint position and vibration senses in the lower limbs, often in upper limbs also.

At a practical level it is difficult fully to reconcile all these observations: whilst accepting that parallel paths exist, the traditional view of dorsal column function still provides a satisfactory basis for most clinical interpretation.

Pathways to the cerebellum

Note: Symptoms of cerebellar dysfunction are resultant upon damage to that part of the brain. Lesions of spinocerebellar pathways are not recognized clinically.

In contrast to ascending tracts for the cerebrum, those leading to the cerebellum generally provide an *ipsilateral input*, and form a two-neuron chain; all the primary neuron somata are in dorsal root ganglia. There are two functional groups: one group (dorsal spinocerebellar and cuneocerebellar tracts) simply relays proprioceptive input from muscles and joint receptors; the other (ventral and rostral spinocerebellar tracts) conveys pre-integrated information about spinal motor activity and reflexes.

DORSAL SPINOCEREBELLAR TRACT

The cell bodies of primary neurons are in dorsal root ganglia, those of the secondary neurons are in the *thoracic nucleus* (nucleus dorsalis of Clarke). Since this nucleus exists only in cord segments T1–L2, input from below L2 must ascend via the dorsal columns before entering the grey matter: the nucleus is therefore large at its caudal end. Fibres from cervical spinal nerves C5–C8 descend similarly to its upper part. Axons from the thoracic nucleus remain uncrossed, form the dorsal spinocerebellar tract and enter the cerebellum via its inferior peduncle. This tract carries proprioceptive impulses from muscle spindle receptors, Golgi tendon organs and joint capsules, also from some cutaneous pressure receptors. It relays information to the cerebellum about joint movement and muscle contraction, also about external mechanical forces as applied for example to the sole of the foot.

CUNEOCEREBELLAR TRACT

Proprioceptive input from spinal nerves C1–C4 ascends to the *accessory cuneate nucleus*, sited dorsolaterally in the medulla (*see Fig.* 5.8) and thence to the inferior cerebellar peduncle. It should be noted that the cuneate (dorsal column lemniscal) and accessory cuneate nuclei, though adjacent, are on different pathways and subserve different functions.

VENTRAL SPINOCEREBELLAR TRACT

This tract only transmits impulses from the lower limb. Most of its neuron bodies are sited ventrolaterally, a few dorsomedially, in the lumbosacral grey matter: they cannot easily be distinguished from adjacent motor neurons. It conveys integrated information about the internal working of lower motor centres in the lumbosacral cord, including spinal reflexes and motor pattern generators, of general significance in posture and movement of the lower limbs. Many of its fibres ascend contralaterally, recrossing at cerebellar level so that the input, via the superior cerebellar peduncle, is mostly ipsilateral.

ROSTRAL SPINOCEREBELLAR TRACT

This tract, identified physiologically in 1964, is the functional equivalent of a ventral spinocerebellar tract for the upper limb. It ascends uncrossed, enters superior and inferior peduncles and terminates mostly ipsilaterally in the anterior lobe of the cerebellum. The cells of origin have not been clearly identified.

Other tracts

INDIRECT SPINOCEREBELLAR TRACTS

The *spino-olivary tract* is small and ends in the inferior olive, a folded grey mass in the medulla. Most of the olivary input comes from higher centres. The inferior olive integrates information and projects this to the cerebellum via the inferior peduncle.

Spinoreticular fibres pass to the medullary reticular formation; this has an input to the cerebellum via the inferior peduncle. It is a phylogenetically old polysynaptic pathway.

SPINOTECTAL TRACT

This small crossed tract is a supplementary pain pathway ending in the superior colliculus which is sited in the tectum, or roof of the midbrain. It is assumed to arise in dorsal horn cells and ascends in close association with the lateral spinothalamic tract. Reflex head movements in response to visual or auditory stimuli are mediated via the tectum: the spinotectal tract is concerned with similar reactions to pain.

PROPRIOSPINAL TRACTS

The *fasciculus proprius* lies at the periphery of the grey matter and consists of ascending and descending fibres mediating intersegmental reflexes. Some descending branches of dorsal root fibres aggregate in small comma-shaped bundles between the dorsal column funiculi.

Descending tracts (*Fig.* 4.8)

The *pyramidal tract* extends from the cerebral cortex to ventral horn cells of the spinal cord (corticospinal) and to some cranial nerve nuclei in the brainstem (corticobulbar). Relatively recently evolved, it is superimposed upon a phylogenetically more ancient and diverse pattern (*Fig.* 4.13). In lower vertebrates the somatomotor and visceromotor 'control centres' (corpus striatum and hypothalamus) operate through the polysynaptic *reticulospinal* path. Equilibration control is via the archecerebellum and vestibular nuclei to the *vestibulospinal* tract. The tectum, important in visual and auditory motor reflexes, has its *tectospinal* tract. In the primate pattern, the highly developed cerebral cortex has its own direct (pyramidal) path, and also acts indirectly via some brainstem nuclei (e.g. reticular and red nuclei). In humans the corpus striatum influences descending pathways principally

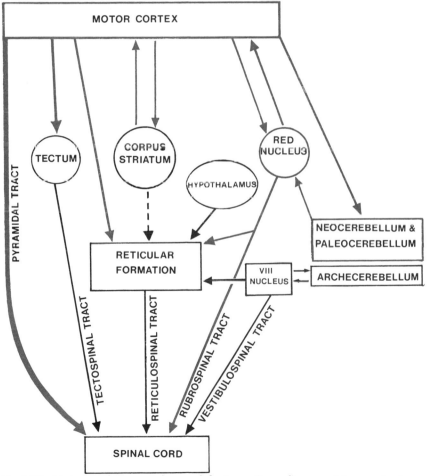

Fig. 4.13 Motor pathways. Advanced features (in red) present in a primate are superimposed on a basic motor system (in black) of lower vertebrates. The human corpus striatum influences descending tracts principally via its cortical connexions; a projection to the midbrain reticular formation is shown by an interrupted line. For more detailed connexions of the corpus striatum see Fig. 9.7.

through its projection to the cortex (via the thalamus). Non-pyramidal tracts originate in the brainstem and are polysynaptic. Pyramidal and non-pyramidal tracts are anatomically and physiologically interlocked and both are involved in the collective clinical term 'upper motor neuron lesion'.

THE PYRAMIDAL TRACT

This is so named because the corticospinal tract traverses the medullary pyramid, but it also includes corticobulbar (corticonuclear) fibres to motor nuclei of cranial nerves (*Fig.* 4.14).

Anterior to the central sulcus of each cerebral hemisphere, the primary motor area (precentral gyrus) and the premotor area (*see Fig.* 12.8) are the source of 60% of the pyramidal fibres; the remainder arise in the parietal cortex. The neuronal somata are pyramidal in shape and 3% are the so-called 'giant pyramidal' or Betz cells, up to 120 μm in height with thick, fast-conducting axons.

In the cortical motor representation of the body the lower limbs are superomedial and the face inferolateral (*see Fig.* 12.9). Moreover the area of motor cortex innervating an individual part is related to its functional motor significance, delicacy of control and innervation density rather than its actual size. Neurons to the face, tongue, larynx and hand are necessarily numerous and their somata occupy large cortical areas; they are associated, via ventral horn cells, with small motor units of neuromuscular innervation.

The pyramidal tract, of about a million fibres, descends through the posterior limb of the internal capsule, occupies the middle three-fifths of the basis pedunculi in the midbrain, separates into bundles in the pons and forms the pyramid on the ventral aspect of the medulla, where the two tracts are adjacent, flanking the midline. In the lower medulla 85–90% of the fibres cross in the *pyramidal decussation* to form a *lateral corticospinal tract* in each lateral funiculus. Most of the remainder continue as a *ventral corticospinal tract*, descending to the cervical and upper thoracic regions, the majority crossing in the white commissure prior to termination. **The corticospinal projection is essentially contralateral:** thus the left cerebral hemisphere controls the right side of the body. A few fibres, about 2%, continue ipsilaterally into the lateral tract and do not cross. Corticospinal axons synapse, mostly via interneurons, with α and γ motor neurons of the ventral grey column; 55% terminating in cervical segments (mostly for upper limbs), 20% in thoracic segments, 25% in lumbosacral segments. In primates some axons synapse directly on α motor neurons, particularly those which innervate digital muscles and this conduces to specificity and delicacy of control.

As the pyramidal tract traverses the brainstem, corticobulbar fibres supply motor nuclei of cranial nerves. Some cross the midline, others do not. Some cranial nerves receive a bilateral cortical innervation.

The principal feature of pyramidal tracts is that axons descend from their cortical origins to their spinal or bulbar terminations without interruption. Some pyramidal axons are the longest in the central nervous system: a 100 μm Betz cell reaching to the lowest part of the spinal cord has an axon about

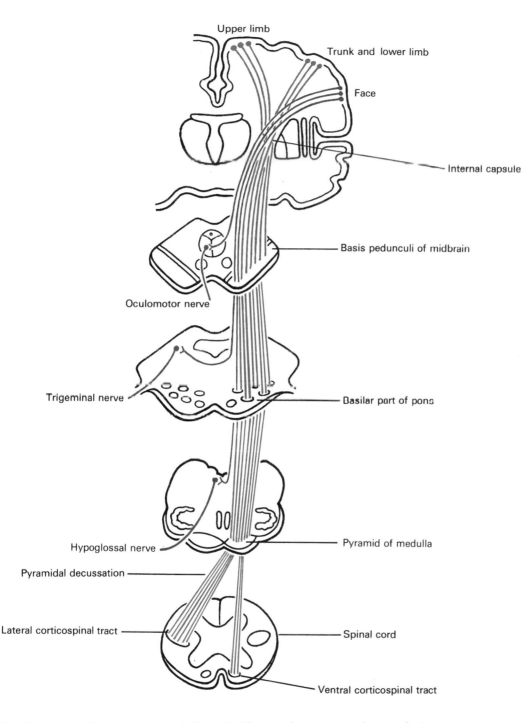

Fig. 4.14 Pyramidal tracts, corticobulbar (in blue) and corticospinal (in red). In addition to the cranial nerves shown, corticobulbar fibres innervate the motor nuclei of the trochlear, abducent and facial nerves and the nucleus ambiguus (of the glossopharyngeal, vagus and cranial accessory nerves).

60 cm long, or 6000 times its cell body height. To illustrate this relationship, imagine the latter as one metre, then the axon would be 6 km long! By contrast, motor tracts arising in the brainstem have many intermediate synapses in their courses.

The cortical areas from which the pyramidal tract arises also project to subcortical motor centres such as the red nucleus and reticular formation partly via corticospinal collaterals and partly via separate neurons. Corticospinal fibres arising from the postcentral 'sensory' cortex give off branches to secondary sensory neurons such as those in the nucleus proprius, the cuneate and gracile nuclei and thereby influence the central transmission of sensory impulses. During periods of intense physical activity unwanted forms of input can be suppressed.

VESTIBULOSPINAL TRACTS

The vestibular nuclei receive afferents via the eighth nerve from the vestibular apparatus of the inner ear and have intimate cerebellar connexions but have no direct control from the cerebral cortex. The main (ventrolateral) *vestibulospinal tract* starts in the lateral vestibular (Deiter's) nucleus and descends uncrossed throughout the cord's ventral funiculus. It facilitates extensor muscle action in the anti-gravity maintenance of posture and in locomotion. A much smaller tract, the *medial longitudinal fasciculus* receives input from the medial and inferior vestibular nuclei and descends as a *medial vestibulospinal tract* to cervical segments, conveying vestibular influences to the neck and forelimb muscles. Continued rostrally throughout the brainstem to cranial nerve nuclei supplying eye muscles, this fasciculus also coordinates movement of head and eyes (*see Fig.* 6.10).

RETICULOSPINAL TRACTS

The reticular formation is a phylogenetically primitive network of small neurons extending throughout the brainstem and into the spinal cord. It has a diverse input; its descending connexions are mostly from the cerebral cortex, cerebellum and red nuclei. Spinal projections terminate on α and γ motor neurons, the latter influencing muscle tone. Its tracts are not well localized in the spinal cord: our understanding of them is derived mainly from animal study, direct information about their human anatomy is very limited. They comprise long and short polysynaptic routes. The *medullary (lateral) reticulospinal tract*, sited deep in the lateral funiculus, descends bilaterally from an inhibitory area of the medullary reticular formation. The smaller *pontine (medial) reticulospinal tract* consists of scattered fibres in the ventral funiculus which descend, mostly uncrossed, from a facilitatory area of the pontine reticular formation. Precise functional inter-relationships between the two tracts is not clearly defined and during normal activity (as distinct from experimental stimulation) it probably varies with the complex input to the reticular formation. Reticulospinal tracts innervate axial and proximal limb musculature and are involved in control of muscle tone, posture, locomotion and other stereotyped limb movements. Reticulospinal tracts, like corticospinal, can influence the central transmission of sensory information.

RUBROSPINAL TRACT

The red nuclei in the midbrain developed at the terrestrial evolutionary stage and their role in an ascending pathway from cerebellum to thalamus increased during phylogeny pari passu with the evolving cerebral cortex. They receive fibres from the motor cortex but the significance of the rubrospinal tracts in limb control varies between species.

Rubrospinal fibres, numerous in quadrupeds, decussate in the midbrain and descend in the lateral funiculus, enhancing flexor muscle activity during locomotion. In cats the cortico-rubrospinal and lateral corticospinal pathways are intermingled and terminate similarly. In monkeys also the red nucleus participates in an indirect corticospinal pathway. In humans the tract is probably small but its precise size and extent are uncertain because of the paucity of clinical evidence.

TECTOSPINAL TRACT

This arises in the superior colliculus of the midbrain tectum. Its fibres decussate at once and descend to cervical segments. The tract is involved in reflex head movements in response to visual, auditory and painful stimuli.

The organization of descending tracts

Cortical control is via *direct* corticospinal and *indirect* cortico-reticulospinal and cortico-rubrospinal routes. Integration of motor activity is dependent upon intrinsic spinal mechanisms: the influence of descending fibres is not simply mediated via motor neurons but also through reflex connexions and *motor pattern generators* in the cord. 'Recent insight into the extremely complex neuronal organization of the spinal cord is compatible with the view that the programmes for learned motor activities may be "laid down" in the cord. "Higher levels" may have their importance during the learning process mainly by correcting and refining the first crude programmes.' (Brodal, 1981).

Muscle tone is maintained by continuous muscle spindle activation of α motor neurons: corticospinal, cortico-reticulospinal and -rubrospinal tracts exert an inhibitory control over this. Vestibular nuclei are largely independent of cortical control; they facilitate antigravity extensor muscle action. Section of the brainstem rostral to the vestibular nuclei produces *decerebrate rigidity*. Following a stroke there is spasticity of lower limb extensor muscles.

Corticospinal and rubrospinal fibres predominantly activate flexor muscles. Vestibulospinal tracts facilitate extensors and, together with reticulospinal tracts, they are important in equilibration, maintenance of an upright posture and locomotion. Reticulospinal innervation is mostly to axial and proximal limb musculature, corticospinal to distal limb muscles.

Experimental transection of the medullary pyramids in a monkey abolishes discrete movements of the fingers and toes and also results in hypotonia, loss of cremasteric and abdominal wall reflexes. No such isolated lesion occurs clinically in humans whereby we might evaluate detailed function but the human pyramidal tract is evidently highly evolved and essential for rapid, precise skilled movements. The pyramidal and the other motor tracts are functionally coordinated: the widely used clinical terms 'pyramidal tract syndrome' or 'pyramidal signs' are misleading because many features, such as spasticity, are partly resultant on damage to non-pyramidal motor tracts, e.g. reticulospinal, also involved in an 'upper motor neuron lesion'.

Descending autonomic fibres

Visceromotor fibres descend from the hypothalamus and from regulatory cardiovascular and respiratory centres in the medulla and pons via a polysynaptic visceral efferent pathway, interspersed with reticulospinal fibres in the lateral funiculus. Its multisynaptic nature makes experimental localization difficult. It controls the sympathetic (T1–L2) and sacral parasympathetic (S2–S4) spinal outflow. For the thoracic and most of the non-pelvic viscera the parasympathetic supply emerges from the brainstem in the vagus nerve.

APPLIED ANATOMY

SENSORY ATAXIA

Ataxia is incoordination of movement and occurs in diseases of the cerebellum (cerebellar ataxia), or damage to the dorsal spinal columns (sensory ataxia). The spinal cord diameter is greatest in the lower cervical region, a very mobile part of the vertebral column. Collagenous degeneration associated with arthritis can cause ligamenta flava to deform and buckle when the neck extends: *cervical compression* of the dorsal columns ensues.

Subacute combined degeneration of the cord is caused by vitamin B_{12} deficiency. Ataxia and paraesthesia are symptoms of dorsal column demyelination. The term 'combined' is used because motor pathways are also affected. *Tabes dorsalis* (locomotor ataxia), an advanced form of syphilis, causes atrophy of the dorsal columns and also affects dorsal spinal roots, leading to proprioceptive and general sensory loss (*Fig. 4.15*).

PAIN PATHWAYS

Syringomyelia is congenital cystic cavitation of the central canal, which destroys commissural fibres of the spinothalamic tracts. 'Dissociated anaesthesia' ensues: pain sensation is lost but tactile paths in dorsal columns are unaffected.

Referred pain is pain from a visceral source referred to an area of the body surface with the same segmental innervation. Thus the early pain in appendicitis is referred to the peri-umbilical region. Spinal and supraspinal paths are involved and there is proximity between these visceral and somatic

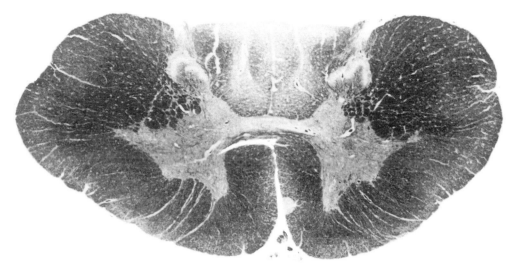

Fig. 4.15 Tabes dorsalis: a transverse section of the cervical spinal cord shows degeneration and atrophy of the dorsal white columns. (Weigert stain, × 12.8.)

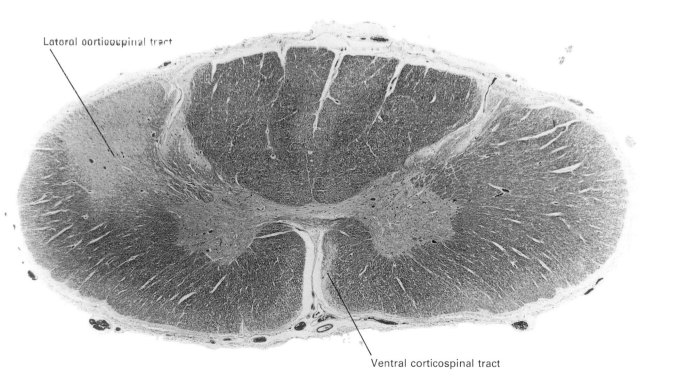

Lateral corticospinal tract

Ventral corticospinal tract

Fig. 4.16 Transverse section of the cervical spinal cord, viewed from below, showing pyramidal tract degeneration following a left-sided cerebral thrombosis. (Weigert stain, × 12.8.)

afferents at thalamic level. The abdominal wall rigidity of peritonitis involves only a spinal reflex.

The Brown-Séquard syndrome follows spinal hemisection. Pain and temperature sensation are lost contralateral to the lesion. Touch sensation is little affected because it has both ipsilateral (dorsal column) and contralateral (ventral spinothalamic) paths. There is also ipsilateral motor loss.

MOTOR PATHWAYS

It has been noted that thousands of axons may converge on a single ventral horn cell (*see Fig.* 2.6). The collective term *upper motor neuron lesion* usually indicates generalized damage to descending fibres, not only to pyramidal tracts. This condition is characterized by spasticity and exaggerated tendon reflexes, but there is little atrophy of affected muscles: stretch reflex arcs are intact but no longer under inhibitory supraspinal control. The *plantar reflex* becomes extensor: when the lateral part of the sole is firmly stroked the great toe is dorsiflexed and the other toes fan out; this is the *Babinski sign*. The superficial *abdominal reflex* (stroking the anterior abdominal wall normally causes contraction of underlying muscles) and the male *cremasteric reflex* (elicited by stroking the medial side of the thigh) are lost. The precise anatomical mechanism for these changes in superficial reflexes is unclear.

Following cord injury there is initially a state of *spinal shock*, characterized by flaccid paralysis below the lesion, loss of tendon reflexes and retention of urine. As this subsides spastic paralysis ensues, with uninhibited flexor reflexes; slight stimulation of the foot provokes gross flexor spasms. An *automatic bladder* usually develops whereby, through sacral reflexes, it empties when distended. Lesions of the conus medullaris or cauda equina interrupt the central connexions of the bladder which then becomes *atonic*, distension causing incontinence.

Transection at spinal cord level C4 results in loss of diaphragmatic and intercostal muscle action, with respiratory paralysis. A lesion between cord segments C4 and T1 paralyses all four limbs (quadriplegia), the severity of paralysis in the upper limbs depending on the level of section. Damage to segment T1 affects small muscles in the hands. Section at T1 or above interrupts the sympathetic efferent pathway, and its outflow at this level to the head. Signs of sympathetic denervation of the head are included in *Horner's syndrome:* on the side of lesion there is pupillary constriction (miosis), loss of sweating of the face (anhidrosis), drooping of upper eyelid (ptosis–levator palpebrae superioris contains some smooth muscle), and apparent enophthalmos. Damage at midthoracic level results in paralysis of the lower limbs (paraplegia). Section at S1 causes loss of sacral parasympathetic control over the bladder and rectum. It is sometimes wrongly assumed that paraplegia in the male must be accompanied by sexual impotence: although psychogenic influences are rendered inoperative, relevant reflexes should be intact in high lesions, though probably lost in damage to sacral cord or cauda equina. Erection is mediated through parasympathetic fibres from S2–4, seminal emission through sympathetic fibres from T11–L2 cord segments. Recovery may not begin for 3 months after injury and can continue for up to two years.

If ventral horn cells are destroyed, as in poliomyelitis, or peripheral nerves are damaged, a *lower motor neuron lesion* results. There is severe atrophy of muscles, loss of muscle tone and tendon reflexes.

Chapter 5

Brainstem

Transition from Spinal Cord to Medulla Oblongata

As an introduction to a study of the brainstem it is helpful to consider how the grey and white matter of the cervical spinal cord are rearranged in the medulla. This transition is illustrated diagrammatically in *Fig.* 5.1 and by sections in *Figs.* 5.6 to 5.8.

White matter

On each side of the medulla, *corticospinal fibres* are located ventrally in the pyramids. As they descend through the *pyramidal decussation*, fibres forming a *lateral corticospinal tract* incline dorsolaterally into the lateral funiculus, and thus cut through the grey matter, isolating the ventral horn.

The nuclei gracilis and cuneatus, on the dorsal aspect of the medulla, mark the rostral extent of the spinal dorsal columns. Their axons arch ventromedially as *internal arcuate fibres* of the *sensory decussation*, crossing to form the opposite *medial lemniscus*, dorsal to the pyramid. This decussation also intersects grey matter, separating the medullary equivalent of the dorsal horn (trigeminal spinal nucleus) from the central grey. Traced rostrally, the grey matter around the central canal opens out into the floor of the fourth ventricle.

Two tracts in the spinal ventral funiculus are displaced dorsally in the medulla by the pyramid and medial lemniscus; these are the *tectospinal tract* and the *medial longitudinal fasciculus* (medial vestibulospinal tract).

Tracing the tracts of the lateral funiculus rostrally, the *dorsal spinocerebellar tract* enters the inferior cerebellar peduncle, and the *ventral spinocerebellar tract* passes through the medulla and pons to enter the superior peduncle. The remaining tracts (excluding corticospinal fibres, already described) are grouped dorsal to the inferior olivary nucleus. The *lateral* and *ventral spinothalamic* and *spinotectal tracts* are close to one another, and are sometimes collectively termed the 'spinal lemniscus'. The *reticulospinal, rubrospinal, main vestibulospinal tracts* and the *visceral efferent pathway* are also located here.

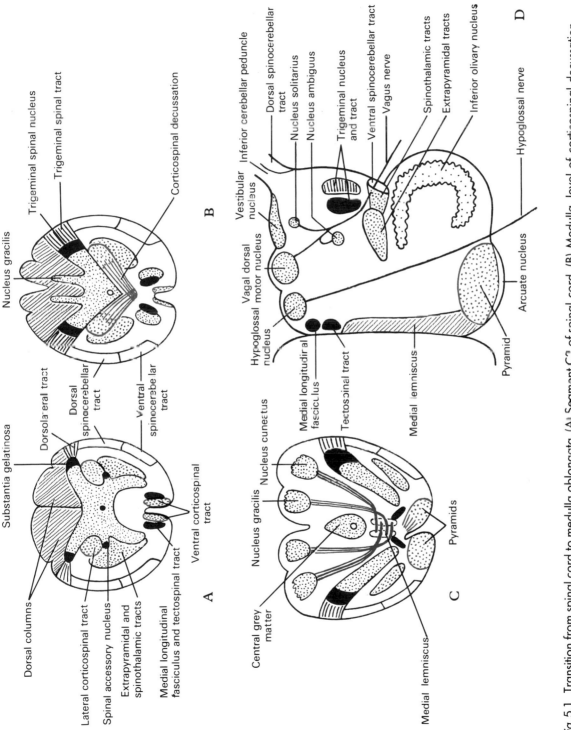

Fig. 5.1 Transition from spinal cord to medulla oblongata. (A) Segment C2 of spinal cord. (B) Medulla, level of corticospinal decussation. (C) Medulla, level of sensory decussation. (D) Medulla, level of olive.

Grey matter

Although the spinal pattern of grey matter is altered in the medulla, there are functional similarities (see *Table* 5.1). Motor nerve roots emerge from the upper cervical cord in two separate rows for muscles of dissimilar developmental origin. The ventral nerve roots supply myotomal muscles. Other fibres emerge more dorsally from the lateral surface of the cord to form the *spinal accessory (XI)* nerve, ascending through the foramen magnum to supply branchial arch musculature. The *hypoglossal (XII)* nerve rootlets are in series with, and equivalent to spinal ventral roots. The *cranial roots of the accessory (XI)*, the *vagus (X)* and *glossopharyngeal (IX)* nerves supply branchial arch muscles: their roots emerge from the medulla in series with the spinal accessory nerve and are therefore dorsolateral to the hypoglossal roots.

In the first cervical spinal segment the nucleus proprius, substantia gelatinosa and tract of Lissauer are replaced by the *spinal nucleus and tract of the trigeminal (V) nerve* (hence there is no C1 dermatome). The trigeminal tract, external to the nucleus, contains input fibres from the facial region, concerned with pain and temperature sensation. The thoracic nucleus has its medullary equivalent in the *accessory cuneate nucleus*.

Visceral (parasympathetic) components of cranial nerves are represented in the medulla by vagal and glossopharyngeal nuclei. The vagus provides a

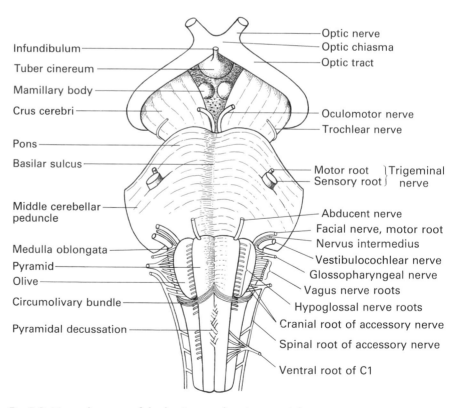

Fig. 5.2 Ventral aspect of the brainstem showing cranial nerves.

parasympathetic supply to thoracic and abdominal viscera, the latter supplemented by the sacral parasympathetic. In contrast to the spinal cord, there is no sympathetic outflow in cranial nerves. Sympathetic supply to the head and neck ascends from upper thoracic nerves and relays in cervical ganglia; the intracranial supply comes from the superior cervical ganglion via a plexus around the internal carotid artery.

Table 5.1 Comparison of grey matter in the spinal cord and lower medulla

	Grey matter of spinal cord	Medulla
Dorsal column	Nucleus proprius Thoracic nucleus Visceral afferent	Trigeminal spinal nucleus Accessory cuneate nucleus Vagal sensory nucleus
Lateral column	Sympathetic efferent Parasympathetic efferent	Nil Vagal dorsal motor nucleus
Ventral column	Somatomotor Branchiomotor-cervical (spinal accessory)	Hypoglossal Nucleus ambiguus (cranial accessory)

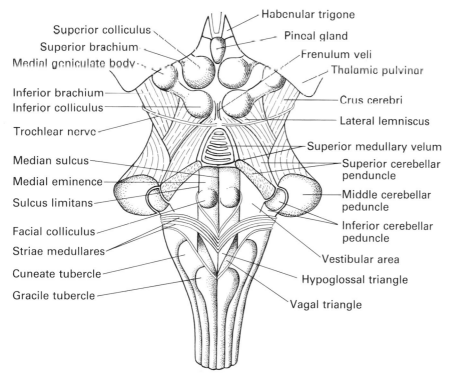

Fig. 5.3 Dorsal aspect of the brainstem and the floor of the fourth ventricle.

General Topography of the Brainstem

The brainstem comprises the medulla, pons and midbrain (*Figs.* 5.2 and 5.3).

The medulla

This is slightly conical, wider rostrally. It is in continuity with the spinal cord immediately below the foramen magnum and extends to the lower border of the pons. The very small central canal of the spinal cord continues through the lower half of the medulla and then opens out as the *fourth ventricle*. From the dorsal aspect the medulla is seen to have a *lower closed part*, and an *upper open part* in the floor of the fourth ventricle.

The *ventral median fissure* of spinal cord continues to the lower border of pons, but in the lower medulla it is interrupted by the *decussation of the pyramids*. The spinal *dorsal median sulcus*, between the two fasciculi gracilis, extends into the lower medulla. Fibres of the hypoglossal nerve emerge from a *ventrolateral sulcus*. The cranial accessory, vagus and glossopharyngeal nerves emerge as a row of rootlets in a *dorsolateral sulcus*. On each side the medulla may be subdivided by these sulci into ventral, lateral and dorsal regions.

Ventrally, on each side of the median fissure, is the longitudinal elevation of the *pyramid*, composed of corticospinal fibres, most crossing in the pyramidal decussation to form a lateral corticospinal tract in the lateral funiculus of the cord, the rest continuing into the ventral funiculus as the ventral corticospinal tract. The *abducent (VI)* nerve emerges between the pyramid and pons.

Lateral to each pyramid, and separated from it by rootlets of the *hypoglossal (XII)* nerve, is the *olive*, an oval bulge made by a crumpled mass of grey matter, the *inferior olivary nucleus*. A few fibres emerge from the ventral median fissure, curving round the olive as the *circumolivary bundle* en route to the inferior cerebellar peduncle; these arise in the *arcuate nucleus*, sparse grey matter superficial to the pyramid. Lateral to the olive, rootlets of the *glossopharyngeal (IX)*, *vagus (X)* and *cranial accessory (XI) nerves* emerge, the last being joined by the spinal accessory nerve. In the angle between the lateral medulla and lower pontine border, the *facial (VII)* and *vestibulocochlear (VIII) nerves* appear: the facial is the more medial of the two and between them is the *nervus intermedius*, the so-called 'sensory root' of the facial nerve.

On each side of the dorsal surface of the lower half of medulla the fasciculi gracilis and cuneatus terminate in two ovoid *gracile and cuneate tubercles*, produced by the corresponding nuclei. Dorsal to each olive an *inferior cerebellar peduncle* appears and ascends to the lateral angle of the fourth ventricle, where it arches backwards into the cerebellum between superior and middle peduncles: here it receives the *striae medullares*, fibres from the arcuate nucleus which pass dorsally through the midline of the medulla and then cross the ventricular floor. Efferent fibres from the arcuate nucleus to cerebellum are hence visible on the medullary surface both ventrally (circumolivary bundle) and dorsally (striae medullares).

The pons

The pons is between the medulla and midbrain. Its prominent, convex, ventral, basilar surface is marked by transverse fibres, arising in numerous *pontine nuclei* and forming a *middle cerebellar peduncle* on each side. The junction of pons and peduncle is arbitrarily set at the attachment of the *trigeminal (V) nerve*. This nerve has two components; a small motor root is anteromedial to a larger sensory root. On the ventral surface there is a shallow midline *basilar sulcus* which is occupied by the basilar artery. The dorsal surface of pons forms the rostral half of the fourth ventricle's floor. When the internal pontine structure is described it will be evident that its dorsal region, or *tegmentum*, and its ventral *basilar part* are quite different in content. The tegmentum is continuous rostrally with the tegmentum of the midbrain, caudally with the medulla; it contains cranial nerve nuclei, reticular formation and slender association tracts. Pyramidal tracts descend through the basilar region, broken into bundles by transverse pontocerebellar fibres.

The fourth ventricle

During hindbrain development, combined ventral flexure and dorsal cerebellar growth cause the neural tube to widen and flatten. The alar laminae of its lateral walls are splayed apart, like opening a book, and the roof plate is greatly attenuated (*Fig.* 5.4). Grey matter forms its floor; on each side the basal (motor) lamina is medial, the alar (sensory) lamina lateral and the sulcus limitans between them. Thus, in the floor of the fourth ventricle, somatic motor nuclei of the cranial nerves are near the midline, somatic sensory nuclei are lateral, and visceral components are intermediate around the sulcus limitans.

The *rhomboid fossa*, or floor of the fourth ventricle, is formed by the dorsal surfaces of pons and the open part of medulla. Between the midbrain aqueduct rostrally and central canal of medulla caudally, its lateral boundaries are formed by the superior cerebellar peduncles, inferior peduncles,

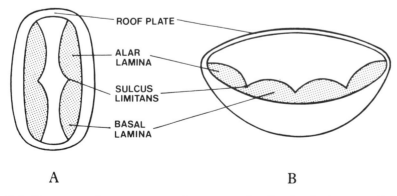

ROOF PLATE

ALAR LAMINA

SULCUS LIMITANS

BASAL LAMINA

A   B

Fig. 5.4 Diagrammatic transverse sections comparing the developing neural tube in the spinal cord (A) and in the region of the fourth ventricle (B).

cuneate and gracile tubercles (*Fig.* 5.3). At its widest level it has a *lateral recess* on each side. The floor is divided longitudinally by a *median sulcus*, from which *striae medullares* cross into lateral recesses, their position dividing the floor into pontine and medullary regions. Rostral to the striae on each side, between median sulcus and sulcus limitans, is the *medial eminence*, in whose lower part a slight swelling, the *facial colliculus*, is produced by facial nerve motor fibres looping over the abducent nucleus. The sensory region lateral to the sulcus limitans overlies the vestibular nuclear complex, and is termed the *vestibular area*. Caudal to the striae are two motor nuclei: adjacent to the midline is the *hypoglossal triangle;* lateral to this the *vagal triangle* is a shallow depression like an inverted 'V'. These features, likened to a tip of a pen, are collectively termed the 'calamus scriptorius'. These triangles mark the rostral ends of the hypoglossal and vagal motor nuclei.

The roof of the fourth ventricle is angled in sagittal section (*Fig.* 5.5) and closely related to the cerebellum. Rostrally the *superior medullary velum* extends between the two superior cerebellar peduncles and meets the midbrain tectum. The cerebellum's lingula is fused with the dorsal surface of the velum. The caudal part of the roof is a very thin lamina of fused pia and ependyma, the *inferior medullary velum*, attached laterally to the medulla and forming the posterior boundary of each lateral recess. The caudal part of the roof is deficient centrally as the *median aperture of the fourth ventricle* (foramen of Magendie) through which cerebrospinal fluid, formed in the ventricular system, escapes into the subarachnoid space. The lateral recesses lead to two smaller *lateral openings* (foramina of Luschka). The *tela choroidea* is a double fold of pia mater between the cerebellum and caudal part of the ventricle's roof, its vascular fringes containing the *choroid plexuses* of the fourth ventricle. Where these invaginate the roof its ependyma becomes

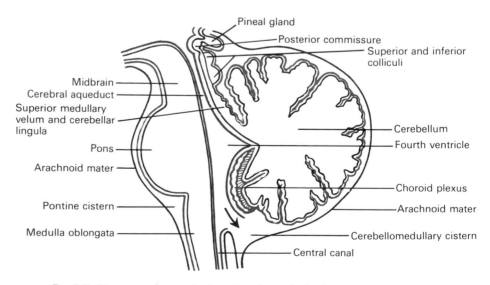

Fig. 5.5 Diagram of a sagittal section through the brainstem and cerebellum. The arrow is in the median aperture of the fourth ventricle. Ependyma in blue, pia mater in red.

secretory epithelium. The plexuses form the shape of a letter T, its vertical limb doubles as a convoluted vascular projection flanking the midline and extending caudally almost to the median aperture. The horizontal part extends into each lateral recess, and often protrudes through the lateral apertures.

The midbrain

The mesencephalon, about 2 cm in length and the shortest brainstem segment, connects the pons and cerebellum to the cerebrum and traverses the tentorial hiatus. For description it is divided sagittally into right and left halves, or *cerebral peduncles*, each consisting of a ventral *crus cerebri* (basis pedunculi), a dorsal *tegmentum* and an intervening stratum of pigmented cells, the *substantia nigra*.

Each crus cerebri contains axons descending ipsilaterally from the cerebral cortex, namely corticospinal, corticobulbar and corticopontine fibres. A *lateral sulcus* grooves the side of each peduncle. Between the crura is the *interpeduncular fossa*, the floor of which is known as the *posterior perforated substance*, because it is penetrated by small arteries: the two *oculomotor (III) nerves* emerge from the sides of the fossa.

The *cerebral aqueduct* traverses the tegmentum, connecting the third and fourth ventricles. The region dorsal to the plane of the aqueduct is the *tectum*, or roof, occupied externally by four paired, round elevations, the *superior* and *inferior colliculi* (corpora quadrigemina). From the caudal end of the tectum a white median fold, the *frenulum veli*, extends to the superior medullary velum. On each side of the frenulum a slender *trochlear (IV) nerve* emerges and curves ventrally round the midbrain. The inferior colliculi are relay stations on auditory pathways. From each inferior colliculus, ascending fibres form an elevated *inferior brachium* as they pass to a thalamic nucleus, the *medial geniculate body*. The superior colliculi are concerned with visual reflexes. A *superior brachium* extends to each superior colliculus from a *lateral geniculate body;* it comprises descending fibres from the optic tract and visual cortex (retinocollicular and corticocollicular).

Internal Structure of the Brainstem

The locations of the cranial nerve nuclei will be detailed later; we are here concerned with the general internal plan, best studied in representative sections to construct a three-dimensional concept. For convenience, each photograph has been bisected and half is shown diagrammatically (*Figs.* 5.6 to 5.16). The transition from spinal cord to brainstem is demonstrated by diagrams in *Fig.* 5.1; the arrangement of tracts at C2 cord level is shown in *Fig.* 5.6. The nucleus proprius is in continuity rostrally with the trigeminal spinal nucleus.

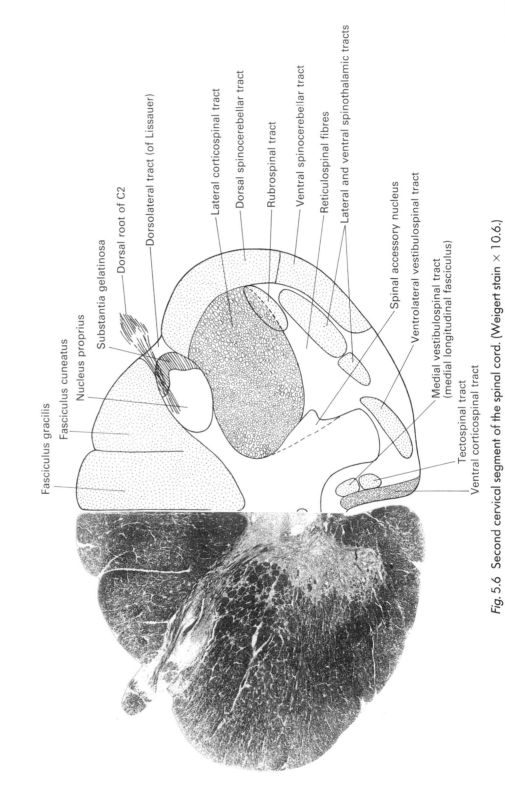

Fig. 5.6 Second cervical segment of the spinal cord. (Weigert stain × 10.6.)

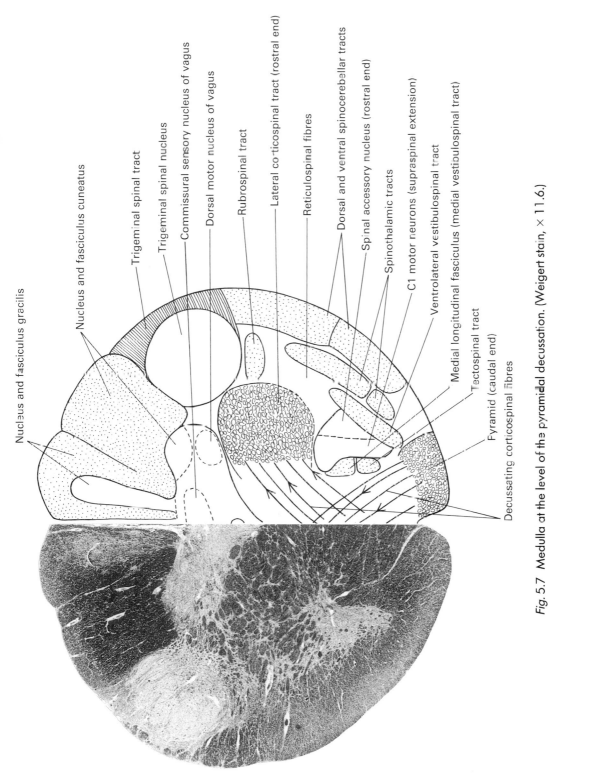

Nucleus and fasciculus gracilis

Nucleus and fasciculus cuneatus

Trigeminal spinal tract

Trigeminal spinal nucleus

Commissural sensory nucleus of vagus

Dorsal motor nucleus of vagus

Rubrospinal tract

Lateral corticospinal tract (rostral end)

Reticulospinal fibres

Dorsal and ventral spinocerebellar tracts

Spinal accessory nucleus (rostral end)

Spinothalamic tracts

C1 motor neurons (supraspinal extension)

Ventrolateral vestibulospinal tract

Medial longitudinal fasciculus (medial vestibulospinal tract)

Tectospinal tract

Pyramid (caudal end)

Decussating corticospinal fibres

Fig. 5.7 Medulla at the level of the pyramidal decussation. (Weigert stain, × 11.6.)

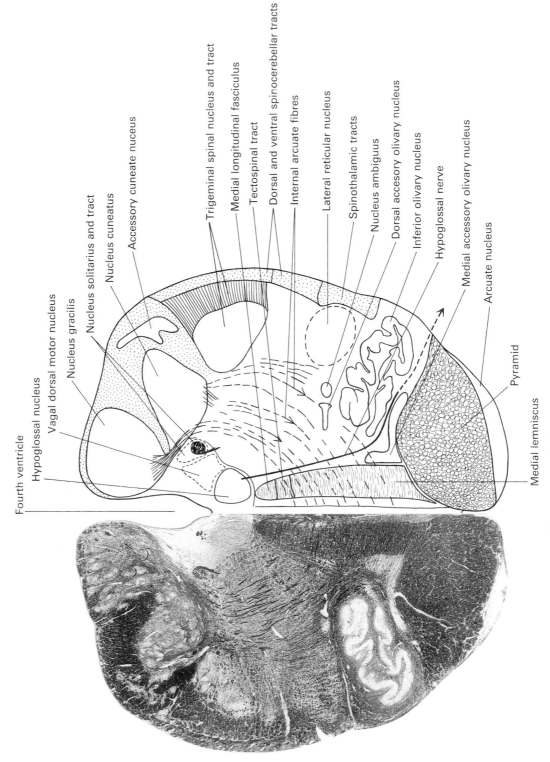

Fig. 5.8 Medulla at the level of the sensory decussation. (Weigert stain, × 8.2.)

Fourth ventricle

Hypoglossal nucleus

Vagal dorsal motor nucleus

Nucleus gracilis

Nucleus solitarius and tract

Nucleus cuneatus

Accessory cuneate nuceus

Trigeminal spinal nucleus and tract

Medial longitudinal fasciculus

Tectospinal tract

Dorsal and ventral spinocerebellar tracts

Internal arcuate fibres

Lateral reticular nucleus

Spinothalamic tracts

Nucleus ambiguus

Dorsal accesory olivary nucleus

Inferior olivary nucleus

Hypoglossal nerve

Medial accessory olivary nucleus

Arcuate nucleus

Pyramid

Medial lemniscus

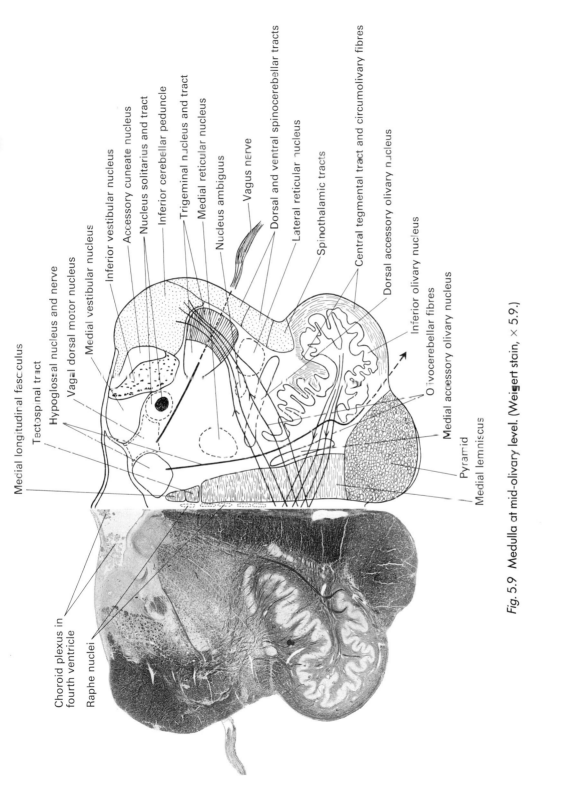

Medial longitudinal fasciculus

Tectospinal tract

Hypoglossal nucleus and nerve

Vagal dorsal motor nucleus

Medial vestibular nucleus

Inferior vestibular nucleus

Accessory cuneate nucleus

Nucleus solitarius and tract

Inferior cerebellar peduncle

Trigeminal nucleus and tract

Medial reticular nucleus

Nucleus ambiguus

Vagus nerve

Dorsal and ventral spinocerebellar tracts

Lateral reticular nucleus

Spinothalamic tracts

Central tegmental tract and circumolivary fibres

Dorsal accessory olivary nucleus

Inferior olivary nucleus

Olivocerebellar fibres

Medial accessory olivary nucleus

Pyramid

Medial lemniscus

Choroid plexus in fourth ventricle

Raphe nuclei

Fig. 5.9 Medulla at mid-olivary level. (Weigert stain, × 5.9.)

The medulla

In the lowest medullary levels (*Fig.* 5.7) the ventral grey column is separated from the central grey matter by decussating corticospinal fibres; as these descend, most pass dorsolaterally in the pyramidal decussation. The 'detached' ventral grey column contains supraspinal extensions of the *spinal accessory nucleus* laterally and *first cervical motor neurons* medially. Traced rostrally these continue into the nucleus ambiguus and hypoglossal nuclei respectively. The *dorsal motor vagal nucleus* (parasympathetic), which supplies smooth muscle, is located in the central grey matter. The general visceral afferent components of both vagus nerves meet dorsal to the central canal as the median *commissural nucleus*. Upward continuation of the dorsal grey horn of the spinal cord is represented here by the *spinal trigeminal nucleus*, bounded peripherally by its afferent tract. The *nucleus gracilis* is beginning to appear in the corresponding funiculus.

A transverse section just above the pyramidal decussation (*Fig.* 5.8) shows a development of these features, and some new structures. The *sensory decussation* of internal arcuate fibres streams ventromedially from the nucleus gracilis and nucleus cuneatus, crossing the midline to form the contralateral *medial lemniscus*. The somatotopic arrangement in the lemniscus is such that input from the lower half of the body, via the fasciculus gracilis, is ventral to that from the nucleus cuneatus. The *trigeminal nucleus* is separated from the central grey matter by the sensory decussation. The *medial longitudinal fasciculus* and the *tectospinal tract* lie dorsal to the medial lemniscus. The *accessory cuneate nucleus* receives proprioceptive input from upper cervical segments, and projects to the cerebellum via the inferior peduncle. The central canal has inclined dorsally, prior to its junction with the fourth ventricle. The central grey matter contains the *hypoglossal nucleus* medially, lateral to which are the vagal *dorsal motor nucleus* (parasympathetic) and the *nucleus solitarius* (gustatory). The latter is characterized by a prominent afferent tract. There are additional areas of grey matter: the *arcuate nucleus* overlies the pyramid, and represents 'displaced' pontine nuclei in the cortico-ponto-cerebellar pathway; the *inferior olivary nucleus* is dorsolateral to the pyramid. The *reticular formation*, a diffuse network of cells and fine fibres, extends throughout the medulla and will be described later.

In the next section (*Fig.* 5.9), the central grey matter has opened out into the fourth ventricle. The *hypoglossal nucleus* is flanked by the vagal *dorsal motor nucleus* and the *nucleus solitarius* and its tract. The medial and inferior *vestibular nuclei* are in the lateral part of the ventricular floor. The *inferior cerebellar peduncle* has received the dorsal spinocerebellar tract, and overlies the trigeminal nucleus and tract. The rostral end of the *accessory cuneate nucleus* adjoins the peduncle. The *inferior olivary nucleus* is a large folded grey mass with a mesial opening from which *olivocerebellar fibres* pass to the opposite inferior cerebellar peduncle. The dorsal and medial *accessory olivary nuclei* are phylogenetically more ancient. The inferior olivary complex is an integration centre for certain cerebellar afferents. The *hypoglossal nerve* passes lateral to the medial lemniscus and emerges between the pyramid and olive. The *vagus nerve* traverses the trigeminal nucleus to emerge dorsal to

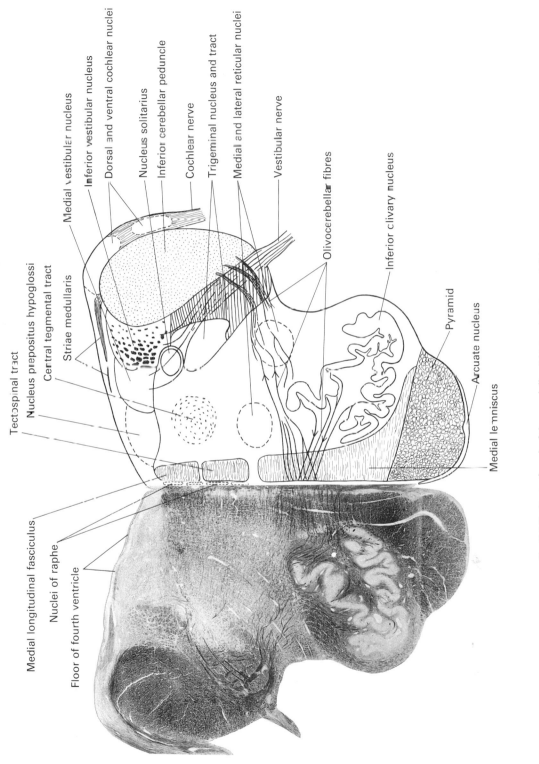

Tectospinal tract

Nucleus prepositus hypoglossi

Central tegmental tract

Striae medullaris

Medial vestibular nucleus

Inferior vestibular nucleus

Dorsal and ventral cochlear nuclei

Nucleus solitarius

Inferior cerebellar peduncle

Cochlear nerve

Trigeminal nucleus and tract

Medial and lateral reticular nuclei

Vestibular nerve

Olivocerebellar fibres

Inferior olivary nucleus

Pyramid

Arcuate nucleus

Medial lemniscus

Medial longitudinal fasciculus

Nuclei of raphe

Floor of fourth ventricle

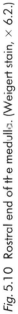

Fig. 5.10 Rostral end of the medulla. (Weigert stain, × 6.2.)

the olive. The hypoglossal nerve demarcates the medulla into areas of different blood supply; the area medial to it is supplied by the anterior spinal artery, the area dorsolateral to it by the posterior inferior cerebellar artery. In the area dorsal to the inferior olivary nucleus there are the *spinothalamic, reticulospinal, rubrospinal* and *vestibulospinal tracts*, the *visceral efferent pathway* and *nucleus ambiguus*. Together with the vestibular and trigeminal nuclei, these are damaged in thrombosis of the posterior inferior cerebellar artery, a well recognized clinical entity. Within the reticular formation there are nuclear aggregations, situated laterally, medially and in the midline raphe.

A section at the cranial end of the medulla (*Fig.* 5.10) shows some features already noted. The ventricular floor has widened and *striae medullares* traverse it at the pontomedullary junction. The *cochlear division* of the eighth nerve passes lateral, the *vestibular division* enters medial to the inferior cerebellar peduncle. The *dorsal* and *ventral cochlear nuclei* are on the surface of the peduncle. The medial lemniscus is beginning to extend laterally between the pyramid and inferior olive; at the pontomedullary junction it rotates through 90° into a transverse plane. The *nucleus prepositus hypoglossi* is sited rostral to the hypoglossal nucleus, between it and the abducent nucleus; functionally it is interposed between the cerebellum, vestibular nuclei, superior colliculi and the oculogyric nuclei (III, IV, VI) in the reflex control of eye movements.

The pons

The next four sections (*Figs* 5.11 to 5.14) are at levels through the facial nucleus, trigeminal nerve, rostral pons and junction with midbrain. In each, the basilar region contains *descending fasciculi* (corticospinal, corticobulbar and corticopontine). These are interspersed with *transverse fibres* which arise from numerous nuclei pontis and form the *middle cerebellar peduncles*. The fourth ventricle is flanked by the *superior cerebellar peduncles* and roofed by the superior medullary velum, overlain by the cerebellar lingula. The superior peduncles are efferent from the dentate nuclei of the cerebellum, each peduncle projecting to the opposite red nucleus in the midbrain, and thence to the thalamus. This dentato-rubro-thalamic path is the route whereby the cerebellum influences cerebral cortical motor activity.

In the first section (*Fig.* 5.11), the inferior cerebellar peduncle has turned dorsally and is between the other peduncles. Deep to the ventricular floor, each side of the midline throughout the pons and medulla, is the *medial longitudinal fasciculus*, an internuclear association tract, interconnecting vestibular and oculogyric nuclei. It ascends throughout the midbrain to the level of the posterior commissure, and descends to ventral horn cells in the cervical spinal cord (medial vestibulospinal tract) and the spinal accessory nucleus, coordinating movements of the head, eyes and neck; it will be considered further with the eighth cranial nerve. Throughout most of the brainstem the *tectospinal tract* (including tectobulbar fibres) lies immediately subjacent to it. The *facial colliculus* is formed by fibres from the *facial motor*

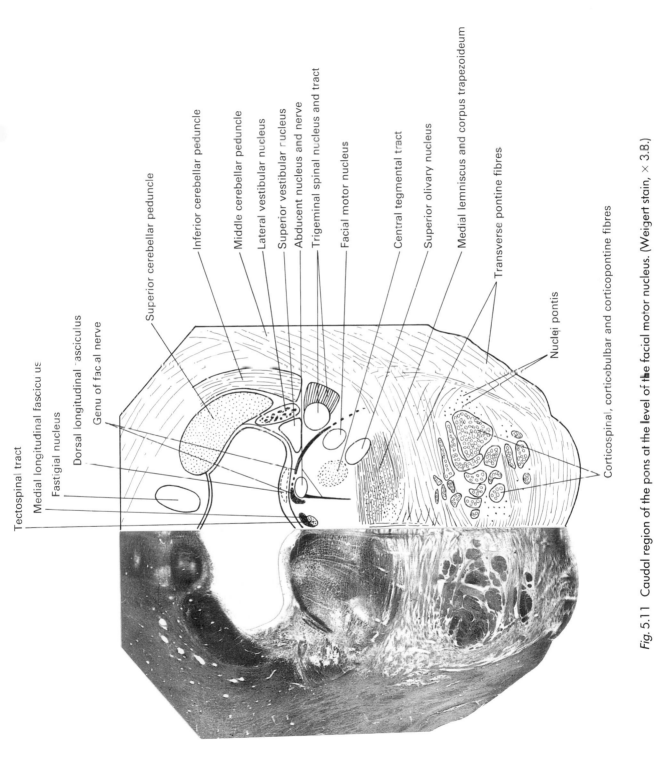

Tectospinal tract
Medial longitudinal fasciculus
Fastigial nucleus
Dorsal longitudinal fasciculus
Genu of facial nerve
Superior cerebellar peduncle
Inferior cerebellar peduncle
Middle cerebellar peduncle
Lateral vestibular nucleus
Superior vestibular nucleus
Abducent nucleus and nerve
Trigeminal spinal nucleus and tract
Facial motor nucleus
Central tegmental tract
Superior olivary nucleus
Medial lemniscus and corpus trapezoideum
Transverse pontine fibres
Nuclei pontis
Corticospinal, corticobulbar and corticopontine fibres

Fig. 5.11 Caudal region of the pons at the level of the facial motor nucleus. (Weigert stain, × 3.8.)

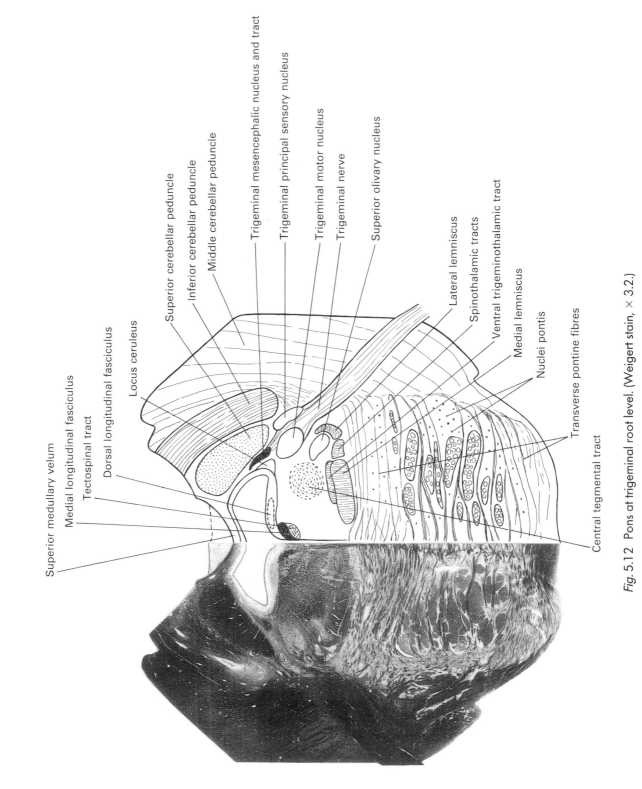

Fig. 5.12 Pons at trigeminal root level. (Weigert stain, × 3.2.)

nucleus curving over the abducent nucleus. The facial nerve's efferent path is between its motor nucleus and the *trigeminal sensory nucleus and tract*. There are *vestibular nuclei* in the lateral angle of the ventricular floor. The *medial lemniscus*, joined by trigemino-thalamic and spinothalamic fibres, lies horizontally and is intersected by transverse auditory fibres which form the *corpus trapezoideum*. The *superior olivary nucleus* is also associated with the auditory path. The *dorsal longitudinal fasciculus* in the ventricular floor is a pathway for visceral and behavioural functions and has olfactory and limbic connexions rostrally.

Fig. 5.12 illustrates a section through the *trigeminal nerve; its motor nucleus* is medial to the *principal sensory nucleus*. The *trigeminal mesencephalic tract* carries proprioceptive fibres, ascending alongside the narrowed ventricular cavity en route to its nucleus in the midbrain. The trigeminothalamic projection consists of a large ventral tract of crossed fibres adjacent to the medial lemniscus, and a smaller uncrossed dorsal tract.

The *reticular formation* is present throughout the pontine tegmentum, and the *central tegmental tract* is a relatively dense group of association fibres in it, ascending to the thalamus and descending from midbrain tegmentum and red nucleus to the inferior olivary nucleus. Two reticular nuclei have particular significance. The *locus ceruleus* lies ventral to the mesencephalic trigeminal nucleus (*Figs.* 5.12–5.14). It is a source of noradrenaline (nor-epinephrine), and has remarkably widespread projections throughout the central nervous system. Its thalamic and cortical connexions play a role in 'paradoxical sleep'. The *raphe nuclei* produce serotonin (5–IIT) which, in general, has an inhibitory effect. They comprise small midline aggregations of neurons in medulla and pons; in the midbrain there is a relatively large *dorsal nucleus of the raphe* in the periaqueductal grey matter (*Fig.* 5.14). Descending raphe-spinal fibres inhibit pain transmission; ascending fibres are associated with 'slow wave sleep'; destruction of the raphe nuclei produces insomnia. The cells of the locus ceruleus and raphe nuclei are readily distinguished by the formaldehyde-fluorescence technique: noradrenaline fluoresces pale green and serotonin yellow.

At the junction of the pons and midbrain (*Fig.* 5.14), where the fourth ventricle and aqueduct join, the *superior cerebellar peduncles* decussate. The *medial lemniscus* has moved away from the midline and the *lateral lemniscus* inclines dorsally to enter the inferior colliculus. In the basilar region descending fibres are massed together rather than scattered in bundles.

The midbrain

Each *crus cerebri* (basis pedunculi) is separated from the tegmentum by the *substantia nigra*, which extends from the lateral midbrain sulcus to the interpeduncular fossa. The black colour seen in unstained sections is due to melanin, a by-product of dopamine metabolism. The substantia nigra has functional links with the corpus striatum and influences motor activity. These motor quality control centres, or basal ganglia, are often termed 'extrapyramidal nuclei', a nomenclature which persists because their clinical

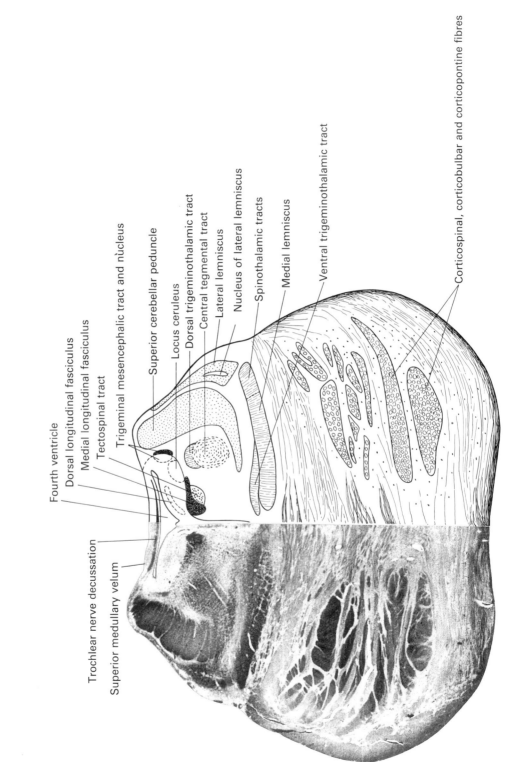

Fig. 5.13 Upper third of pons near the junction between fourth ventricle and cerebral aqueduct. (Weigert stain, × 4.)

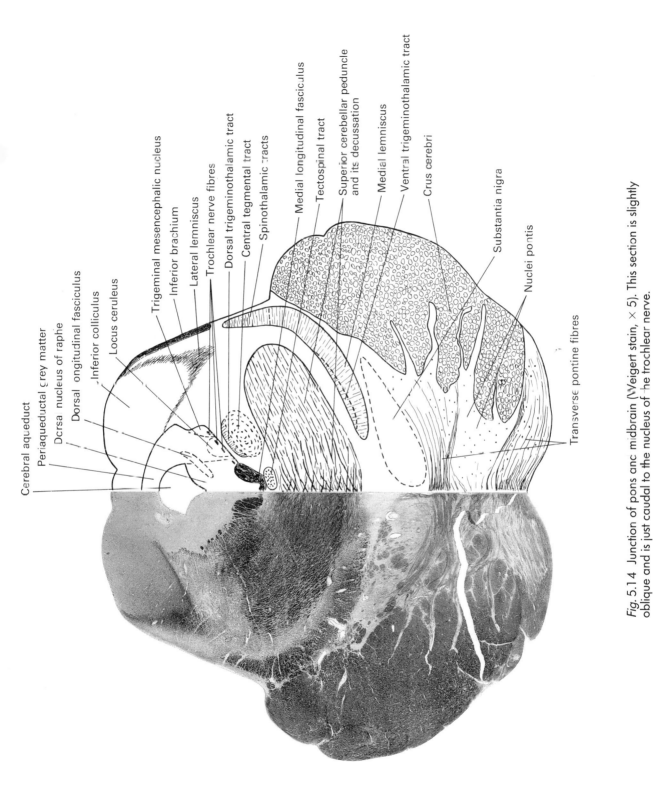

Cerebral aqueduct

Periaqueductal grey matter

Dorsal nucleus of raphe

Dorsal longitudinal fasciculus

Inferior colliculus

Locus ceruleus

Trigeminal mesencephalic nucleus

Inferior brachium

Lateral lemniscus

Trochlear nerve fibres

Dorsal trigeminothalamic tract

Central tegmental tract

Spinothalamic tracts

Medial longitudinal fasciculus

Tectospinal tract

Superior cerebellar peduncle and its decussation

Medial lemniscus

Ventral trigeminothalamic tract

Crus cerebri

Substantia nigra

Nuclei pontis

Transverse pontine fibres

Fig. 5.14 Junction of pons and midbrain (Weigert stain, × 5). This section is slightly oblique and is just caudal to the nucleus of the trochlear nerve.

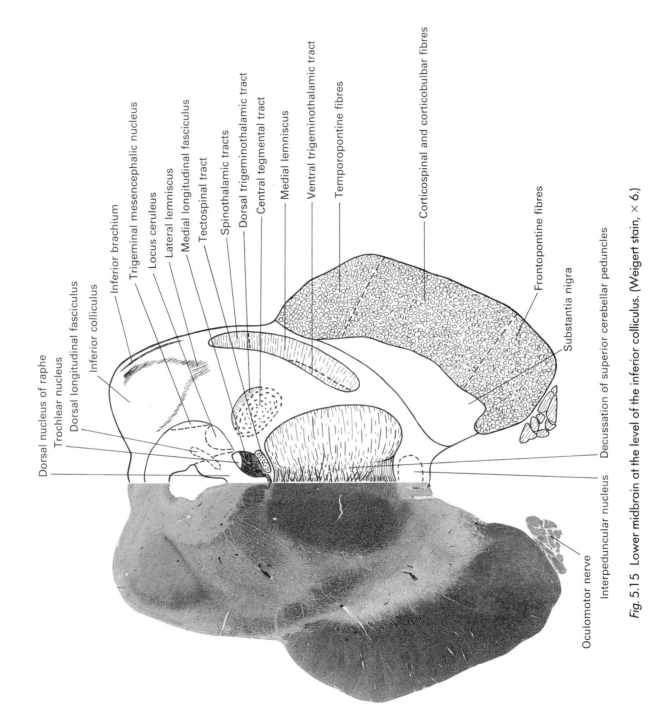

Fig. 5.15 Lower midbrain at the level of the inferior colliculus. (Weigert stain, × 6.)

derangements are known as 'extrapyramidal disorders'. One such condition, Parkinson's disease, results from degeneration in cells of the substantia nigra and is associated with dopamine deficiency; it is described in Chapter 9. Each crus cerebri consists of descending fibres, *corticospinal* and *corticobulbar* fibres occupying its middle three fifths, the latter mostly comprising cortico-nuclear fibres to cranial nerve motor nuclei. Here the somatotopic arrange-ment is such that the head is medial and the feet lateral. *Corticopontine* fibres have extensive origins in the cerebral cortex and descend to synapse ipsilaterally with the nuclei pontis; in the crus cerebri they are in two main groups, temporopontine laterally and frontopontine medially.

A section at inferior collicular level (*Fig.* 5.15) shows features which differ from sections through the superior colliculus (*Fig.* 5.16). In the more caudal section (*Fig.* 5.15) the *lateral lemniscus* is passing into the *inferior colliculus*, a relay station on the auditory path. The *medial lemniscus* inclines dorsally en route to the thalamus. The *decussation of the superior cerebellar peduncles* is a prominent central feature. The *trochlear nucleus* is ventral in the periaque-ductal grey matter, contiguous with the *medial longitudinal fasciculus;* it supplies the superior oblique muscle of the eye and its fibres pass dorsally, crossing the midline before emerging from the superior medullary velum. The *mesencephalic trigeminal tract*, being sensory, is more dorsal in the grey matter. The *mesencephalic nucleus* of the trigeminal nerve consists of unipolar cells which are *primary sensory neurons*, a uniquely central location (cf. spinal dorsal root ganglion). Sited also in the periaqueductal grey matter are the *dorsal longitudinal fasciculus, locus ceruleus* and *dorsal nucleus of the raphe.*

At the level of the *superior colliculus* (*Fig.* 5.16) is the *red nucleus*, a large round mass on each side, pinkish in colour in fresh sections. It is continuous with the crossed superior cerebellar peduncle; some fibres of the dentato-rubro-thalamic tract terminate in it, while others surround it in their onward path to the thalamus. The red nucleus is classed as an extrapyramidal nucleus because descending motor fibres arise in it, cross in the *ventral tegmental decussation* and form the rubrospinal tract; the nucleus also provides a large input to the reticular formation and central tegmental tract. The *superior colliculi* have a complex, six-layered structure of grey and white matter, reflecting their derivation from the optic lobes of lower vertebrates. In humans they are concerned in visual reflexes and eye movements, integrating afferents from diverse sources — cortical, retinal (via the superior brachium), auditory (from the inferior colliculus) and spinal. Descending fibres, originating in the superior colliculus, cross in the *dorsal tegmental decussation* to form tectospinal and tectobulbar tracts. Tectobulbar con-nexions influence the oculogyric nuclei (reflex eye movements) and the facial motor nuclei (reflex closure of the eyelids). Interconnexions between the superior colliculi form part of the *posterior commissure.* The pretectal nucleus, not seen in this section, is slightly rostral to the superior colliculus and participates in the pupillary reflex response to light. These structures will be described with the oculogyric nuclei (III, IV, VI). The *inferior brachium*, ascending from inferior colliculus to medial geniculate body, forms a dorsolateral ridge on the surface of the intact midbrain. The *oculomotor*

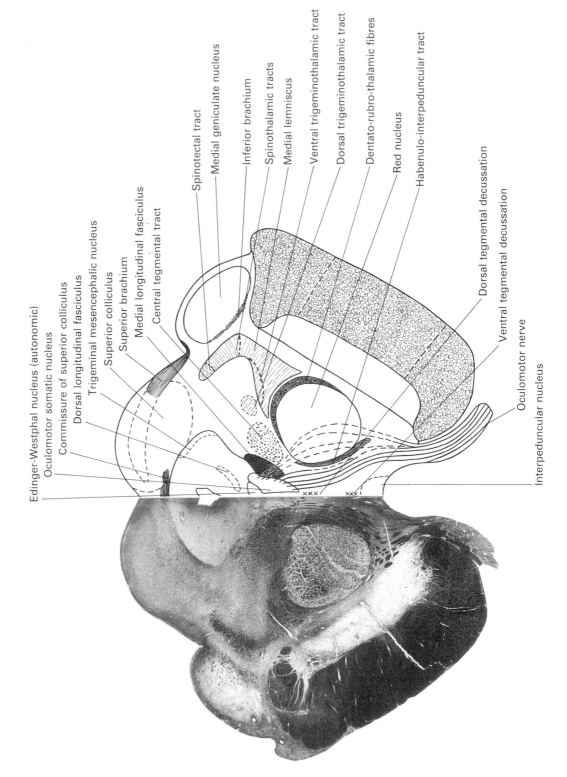

Edinger-Westphal nucleus (autonomic)
Oculomotor somatic nucleus
Commissure of superior colliculus
Dorsal longitudinal fasciculus
Trigeminal mesencephalic nucleus
Superior colliculus
Superior brachium
Medial longitudinal fasciculus
Central tegmental tract

Spinotectal tract
Medial geniculate nucleus
Inferior brachium
Spinothalamic tracts
Medial lemniscus
Ventral trigeminothalamic tract
Dorsal trigeminothalamic tract
Dentato-rubro-thalamic fibres
Red nucleus
Habenulo-interpeduncular tract

Dorsal tegmental decussation
Ventral tegmental decussation
Oculomotor nerve
Interpeduncular nucleus

Fig. 5.16 Upper midbrain at the level of the superior colliculus. (Weigert stain, × 3.8.)

nucleus is in the ventral region of the periaqueductal grey matter, near the *medial longitudinal fasciculus;* it supplies four extra-ocular muscles and striated muscle of the levator palpebrae superioris. Its dorsal region is the parasympathetic *Edinger-Westphal nucleus*, which innervates the ciliary muscle and constrictor pupillae. Oculomotor fibres traverse the red nucleus to emerge in the interpeduncular fossa.

Autonomic pathways descend from the hypothalamus through the mid-brain. From the hypothalamic mamillary bodies, the *mamillotegmental tract* enters the tegmental reticular formation and thence, via polysynaptic fibres, extends through the brainstem to spinal cord. The *dorsal longitudinal fasciculus* consists of non-myelinated fibres in the periaqueductal grey matter, descending to autonomic nuclei of the brainstem. The *interpeduncular nucleus* of the midbrain is in an efferent path from the habenular nucleus (*see Figs* 5.3 and 8.8) which has an input from the limbic system.

The Reticular Formation

The reticular formation comprises a phylogenetically ancient network of small neurons throughout the brainstem, extending to the thalamus cranially and blending caudally into the intermediate grey matter of the spinal cord. Their dendritic fields are orientated across the brainstem's axis, and inter-spersed with long ascending and descending reticular axons, allowing diffuse interactions. Their pathways are polysynaptic, crossed and uncrossed, and serve somatic and visceral functions.

Ascending connexions to the brainstem reticular formation are diffuse, somatic and visceral in origin, and relate to intensity and quality rather than to location. Spinal input is from spinoreticular tracts and a via a few collaterals of long ascending tracts (except the dorsal column–medial lemnis-cal path which is discrete and discriminatory). Bulbar input is from the sensory components of all cranial nerves, somatic afferents (trigeminal, vestibular, and cochlear nuclei), gustatory (nucleus solitarius), olfactory (medial forebrain bundle), and visual (superior colliculus).

Descending connexions from the cerebral cortex are mostly through cortico-reticular fibres and also via a few collaterals from corticospinal and cortico-bulbar tracts. The cerebellum and medullary reticular formation are reciprocally connected via the inferior cerebellar peduncles. The hypothala-mus, limbic system and some extrapyramidal nuclei such as the red nucleus also produce effects via the reticular formation.

In the brainstem reticular formation, groups of neuronal somata, referred to as nuclei, have been classified in two ways, either by their locations and morphology or by their known neurotransmitter content. Morphologically they comprise three main groups:

A **median column** includes all the *raphe nuclei* and extends throughout the brainstem.

A **medial column** extends from mid-medulla to lower midbrain. Caudally a medial reticular *magnocellular nucleus* lies near the central tegmental tract.

Alongside the abducent nucleus there is the *paramedian pontine reticular formation*. The *nucleus ceruleus* extends rostrally from the upper pons into the midbrain. In the midbrain also there are *tegmental nuclei, periaqueductal nuclei* and the *cuneiform nucleus*.

A **lateral column** comprises scattered small (parvocellular) neurons throughout the brainstem; the *lateral reticular nucleus* of the medulla is dorsolateral to the inferior olivary nucleus.

Neurotransmitter pathways, described in Chapter 15, include monoamine, cholinergic and amino acid systems of reticular neurons which serve to *modulate synaptic transmission*. Neurons of the locus ceruleus contain *noradrenaline* and project throughout the central nervous system, enhancing or diminishing the effects of other transmitters at synapses, influencing capillary blood flow and generally responsive to alerting or emergency situations. Raphe nuclei contain 5–HT: descending fibres synapse with enkephalin-containing neurons of the substantia gelatinosa, inhibiting transmission of nociceptor stimuli. Raphe nuclei and the locus ceruleus are involved in sleep mechanisms (*see* p.232). *Dopamine* reticular neurons project to the hypothalamus, influencing endocrine secretion, and, via the limbic system, have profound psychological effects. There are *cholinergic* projections from the basal forebrain to the entire cerebral cortex and if deficient, Alzheimer's senile dementia results. Of the amino acid systems, *γ-aminobutyric acid* (*GABA*) is in highest concentration, its inhibitory neurons projecting to the cerebrum and cerebellum.

The ascending *reticular activating system* projects through thalamic nuclei to the cerebral cortex and is involved in arousal, alerting reactions and heightened perception, Pain, loud noise or strong psychic stimuli thereby inhibit sleep. Prolonged coma may follow damage to this system. Anaesthesia or barbiturates block transmission through the polysynaptic reticular paths and the cortex thus becomes unresponsive to impulses which may continue to arrive via specific sensory pathways. Natural sleep should not, however, be regarded as simply passive; it involves complex interactions which are briefly described on p.232.

Descending *reticulospinal tracts* influence activity in α and γ motor neurons. Experimentally there are inhibitory zones in the medial part of the medulla, facilitatory areas in the lateral medulla and caudal pons but during normal activity these effects fluctuate. Reticulospinal tracts act on axial and proximal limb musculature and are significant in the control of muscle tone, posture and stereotyped action such as walking. The cuneiform nuclei, sited ventral to the inferior colliculi are central 'pattern generators' for the organization of the movements of locomotion, largely a subconscious activity.

The *paramedian pontine reticular formation*, sometimes termed the 'para-abducent nucleus', is a centre for conjugate lateral gaze; if damaged there is inability to look to the side of the lesion (damage to an abducent nerve only affects lateral movement of one eye). Its connexions are described on p. 141.

Respiratory and *cardiovascular* functions are regulated by so-called 'vital centres' in the medullary and lower pontine reticular formation. These are influenced by the hypothalamus and by visceral afferents, including those from receptors in the carotid body, carotid sinus and bronchial tree. Trauma

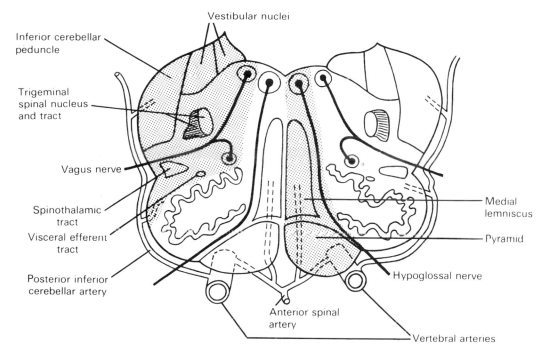

Vestibular nuclei

Inferior cerebellar
peduncle

Trigeminal
spinal nucleus
and tract

Vagus nerve

Spinothalamic
tract

Visceral efferent
tract

Posterior inferior
cerebellar artery

Anterior spinal
artery

Medial
lemniscus

Pyramid

Hypoglossal nerve

Vertebral arteries

Fig. 5.17 Medullary infarction: (on left) of the posterior inferior cerebellar artery (lateral medullary syndrome); (on right) of the anterior spinal artery (medial medullary syndrome).

to the brainstem is lethal if vital centres are damaged. (For further reading *see* Brodal 1981, FitzGerald 1985, Williams et al., 1989.)

APPLIED ANATOMY

Vascular lesions of the brainstem illustrate the location of nuclei and tracts. The main blood supply is from the two vertebral arteries, joining at the pontomedullary junction to form the basilar artery, which extends rostrally to divide into two posterior cerebral arteries. The vertebral arteries each give a medial branch to form the anterior spinal artery: this supplies the medial part of the medulla before passing to the spinal cord. From the lateral aspect of each vertebral artery, a posterior inferior cerebellar artery winds round the side of the medulla to supply the dorsolateral region.

The *medial medullary syndrome* is a result of blockage of the anterior spinal artery or medial medullary branches of the vertebral artery. It affects the pyramid, medial lemniscus and hypoglossal nerve (*Fig.* 5.17), resulting in contralateral hemiparesis of the limbs, ipsilateral lingual paralysis, and contralateral impaired perception of joint position, vibration and discriminative touch.

The *lateral medullary syndrome* (*Fig.* 5.17) results from thrombosis of a

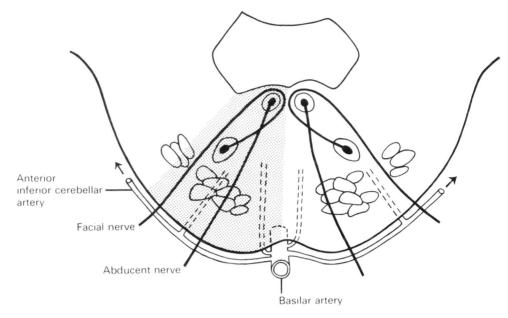

Fig. 5.18 Paramedian pontine infarction.

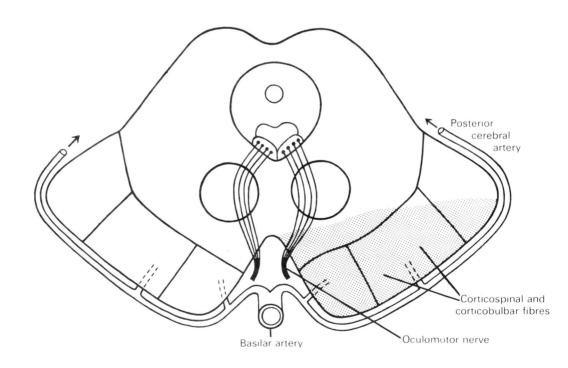

Fig. 5.19 Basal midbrain infarction.

posterior inferior cerebellar artery or a vertebral artery. This leads to severe dizziness, vomiting and nystagmus (infarction of vestibular nuclei), ataxia of limbs on the side of the lesion (inferior cerebellar peduncle and cerebellum), difficulty in swallowing and speaking (nucleus ambiguus), ipsilateral facial loss of pain and temperature sensation (trigeminal spinal nucleus), contralateral loss of pain and temperature sensation in the body (lateral spinothalamic tract), and Horner's syndrome (visceral efferent pathway).

Basal infarction of the pons (*Fig.* 5.18) follows occlusion of pontine branches of the basilar artery. Corticospinal fibres are dispersed at this level and partial contralateral hemiplegia results. Abducent nerve damage paralyses the lateral rectus muscle. If the lesion extends dorsally the facial nerve may be affected.

A *basal midbrain lesion* (*Fig.* 5.19) results from thrombosis of central branches of the posterior cerebral artery, involving corticospinal and corticobulbar fibres in the basis pedunculi, with contralateral hemiplegia. Destruction of the oculomotor nerve causes severe ipsilateral ophthalmoplegia, only the lateral rectus and superior oblique muscles escaping.

Internuclear ophthalmoplegia arises when the medial longitudinal fasciculus is involved either in a vascular lesion or in a demyelinating disease such as multiple sclerosis.

Chapter 6

Cranial nerves

The cranial nerves are numbered in rostrocaudal order:

I	–	Olfactory	VII	–	Facial
II	–	Optic	VIII	–	Vestibulocochlear
III	–	Oculomotor	IX	–	Glossopharyngeal
IV	–	Trochlear	X	–	Vagus
V	–	Trigeminal	XI	–	Accessory
VI	–	Abducent	XII	–	Hypoglossal

They may be classified into three main morphological groups:

1. Those supplying muscles derived from *cranial myotomes*, namely the oculomotor (III), trochlear (IV) and abducent (VI) which supply the eye muscles, and the hypoglossal (XII) supplying the tongue.
2. Those innervating muscles of *branchial arch* origin, namely the trigeminal (V), facial (VII), glossopharyngeal (IX), vagus (X) and accessory (XI).
3. Those serving *special senses*, namely the olfactory (I), optic (II) and vestibulocochlear (VIII). The olfactory and optic nerves are described separately in Chapters 10 and 11. Developmentally, the optic nerve is an outgrowth of the forebrain.

A summary table of cranial nerve components and functions is provided at the end of this chapter.

Components

As noted in Chapter 1, spinal nerves have four 'general' components: somatic afferent ('general' sensation), visceral afferent (visceral sensation), visceral efferent (autonomic), somatic efferent (to skeletal muscles) (*Fig. 6.1A*). These are present singly or in combination in some cranial nerves; their visceral components are parasympathetic. In addition, three 'special' components are found in some cranial nerves (*Fig. 6.1B*):

1. *Special somatic afferent*, equilibration and auditory (VIII).
2. *Special visceral afferent*, gustatory (taste) (VII, IX, X).
3. *Special visceral efferent*, branchiomotor (V, VII, IX, X, XI).

Note: branchial arch musculature of face, mouth, pharynx and larynx, though striated and under voluntary control, is associated with visceral

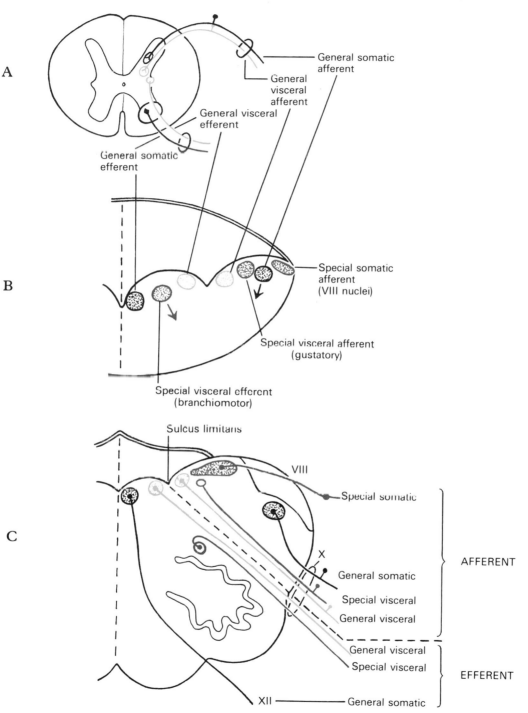

Fig. 6.1 Components of nerves. Compare spinal cord (A) with developing brainstem (B). (C) illustrates components of cranial nerves and their nuclei in the medulla. Black: general somatic. Green: general visceral. Red: special afferent. Blue: special efferent.

functions such as eating and breathing; hence its innervation is classified as 'special visceral'.

There are therefore seven possible components in cranial nerves, though no nerve contains all of these. Proprioceptive afferents in the cranial nerves probably all converge on a mesencephalic nucleus which is part of the trigeminal sensory nuclear complex. Nerves supplying striated muscle generally carry proprioceptive afferents but these will not be separately described.

As already noted, grey matter forms the floor of the fourth ventricle, divided on each side by a sulcus limitans into a lateral sensory and a medial motor area (*see Fig.* 5.4). The disposition of the seven functional components of the cranial nerves during development is shown in *Fig.* 6.1B and their final locations in *Fig.* 6.1C. A large vestibular nuclear complex occupies the lateral angle of the ventricular floor: this and the inferior cerebellar peduncle displace the trigeminal sensory nucleus ventrally in the medulla and pons. Most of the branchiomotor column migrates ventrolaterally during development and its caudal part, the nucleus ambiguus, lies just dorsal to the medial part of the inferior olive. The distributions of the sensory and motor nuclei are shown in *Figs.* 6.2 and 6.3: these are described with their cranial nerves.

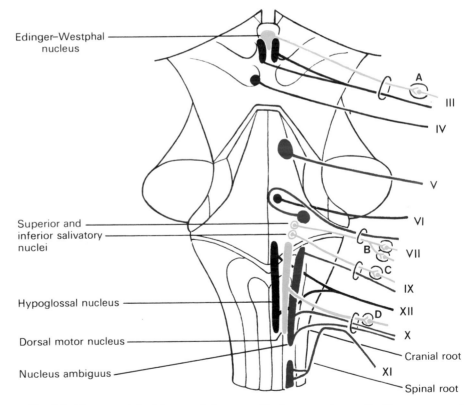

Fig. 6.2 Motor nuclei of the cranial nerves. Black: general somatic. Green: general visceral (parasympathetic). Blue: special visceral (branchiomotor). Parasympathetic ganglia: **A**, ciliary; **B**, pterygopalatine and submandibular; **C**, otic; **D**, peripheral visceral ganglia in thorax and abdomen.

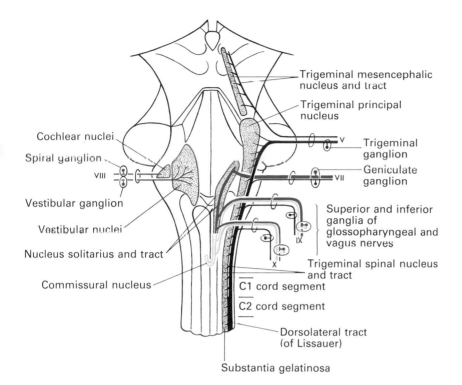

Fig. 6.3 Sensory nuclei and ganglia of the cranial nerves. Black: somatic. Green: general visceral. Red: special somatic, special visceral.

General comparison of cranial and spinal nerves

It is useful to summarize certain generalizations at this stage:

1. **Components.** Each typical spinal nerve contains four general components, but cranial nerves vary in both the number and the functional type of their components. Cranial nerves may contain 'special' components, not present in spinal nerves.

2. **Grey columns.** In the spinal cord there are four continuous columns of nuclei in the grey matter. In the brainstem the motor 'column' is in separated nuclei (*Fig.* 6.2) The trigeminal sensory nuclei, however, form a continuous column extending from midbrain to upper cervical spinal cord (*Fig.* 6.3).

3. **Afferent ganglia.** Spinal dorsal root ganglia contain the cell bodies of visceral and somatic afferent neurons. In cranial nerves the somata of primary sensory neurons are also in ganglia, but these are usually *either somatic or visceral*. Thus the trigeminal ganglion is purely somatic afferent. The vagus and glossopharyngeal nerves each have two ganglia, a superior (mostly somatic) and an inferior (mostly visceral). The facial nerve's geniculate ganglion consists mostly of cell bodies of special visceral afferent neurons subserving taste: very few of its cells mediate general somatic afferents. Spinal ganglia are sited in intervertebral foramina or

just inside the vertebral canal; similarly, cranial afferent ganglia are located in the skull (V, VII) or in its foramina (IX, X). The proprioceptive trigeminal input is unique: the cell bodies of the primary sensory neurons are in the midbrain (mesencephalic nucleus).

4. **Efferent ganglia**. In cranial nerves the intrinsic autonomic components are parasympathetic (sympathetic input is from the superior cervical ganglion via the internal carotid plexus). Visceral efferent fibres both in spinal and cranial nerves originate in central nuclei and comprise two-neuron chains of pre- and post-ganglionic neurons. Autonomic efferents of spinal nerves synapse in ganglia outside the vertebral canal (e.g. paravertebral). Similarly, parasympathetic axons of cranial nerves synapse in ganglia outside the bony confines of the skull (*Fig.* 6.2) (e.g. ciliary ganglion in the orbit, vagal ganglia in enteric plexuses).

The following descriptions of cranial nerves deal with their nuclear origins, central connexions, general course and distribution, function and dysfunction. They will be described in an ascending regional order in conformity with the sequence adopted in the account of the brainstem in Chapter 5.

The Hypoglossal (XII) Nerve

The hypoglossal nerve is motor to the tongue muscles. Its nucleus, somatic efferent, in series with the spinal ventral grey, forms a longitudinal column in the medulla, adjacent to the midline. Rostrally it underlies the hypoglossal triangle in the floor of the fourth ventricle; it extends caudally into the ventral grey matter of the closed part of the medulla (*Fig.* 6.4). Fibres pass ventrally from the nucleus, emerging as a row of 10–15 rootlets in the sulcus between the pyramid and olive. The rootlets form two bundles which pierce the dura mater separately, uniting as they traverse the hypoglossal canal in the occipital bone. Since this canal is medial to the jugular foramen, the emerging nerve is deep to the internal jugular vein and associated cranial nerves (IX, X, XI). It passes laterally behind these nerves, descends between the internal jugular vein and internal carotid artery, hooks round the origin of the occipital artery and finally courses forwards superficial to internal and external carotid arteries to reach the lingual muscles (*Fig.* 6.4). It supplies the lingual intrinsic muscles and the extrinsic styloglossus, hyoglossus and genioglossus. It is joined by a communication from the ventral primary ramus of C1, which the hypoglossal distributes to geniohyoid and thyrohyoid; descending C1 fibres constitute the upper root of the *ansa cervicalis*, C2 and C3 fibres forming its lower root.

Central connexions of the hypoglossal nerve exemplify those of somatomotor nuclei of cranial nerves:

1. *Corticonuclear innervation*. This is bilateral, usually on a 50:50 ratio but with a bias towards contralateral cortical control in a few people. Control of the genioglossus is predominantly contralateral. As with spinal motor neurons, cortical innervation is both direct (pyramidal) and indirect (corticoreticular). Qualitative cortical control is influenced by the cerebellum and by extrapyramidal nuclei such as the corpus striatum.

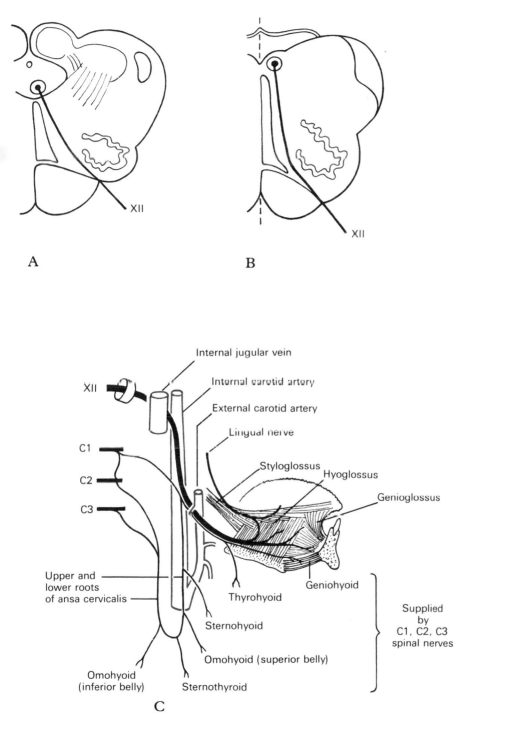

Fig. 6.4 The hypoglossal nerve. (A) Lower medulla. (B) Upper medulla. (C) Course and relationships.

2. *Associated sensory nuclei:* Reflex links with sensory input are comparable to spinal reflex arc connexions. For example, tongue movements may be in response to gustatory stimuli (via nucleus solitarius) or to tactile oral stimuli (via trigeminal sensory nuclei).
3. *Associated motor nuclei:* Movements of the masticatory, facial, pharyngeal and laryngeal muscles require a correlated control of the motor nuclei of cranial nerves V, VII, IX, X, XI (cranial root), and XII.

APPLIED ANATOMY

As with lesions of spinal nerves, the results of lower motor neuron lesions (nuclear or infranuclear) differ from those of upper motor neuron (supranuclear) lesions.

The hypoglossal nucleus may be paralysed in poliomyelitis or in motor neuron disease (bulbar palsy). Both the nucleus and the nerve are affected by vascular occlusion in the medial medullary syndrome (*see Fig.* 5.17). When the hypoglossal *nerve* is damaged, that half of the tongue atrophies; if protruded, the tongue deviates towards the side of the lesion as the unopposed action of the opposite genioglossus pulls it forward.

Supranuclear damage is usually due to vascular occlusion, either of the cortex or internal capsule. In most patients who have had a stroke on one side of the brain there is little or no weakness or atrophy of the tongue because of its bilateral cortical motor innervation. There is individual variation: the protruded tongue may be midline or may deviate towards the side of limb paralysis due to the unopposed action of the opposite genioglossus (Willoughby and Anderson, 1984). Tremor or involuntary movements of the tongue often feature in extrapyramidal disorders, such as Parkinson's disease.

The Accessory (XI) Nerve

The accessory nerve (*Fig.* 6.5) is branchiomotor and has *spinal* and *cranial* roots, which have separate origins and destinations, and are joined together for a short distance only in the jugular foramen. Beyond this the *cranial* root fuses with the vagus and is distributed by its pharyngeal and laryngeal branches to the soft palate, pharynx and larynx. It arises in the caudal part of the *nucleus ambiguus*, its rootlets emerging in line with those of the vagus, which it joins. The vagus and cranial accessory nerves will be described together.

The *spinal accessory* nerve starts from the *accessory nucleus*, a column of nerve cells in the dorsolateral part of the ventral horn of the first five cervical segments (*see Fig.* 5.6). Morphologically, the rostral end of the accessory nucleus is probably in series with the nucleus ambiguus: whether the sternomastoid and trapezius muscles are of branchial arch origin is debatable. The nerve roots traverse the lateral funiculus, emerge between the dorsal and ventral spinal roots, and ascend posterior to the denticulate ligament.

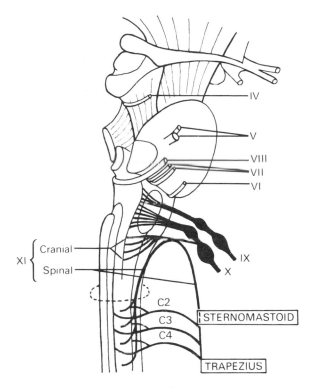

Fig. 6.5 Lateral view of the brainstem and upper cervical spinal cord. Note the cranial and spinal roots of the accessory nerve and the relationships of the former to the vagus. Cervical nerve fibres to sternomastoid and trapezius are proprioceptive.

The nerve enters the posterior cranial fossa via the foramen magnum behind the vertebral artery, leaving through the jugular foramen, where it briefly adheres to its cranial root. It then descends postero-laterally to the deep surface of sternomastoid, emerges from the middle of its posterior border and crosses the posterior triangle to enter trapezius about 5 cm above the clavicle. The cervical plexus supplies sternomastoid and trapezius with proprioceptive fibres.

APPLIED ANATOMY

The spinal accessory nerve's supranuclear control is unusual: it is ipsilateral for sternomastoid, but contralateral for trapezius. The function of sterno-mastoid in turning the head to the opposite side may explain this arrange-ment. If this pattern of cortical control is overlooked, a unilateral lesion may be misinterpreted as bilateral. In an epileptic fit affecting one side of the body, the head turns to the side of the convulsions.

The spinal accessory nerve may be damaged during surgical excision of malignant lymph glands in the posterior triangle. Such a lower motor neuron lesion results in paralysis and atrophy of affected muscles.

The Vagus (X) and Glossopharyngeal (IX) Nerves

The vagus and glossopharyngeal nerves are so closely alike in their nuclear origins and functional components that they will be considered together, and the cranial root of accessory nerve is included with the vagus. They are predominantly visceral, with only a minor somatic content. Their visceral components may be summarized as follows:

Visceral Components

Motor

Sensory

| Special Visceral Efferent (Branchiomotor to striated muscle) | General Visceral Efferent (Parasympathetic to smooth muscle) | Special Visceral Afferent (Gustatory) | General Visceral Afferent (e.g. from thorax and abdomen) |

Motor components

1. **Branchiomotor**: these fibres arise in the *nucleus ambiguus*, a longitudinal column of motor neurons in the medulla. It moves from its embryonic position (*Fig.* 6.1B) to lie dorsomedial to the inferior olivary nucleus (*Fig.* 6.6). Most of the output enters the vagus, either directly or via the cranial root of the accessory; it supplies muscles of the soft palate (except tensor palati which is supplied by the trigeminal), pharynx, larynx and striated muscle of the upper oesophagus. The contribution to the glossopharyngeal nerve is small, supplying only the stylopharyngeus. The nucleus ambiguus has been termed the 'nucleus of phonation and deglutition'; these functions are impaired when it is damaged.

   Supranuclear control of each nucleus ambiguus is bilateral; on recovery from a unilateral 'stroke' most patients can swallow (but *see* also 'applied anatomy'). Reflex connexions from sensory vagal nuclei are involved in coughing and vomiting; glossopharyngeal afferents via the trigeminal sensory nucleus are tested in the 'gag reflex', excited by touching the soft palate or pharynx.

2. **Parasympathetic components**.

   a. The largest parasympathetic nucleus is the vagal *dorsal motor nucleus*, a column of small nerve cells extending from the vagal triangle in the rhomboid fossa into the grey matter around the central canal of the closed part of the medulla. It is *visceromotor* to involuntary muscle in the bronchi, heart, oesophagus, stomach, small intestine and the proximal two-thirds of the colon. So-called 'vital centres' for cardiac and respiratory control, and reflex centres for swallowing and vomiting, are located in the reticular formation deep to the fourth ventricle's floor. Vagal parasympathetic supply is also *secretomotor* to the gastrointestinal glands and pancreas; the fibres are preganglionic, and synapse in small ganglia and plexuses in or near the walls of viscera. The

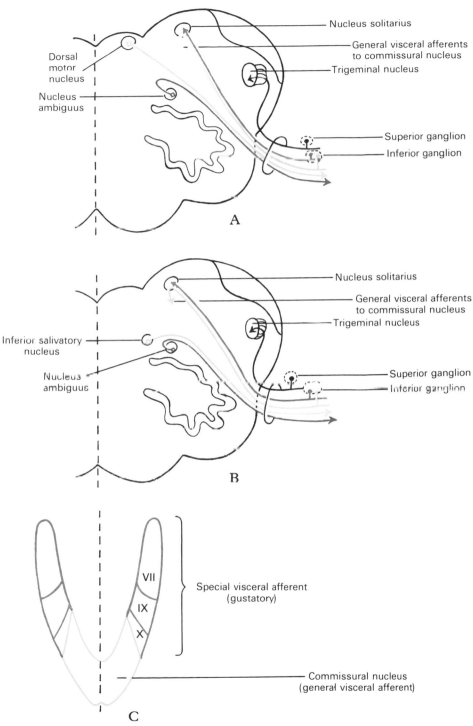

Fig. 6.6 Components of the vagus (A) and glossopharyngeal (B) nerves. Nucleus solitarius (C). Green: general visceral afferent and efferent (parasympathetic). Blue: special visceral efferent (branchiomotor). Red: special visceral afferent (gustatory). Black: general somatic afferent.

nucleus is influenced by gustatory impulses (nucleus solitarius), olfaction and the hypothalamus.

b. The *inferior salivatory nucleus* is the source of parasympathetic fibres in the glossopharyngeal nerve to the otic ganglion, from which postganglionic fibres are *secretomotor* to the parotid gland. Olfaction, taste (nucleus solitarius) and intra-oral general stimuli (trigeminal sensory nucleus) can reflexly induce salivation.

Sensory components

The *nucleus solitarius* receives gustatory (special visceral) afferents from the facial, glossopharyngeal and vagus, their nuclear terminations being in a

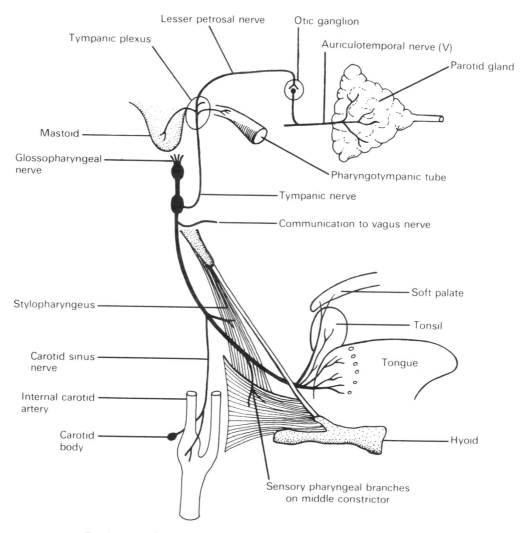

Fig. 6.7 Distribution of the right glossopharyngeal nerve. (After Grant J.C.B. (1949) *Atlas of Anatomy*. London, Baillière Tindall.)

rostrocaudal sequence of decreasing size (*Figs* 6.3 and 6.6). The most caudal region receives general visceral afferents: it reaches the midline dorsal to the central canal in the closed part of medulla, and is aptly termed the '*commissural nucleus*'. The tract containing all these afferent fibres is surrounded by the nucleus, and hence is obvious in Weigert-stained sections. The cell bodies of all the primary visceral afferent neurons are in the inferior glossopharyngeal and vagal ganglia.

1. **Special visceral afferents (gustatory)** in the glossopharyngeal nerve supply the posterior third of tongue, including the vallate papillae. The vagal content of such fibres is very small and limited to the epiglottis.
2. **General visceral afferents** are received from all thoracic and abdominal viscera. Baroreceptors in the carotid sinus monitor changes in blood pressure and chemoreceptors in the carotid body respond to fluctuations of oxygen tension in the blood and these impulses travel in the glosso-pharyngeal nerve.
3. **General somatic afferents** have their primary neuron cell bodies in the superior ganglia of the ninth and tenth nerves. Their dendrites are in the auricular branch of the vagus and the tympanic branch of the glossophar-yngeal; they also conduct impulses of touch and pain in the ninth and tenth nerves from pharynx and posterior third of the tongue. When these afferents reach the medulla they pass to the *spinal trigeminal nucleus*.

Distribution of the glossopharyngeal nerve (*Fig.* 6.7)

The *tympanic nerve* carries sensory fibres from the tympanic plexus of middle ear, from mastoid air cells and pharyngotympanic tube. Parasympathetic fibres travel via the *lesser petrosal nerve* to the otic ganglion, synapse there and join the auriculotemporal branch of the mandibular division of trige-minal to supply secretomotor fibres to the parotid gland. The *carotid sinus nerve* carries afferent fibres from the carotid sinus and body. *Pharyngeal nerves* share in the pharyngeal plexus and supply pharynx, soft palate, tonsil and posterior third of the tongue. The *branchiomotor supply* is to stylopharyngeus.

Distribution of the vagus nerve (*Fig.* 6.8)

Cervical

In the jugular foramen a *meningeal nerve* branches off to supply the dura mater in the posterior cranial fossa. An *auricular* branch supplies the exterior of the ear drum, posterior wall of the external auditory meatus and cranial surface of the auricle. The *pharyngeal nerves* form a plexus with glossophar-yngeal and sympathetic fibres. The branchiomotor supply to pharynx and larynx is derived from the cranial accessory nerve. The *superior laryngeal nerve* has two branches: the *internal laryngeal nerve* pierces the thyrohyoid membrane and is sensory to the mucosa of pharynx and larynx from the level of epiglottis to vocal folds; the *external laryngeal nerve* is motor to

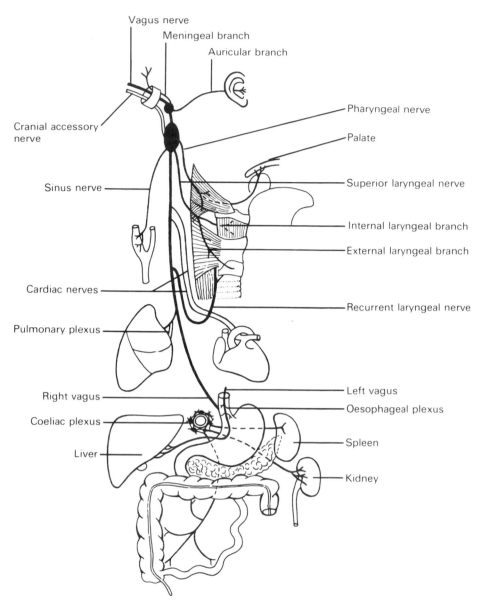

Fig. 6.8 Distribution of the right vagus nerve. (After Grant J.C.B. (1949) *Atlas of Anatomy*. London, Baillière Tindall.)

cricothyroid. The *recurrent laryngeal nerves* loop under the subclavian artery (right) and aortic arch (left) and are motor to all intrinsic laryngeal muscles except cricothyroid; they are also sensory to the mucosa of larynx and pharynx below the level of the vocal folds. The *cardiac nerves* arise in the neck and descend to the cardiac plexuses.

Thoracic

The *bronchial* and *pulmonary nerves* form a plexus with sympathetic fibres, mainly behind the root of each lung, to supply smooth muscle and glands of the bronchial tree, pulmonary blood vessels, the visceral and mediastinal pleura. Afferent fibres are essential to respiratory reflexes. Both vagi contribute motor and sensory fibres to the *oesophageal plexus*, joined by sympathetic fibres from the greater splanchnic nerves.

Abdominal

The anterior and posterior trunks of the vagus descend from the oesophageal plexus as *gastric nerves* supplying the corresponding surfaces of the stomach. The anterior gastric distribution extends through the lesser omentum to the liver. The posterior trunk of the vagus, in addition to its gastric branches, sends rami to the *coeliac*, *superior* and *inferior mesenteric plexuses*, distributed along these articles to the gastrointestinal tract as far as the mid-transverse colon, and to the liver, pancreas, spleen, kidneys and suprarenal glands.

APPLIED ANATOMY

Unilateral supranuclear lesions rarely cause motor disturbance because the nucleus ambiguus has a bilateral cortical innervation. Cortical damage in the 'dominant hemisphere' may involve the language and speech centres which are present there, affecting the understanding and expression of words (dysphasia). Because the muscles of a larynx and pharynx have bilateral cortical control, a unilateral capsular lesion of their corticobulbar fibres may pass unnoticed. If similar fibres in the internal capsule on the *opposite* side are damaged subsequently, suddenly there is difficulty in speaking (dysarthria) and in swallowing (dysphagia), a condition known as 'pseudobulbar palsy', so-named because it mimics a brainstem lesion. Its acute onset is commonly followed by partial recovery. For surveys of the incidence of dysarthria and dysphagia after a stroke *see* Willoughby and Anderson (1984) and Gordon et al. (1987).

The nuclei and nerves may be affected in the brainstem by vascular occlusion (lateral medullary syndrome), by poliomyelitis (acute bulbar palsy) or by degenerative motor neuron disease (chronic progressive bulbar palsy). The prognosis in brainstem lesions is usually poor; it is important therefore to be able to distinguish bulbar (lower motor neuron) palsy from pseudobulbar (upper motor neuron) palsy.

The recurrent laryngeal nerve is close to the inferior thyroid artery and is at risk when this vessel is ligated during thyroidectomy, or it may be subjected to traction during operation on a very large thyroid. A bilateral lesion is particularly serious, because paralysis of the vocal cord abductors ensues, and the only unaffected muscle, the cricothyroid, tenses them. If carcinoma of the lung spreads to tracheobronchial glands on the left side, the nerve may be compressed, making the voice hoarse.

Vagotomy, abdominal division of the vagus nerves, reduces gastric acidity in duodenal ulceration; resultant relative sympathetic overaction would cause pyloric spasm, and this is overcome either by cutting the sphincter (pyloroplasty) or by anastomosing stomach to jejunum (gastrojejunostomy). Sectioning of the nerves just above the cardia (truncal vagotomy) often leads to unpleasant gastrointestinal sequelae, and selective vagotomy of particular gastric branches gives fewer side effects. Advances in medical treatment (e.g. cimetidine) have largely replaced such surgery.

The Vestibulocochlear (VIII) Nerve

The *vestibulocochlear nerve* transmits impulses from the internal ear. It has two components: the vestibular nerve (equilibration) and the cochlear nerve (hearing). Emerging from the internal auditory meatus, the eighth nerve enters the brainstem at the junction of pons and medulla, lateral to the nervus intermedius and facial nerve. This region is often described as the cerebellopontine angle. The cochlear division curves over the lateral surface of the inferior cerebellar peduncle, the vestibular division penetrates the medulla medial to the peduncle (*see Fig.* 5.10).

The vestibular nerve

The vestibular part of the inner ear comprises three *semicircular canals* opening into the *utricle*, which connects with the *saccule*, itself continuous with the *cochlear duct* via the *ductus reuniens* (*Fig.* 6.9). This *membranous labyrinth* is filled with endolymph and separated from its surrounding osseous labyrinth by perilymph. The semicircular canals are at right angles to one another, and at one end of each a dilatation, or *ampulla*, contains a ridge, or *crista*, of neuroepithelial hair cells covered by a gelatinous *cupula*. Movements of the head displace the endolymph and cupula, and this stimulates the hair cells. The utricle and saccule have similar sensory epithelium in their *maculae*, the hair cells of which are in contact with an *otolithic membrane* formed of gelatinous material in which calcareous otoliths or particles are embedded.

The vestibular nerve is formed by the central processes of bipolar cells in the *vestibular ganglion*, located deeply in the internal auditory meatus. The peripheral processes come either from cristae of the semicircular canals (*kinetic labyrinth*), concerned with head *movements* or from maculae of the utricle and saccule (*static labyrinth*), concerned with head *position*. Entering the medulla medial to the inferior cerebellar peduncle, nerve fibres pass to the *vestibular nuclei*, in the floor of the lateral angle of the fourth ventricle; some fibres bypass these nuclei to enter the cerebellum directly via its inferior peduncle, indicating the close functional relationship between labyrinth and cerebellum.

The four vestibular nuclei are the lateral (Deiter's nucleus), superior,

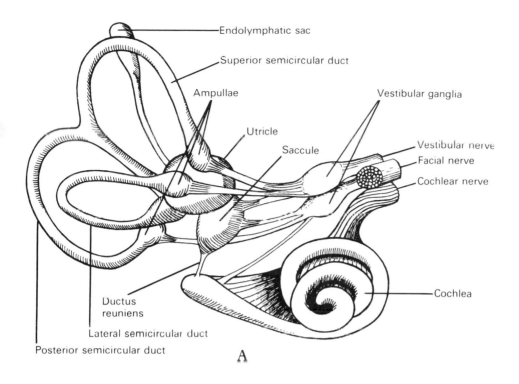

A

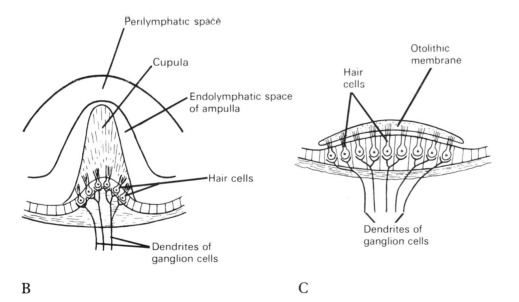

B   C

Fig. 6.9 Distribution of the vestibulocochlear nerve to (A) the membranous labyrinth, (B) the sensory apparatus of a semicircular duct and (C) the utricle.

medial and inferior (*Fig.* 6.10); they influence the cerebellum, spinal cord and oculogyric nuclei, and have cortical connexions. The cerebellar connexions are reciprocal: the archecerebellum is concerned with equilibration and the paleocerebellum with muscle tone, posture and locomotion. The cerebellum receives input from the vestibular nuclei and directly from the vestibular nerve.

Descending paths are via vestibulospinal and reticulospinal tracts. The main (ventrolateral) *vestibulospinal tract* originates in the lateral vestibular (Deiter's) nucleus and descends ipsilaterally throughout the ventral funiculus, synapsing with α and γ motor neurons, supplying anti-gravity extensor muscles. Fibres from the medial and inferior vestibular nuclei of both sides descend in the *medial longitudinal fasciculi*, as small *medial vestibulospinal tracts*, to cervical segments, influencing nerves involved in head movement, including the spinal nucleus of the accessory nerve. This tract facilitates head and eye coordination and effects righting reflexes of the head. There are reciprocal connexions between vestibular nuclei and the reticular formation. *Reticulospinal* tracts influence muscle tone, and are also involved in bodily reactions to vestibular disturbance, as in sea-sickness.

Ascending connexions from vestibular nuclei are with oculogyric (III, IV, VI) nuclei via the *medial longitudinal fasciculi*. These two fasciculi extend throughout the brainstem, flanking the midline, and are interconnected via the posterior commissure. Their associations with individual vestibular nuclei are shown in *Fig.* 6.10. Movements of head and eyes are thereby co-ordinated. The fasciculi also mediate co-ordination between individual oculogyric nuclei, essential to conjugate eye movements and binocular vision. A *centre for lateral gaze* in the paramedian pontine reticular formation (PPRF) correlates the innervation of the lateral rectus (abducent nerve) with that of the contralateral medial rectus (oculomotor nerve). The *interstitial nucleus (of Cajal)* is involved in coordinating reflex vertical head and eye movements, as in walking; it links visual and equilibratory information via inputs from the frontal eye field of the cerebral cortex and from vestibular nuclei.

The precise location of vestibular *cortical projections* is uncertain. Stimulation of the human superior temporal gyrus evokes vertigo. In monkeys the primary cortical representation appears to be adjacent to the face area in the lower part of the postcentral gyrus; the pathway relays near the ventral posterior nucleus of the thalamus.

APPLIED ANATOMY

Vestibular function may be tested by the experimental induction of *nystagmus*, rhythmic lateral ocular movements, the eyes rotating rapidly in one direction and returning more slowly. Nystagmus may be physiological or pathological. In the *rotary test* a patient is spun on a vertical axis about ten times. When body rotation is arrested suddenly, fluid in the semicircular canals continues to move, evoking impulses on the nerve; if it and its connexions are intact, nystagmus occurs. In the *caloric test*, warm or cold water, instilled into the external auditory meatus, causes currents in the

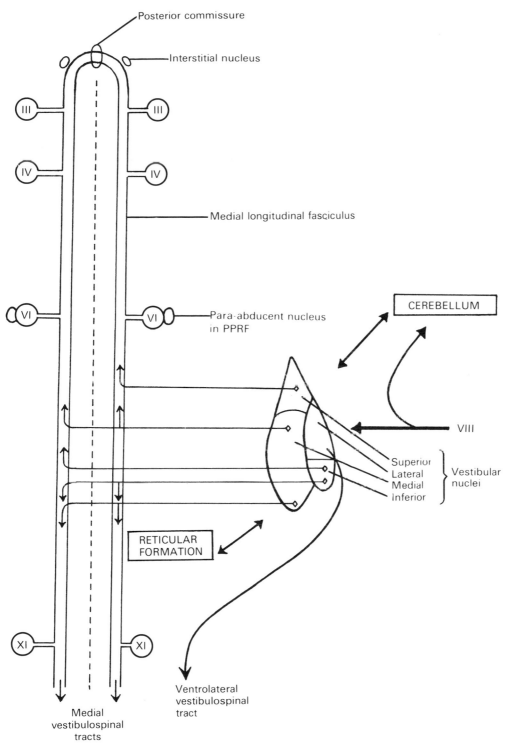

Fig. 6.10 Connexions of the medial longitudinal fasciculi and vestibular nuclei.
PPRF: paramedian pontine reticular formation.

endolymph of the canals, with similar results. The subject is unable to walk along a straight line; in attempting to point at an object the arm deviates or overshoots ('past pointing') (*see* also FitzGerald, 1985).

Dysfunction is accompanied by vertigo, nausea, vomiting and nystagmus, as may occur in the disabling paroxysms of *Ménière's disease*, a disorder of the labyrinth. The medial longitudinal fasciculus is peculiarly susceptible to demyelination in multiple sclerosis: this results in *internuclear ophthalmoplegia*, a loss of conjugate eye movements.

The eighth nerve sometimes develops a primary tumour, an *acoustic neuroma*. The symptoms are instructive of local anatomy. It originates from the vestibular division and compresses the cochlear nerve. Tinnitus (a continuous high pitched sound) is followed by slowly progressive deafness and giddiness. Pressure on the seventh nerve causes facial muscle spasms and much later, facial paralysis. Displacement of the pons puts the fifth nerve under traction: loss of the corneal reflex, an early sign, is followed eventually by more extensive loss of facial sensation. If untreated, brainstem compression results in paralysis of limbs and finally internal hydrocephalus due to blockage of the outflow of cerebrospinal fluid.

The cochlear nerve

The auditory pathways mediate highly discriminative perception of sound at cortical level, and also subcortical reflex reactions to sound.

The *cochlear* part of the labyrinth is a spiral of two and a half turns, divided into three channels by the *basilar* and *vestibular membranes*, forming the *scala vestibuli*, *scala tympani* and *cochlear duct* (*Fig.* 6.11). The stapes fits in an oval window at the base of the scala vestibuli; a round window is closed by a flexible membrane at the base of the scala tympani. At the apex of the bony core, or *modiolus*, the scalae vestibuli and tympani are in continuity by a narrow passage, the *helicotrema*.

The *spiral organ* (of Corti) (*Fig.* 6.11) is an auditory transducer; its *receptor hair cells* are arranged in an inner row and three outer rows, supported on a basilar membrane by phalangeal cells and attached by their hair processes to an overlying *tectorial membrane*. The basilar membrane is not taut and its mobility varies along the cochlea; it is narrowest and most rigid at the cochlear base, widest and slackest at the apex. Stapedial movement transmits sound waves to perilymph in the scala vestibuli, displacing the basilar membrane and bending hair cells attached to the relatively immobile tectorial membrane.

The cochlear nerve consists of central processes from bipolar cells located in the *spiral ganglion*, within the modiolus. Reaching the medulla, the nerve curves over lateral surface of the inferior cerebellar peduncle to two nuclei. The *dorsal cochlear nucleus* forms a small eminence, the *acoustic tubercle*, on the upper surface of the peduncle in the floor of the lateral recess of the fourth ventricle. The *ventral cochlear nucleus* is located on the ventrolateral aspect of the peduncle. There is tonotopic localization throughout the auditory system; high frequencies are received at the base of the cochlea, low frequencies of the apex. Similarly, in a nucleus, neuron bodies respond-

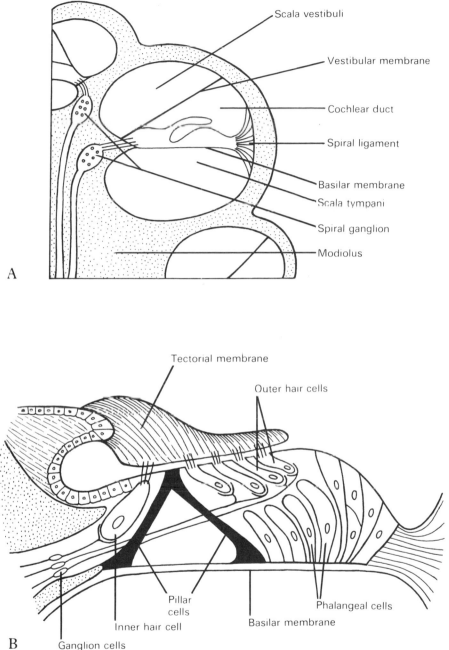

Fig. 6.11 Structure of the cochlea. (A) Section through part of the cochlea. (B) The spiral organ of Corti.

ing to high frequencies are dorsal, those responding to low frequencies are ventral, a pattern transmitted by discrete synapses in neurons of the ventral cochlear nucleus. By contrast, in the dorsal cochlear nucleus there are several types of neurons, their synapses are complex, differing between animal species and evidently involved in processing input; somewhat simpler in humans, the precise functions of this nucleus are unclear. The central projections of both nuclei are shown in *Fig.* 6.12.

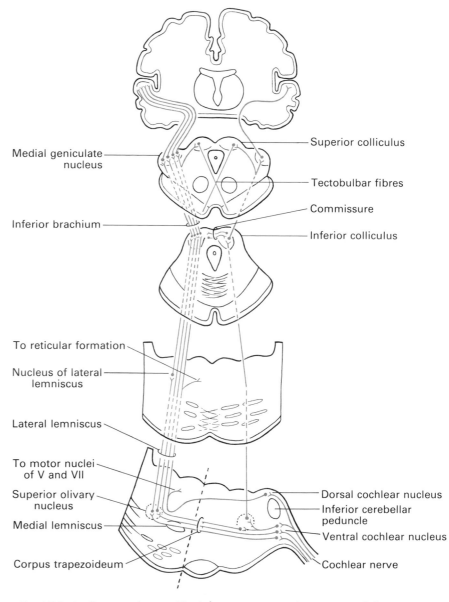

Fig. 6.12 Auditory pathways. The lowest section, at the pontomedullary junction, is oblique, through the pons on the left and medulla on the right.

From the ventral cochlear nucleus fibres decussate in the *trapezoid body* to reach the contralateral *superior olivary nucleus* where some synapse; others have already synapsed in the ipsilateral olivary nucleus and some ascend ipsilaterally, thus providing a bilateral projection. The superior olivary nucleus has functions in the precise localization of sounds in space, an ability dependent on a binaural input, and lost in unilateral deafness (cf. binocular vision). Fibres from the dorsal cochlear nucleus cross more superficially and provide a direct contralateral projection to the opposite inferior colliculus. Fibres from both nuclei form the *lateral lemniscus* which consists of tertiary neurons from both sides. In the small *nucleus of the lateral lemniscus* other scattered synapses occur. Most of the ascending fibres relay in the *inferior colliculus*, and then traverse the inferior brachium to reach the *medial geniculate nucleus*. A few lemniscal fibres bypass the inferior colliculus and continue into the brachium. Through the *auditory radiation* the path reaches the *auditory cortex* of the temporal lobe (Brodmann areas 41, 42), deep in the lateral fissure (transverse temporal gyri) and extending slightly onto the external surface. A tonotopic pattern is maintained in the auditory cortex, low frequency sounds being appreciated anteriorly, high frequency posteriorly.

The auditory pathways are crossed and uncrossed; fibres from one side ascend in both lemnisci and there are commissural connexions between the inferior colliculi. Thus a unilateral cortical lesion would not cause complete deafness, only slight impairment and difficulty in localizing sound. Connexions between the auditory paths and the reticular formation are involved in reflex arousal.

There are *descending fibres* in the auditory pathways, some projecting from the cortex to the medial geniculate nucleus and inferior colliculus. Others descend from the inferior colliculus to cochlear nuclei, concerned with 'neural sharpening' and increased qualitative perception. The *olivocochlear bundle* extends from the superior olivary nucleus through the cochlear nerve to hair cells of the spiral organ of Corti, and can suppress transmission of acoustic stimuli. To some degree auditory stimuli can be ignored or selected; a mother may sleep despite traffic noise, yet awake if her child cries. We need not attend closely to 'background music'. Listening to radio and watching television show differences between the 'control' mechanisms on the auditory and the more compulsive ('hypnotic') visual inputs.

Auditory reflexes

The ears, head and eyes are turned automatically towards an unexpected sound, reflexes mediated via inferior colliculi to superior colliculi, and thence by tectobulbar and tectospinal tracts. Effects via the reticular activating system in arousal from sleep, or its prevention, are commonplace. A loud noise may 'startle'; the extreme percussion of a stun grenade produces a transient motor 'freeze'. A loud noise evokes reflex contractions in tensor tympani (trigeminal nerve) and in stapedius (facial nerve), which prevent excessive vibrations in the tympanic membrane and limit movement of the stapes.

APPLIED ANATOMY

It is necessary to determine whether deafness is due to damage in the middle ear, or in the nerve and its receptors. In middle ear disease, if the nerve is intact, the sound of a tuning fork applied to the mastoid process (bone conduction) is louder than if held near the external ear (air conduction). Cochlear damage often produces permanent tinnitus. The nerve may be the site of a primary tumour (acoustic neuroma, *see* p. 128). In high dosage, drugs such as quinine and streptomycin may damage the nerve.

The Facial (VII) Nerve

The facial nerve emerges at the lower border of pons as two 'roots', a large *motor root*, and a smaller *nervus intermedius* (*Fig.* 6.13). The latter is in an intermediate position between the facial motor root and the vestibulocochlear nerve. The nervus intermedius contains general sensory and gustatory (taste) afferents and also an efferent (parasympathetic) component. Since the facial

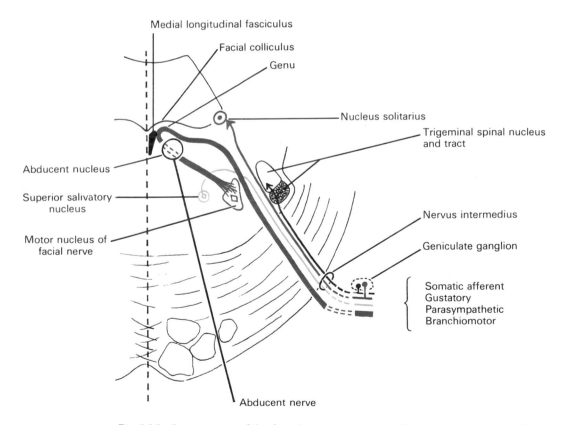

Fig. 6.13 Components of the facial nerve in the pons. Blue: special visceral efferent (branchiomotor). Green: general visceral efferent (parasympathetic). Red: special visceral afferent (gustatory). Black: general somatic afferent.

nerve supplies the second branchial arch, most of its components are classified morphologically as visceral; its somatic sensory input is very minor.

Components

Motor   Sensory

| Branchiomotor (Special Visceral Efferent) | Parasympathetic (General Visceral Efferent) | Special Visceral Afferent (Taste) | General Somatic Afferent |

Nervus Intermedius

Motor components

1. **Branchiomotor**. The *motor nucleus* is situated in the pontine tegmentum (*see Fig.* 5.11). It is rostral to the nucleus ambiguus, in the same special visceral efferent 'column', and medial to the trigeminal spinal nucleus. Evolving in the floor of the fourth ventricle, it has migrated ventrolaterally through the process of 'neurobiotaxis', whereby, during development, functionally associated centres become approximated. Thus the nucleus of VII moves towards that of V, and that of VI towards the medial longitudinal fasciculus. This explains the complex route of the facial motor fibres, which loop dorsally over the abducent nucleus, producing the *facial colliculus*, and then arch ventrally between the nucleus of origin and the trigeminal spinal nucleus to reach the surface. These fibres supply the facial muscles, plus platysma, stylohyoid, posterior belly of digastric and stapedius. Cortical control of lower facial muscles is strictly contralateral, but the upper face (orbicularis oculi and frontalis) has bilateral cortical innervation, a useful fact in distinguishing between upper and lower motor neuron lesions. There is also an influence from subcortical centres concerned with emotion: when this is lost in Parkinson's disease the so-called 'mask-like facies' ensues.

    There are reflex connexions. In the corneal reflex, eyelids close (VII) in response to corneal irritation (V). Loud noises cause reflex contraction of stapedius (VII) via afferents from the superior olivary nucleus (VIII). Tectobulbar fibres from the superior colliculus mediate a protective blink reflex and narrowing of the palpebral fissure in response to bright light.

2. **Parasympathetic**. General visceral efferent fibres from the *superior salivatory nucleus* in the nervus intermedius are preganglionic, secretomotor, and leave the facial nerve as two branches: a) the greater petrosal nerve relays in the pterygopalatine ganglion to innervate the lacrimal gland, nasal and palatine mucosal glands; b) the chorda tympani nerve relays in the submandibular ganglion to supply the submandibular and sublingual salivary glands (*Fig.* 6.14). Salivation is initiated by olfaction and reflexly continued by the taste of food (nucleus solitarius). Oral irritation causes salivation, conjuctival irritation produces lacrimation; in each case the afferents are trigeminal.

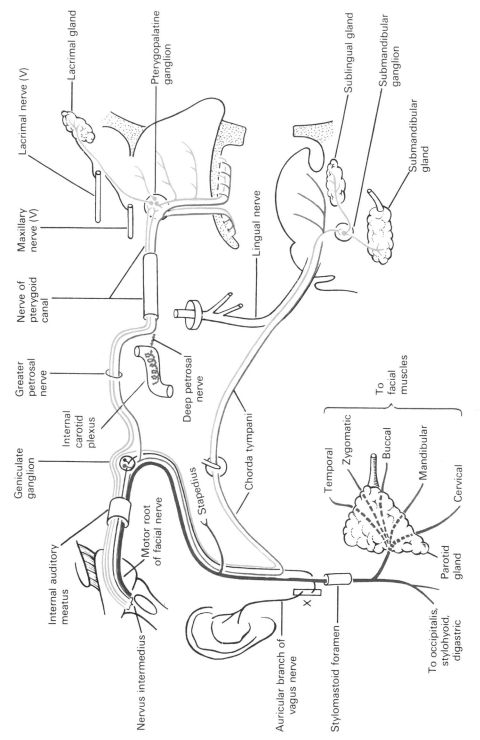

Fig. 6.14 The course and distribution of components of the facial nerve. Blue: branchiomotor. Green: parasympathetic efferent. Beaded red line from internal carotid plexus: sympathetic. Red: afferent gustatory. Black: general somatic afferent.

Sensory components

The afferent fibres are mostly visceral (gustatory); the somatic input is minor. All primary sensory neurons have their cell bodies in the *geniculate ganglion*, at the bend or *genu* of the facial nerve in the medial wall of the middle ear.

1. **Special visceral afferent** (gustatory). Taste afferents from the anterior two-thirds of the tongue leave the lingual nerve (V) to pass centrally in the chorda tympani; from soft palate and palatal arches via palatine nerves (V) to the greater petrosal nerve. The somata are in the geniculate ganglion, and their axons pass via the nervus intermedius to the rostral part of the *nucleus solitarius (Fig.* 6.6). Gustatory impulses relay from here to the hypothalamus and ventral posterior thalamic nucleus, and from the latter to the 'face region' of the sensory cortex. There are reflex connexions to salivatory nuclei; communications with the dorsal motor nucleus of vagus link gustatory stimulation to gastric secretion and gastrointestinal motility.

2. **General somatic afferent**. A small number of fibres from the external auditory meatus, tympanic membrane and skin behind the ear join the facial nerve via the auricular branch of the vagus, traversing the nervus intermedius to end (like similar fibres in glossopharyngeal and vagus nerves) in the *spinal nucleus of the trigeminal nerve*. **The facial nerve is not sensory to the face.**

Course and distribution of the facial nerve

This abbreviated account is supplemented by *Fig.* 6.14. The motor root and nervus intermedius join in the internal auditory meatus, pierce its lateral wall and enter the *facial canal*, where the nerve runs anterolaterally above and between the cochlea and the vestibule. At its *genu* (site of the geniculate ganglion) it turns posteriorly in the middle ear's medial wall and then downwards in the medial wall of the mastoid aditus to exit through the *stylomastoid foramen*. Passing anterolaterally it enters the parotid gland, subdividing into terminal branches.

Leaving the geniculate ganglion, the *greater petrosal nerve* pierces the upper surface of petrous temporal bone, enters the middle cranial fossa, is joined at foramen lacerum by the deep petrosal nerve (sympathetic fibres from internal carotid plexus) to form the *nerve of the pterygoid canal*, which goes to the pterygopalatine ganglion. Secretomotor fibres are carried to the lacrimal gland by the zygomatic and lacrimal nerves (V), and to mucosal glands of nose and palate by nasal and palatine nerves (V). The *nerve to stapedius* branches off in the facial canal. The *chorda tympani* leaves the facial nerve above the stylomastoid foramen, ascends to cross the tympanic membrane and leaves the middle ear via the petrotympanic fissure to join the lingual nerve (V): this carries its taste fibres from the anterior two-thirds of the tongue and its preganglionic secretomotor fibres to the *submandibular ganglion* for sublingual and submandibular salivary glands. A *communicating branch* joins the auricular branch of the vagus.

As the facial nerve leaves the stylomastoid foramen, the *posterior auricular nerve* branches off to supply the occipitalis and posterior auricular muscles, and a *digastric* branch supplies the posterior belly of the digastric and stylohyoid; it then divides into *terminal branches* — temporal, zygomatic, buccal, mandibular and cervical — to the *facial muscles*.

APPLIED ANATOMY

Upper and lower motor neuron lesions differ markedly. Upper motor neuron, or *supranuclear* lesions are usually part of a hemiplegia due to a cerebrovascular accident; only the muscles of the lower half of the face on the opposite side are paralysed; the patient can still close the eyelids and wrinkle the forehead. In cortical or capsular lesions, voluntary and emotional facial activity may be dissociated: the patient may smile if amused but cannot 'show his teeth' on demand. By contrast, loss of emotional expression is very characteristic of Parkinson's disease.

In lower motor neuron lesions (damage to the nucleus or nerve), the upper and lower facial muscles on the same side as the lesion are paralysed. Inability to close the eyelids may lead to corneal ulceration, especially if reflex lacrimation is also lost. The commonest *infranuclear* lesion is *Bell's palsy*, thought to be of viral origin, in which oedema compresses the nerve within its canal. The nerve may be affected by *inflammation of the middle ear* and mastoid air cells, or compressed in the cerebellopontine angle by an *acoustic neuroma*. A *fracture* of petrous temporal bone may involve facial nerve, vestibular apparatus and cochlea. In the *newborn* the nerve is relatively superficial and can be damaged by obstetric forceps.

The extent of loss in a lower motor neuron lesion depends on the level of injury. If this is proximal to the geniculate ganglion, taste is lost in the anterior two-thirds of the tongue and secretion from the submandibular, sublingual and lacrimal glands is impaired. *Hyperacusis* (increased sound perception) is due to paralysis of stapedius. The prognosis is usually good in more distal lesions; in lesions proximal to geniculate ganglion, sensory regeneration is poor and salivatory parasympathetic fibres may be misdirected into the lacrimal gland, producing 'crocodile tears' in response to the smell or taste of food.

If *herpes zoster* affects the geniculate ganglion, vesicles appear on the pinna and sometimes on the soft palate and tongue.

The Abducent (VI), Trochlear (IV) and Oculomotor (III) Nerves

These three nerves will be considered together; they innervate muscles which move the eyes and are often collectively termed 'oculogyric nerves'. Their nuclei of origin are all near the medial longitudinal fasciculus, and are interconnected through it. Each nerve contains general somatic efferent fibres; the oculomotor nerve also has a parasympathetic component. The nerves all traverse the cavernous sinus and superior orbital fissure as shown in *Fig.* 6.15.

The abducent nerve

The abducent nucleus (*Fig.* 6.13) underlies the facial colliculus in the fourth ventricle's floor, where motor fibres of the facial nerve loop over it. The

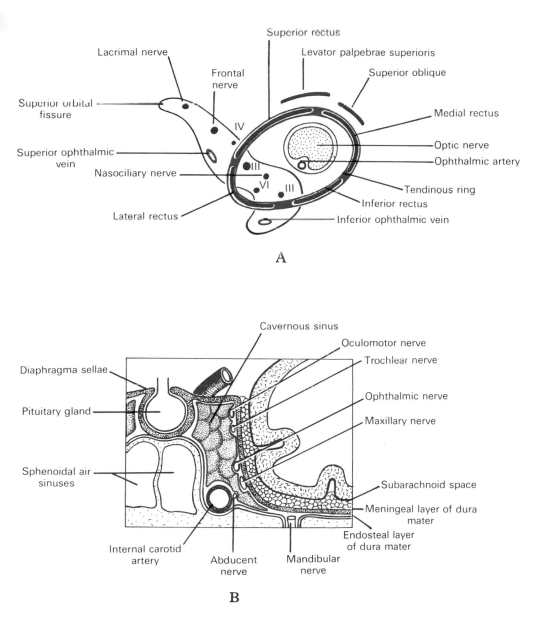

Fig. 6.15 Relationships of nerves in the superior orbital fissure (A) and cavernous sinus (B).

abducent nerve passes ventrally to emerge between the lower border of pons and the pyramid. It supplies the lateral rectus muscle of that side. Near the main nucleus is a group of smaller cells in the *paramedian pontine reticular formation (PPRF)*, sometimes termed the para-abducent nucleus, or the 'centre for lateral gaze', which coordinates activity between the lateral rectus of that side and the contralateral medial rectus (via the medial longitudinal fasciculus and the oculomotor nucleus).

The nerve pierces the dura mater on the dorsum sellae, crosses the apex of the petrous temporal bone and bends forward, running lateral to the internal carotid artery within the cavernous sinus. It enters the orbit through the superior orbital fissure, within the common annular tendon of origin of the rectus muscles (*Fig.* 6.15A).

The trochlear nerve

The trochlear nucleus is in the ventral part of the periaqueductal grey matter of the midbrain at the level of the inferior colliculus, in very close proximity to the medial longitudinal fasciculus (*Fig.* 6.16). It supplies the superior oblique muscle. It has three singular features: it is the most slender cranial nerve, it decussates before emerging, and it emerges on the dorsal aspect. Its emergence is near the midline, through the superior medullary velum just caudal to the inferior colliculus. It curves round the cerebral peduncle, passes between the posterior cerebral and superior cerebellar arteries, pierces

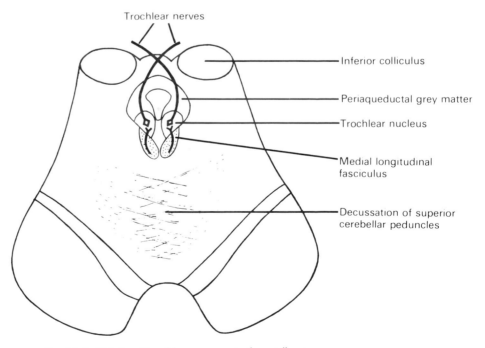

Trochlear nerves

Inferior colliculus

Periaqueductal grey matter

Trochlear nucleus

Medial longitudinal fasciculus

Decussation of superior cerebellar peduncles

Fig. 6.16 Origin of trochlear nerves in the midbrain.

the dura mater just below the tentorial margin, and enters the lateral wall of the cavernous sinus, passing forward into the orbit via the superior orbital fissure, outside the annular tendon (*Fig.* 6.15A).

The oculomotor nerve

The oculomotor nerve contains *somatic efferent* fibres for all the extra-ocular muscles except the superior oblique and the lateral rectus. It also contains *parasympathetic efferents* to the sphincter pupillae and ciliary muscle; it receives postganglionic sympathetic fibres from the internal carotid plexus and distributes them to these intra-ocular muscles. Its terminal branches collect proprioceptive afferents from the ocular muscles, which are transferred by communicating rami to trigeminal branches in the orbit or cavernous sinus. Ocular muscle fibres are thin and their motor units small, and in humans the muscle spindles are numerous, features which are necessary for very delicate and coordinated ocular movements.

From its nucleus the nerve traverses the red nucleus and substantia nigra to emerge in the interpeduncular fossa (*Fig.* 6.17), where it passes between the posterior cerebral and superior cerebellar arteries, pierces the dura mater lateral to the posterior clinoid process to enter the lateral wall of the cavernous sinus. It traverses the superior orbital fissure and annular tendon in superior and inferior divisions (*Fig.* 6.15A), the former supplying the

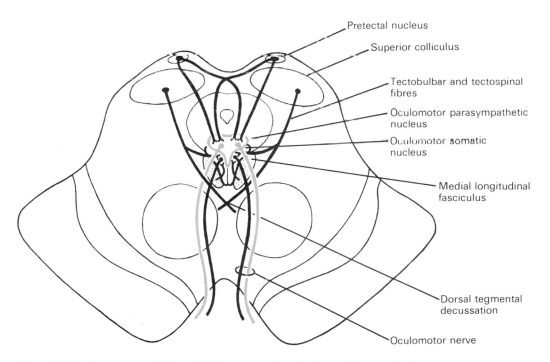

Fig. 6.17 Oculomotor nuclei and their connexions in the midbrain. Oculomotor components shown in black are somatic efferents, those in green are parasympathetic efferents from the Edinger-Westphal nucleus.

superior rectus and levator palpebrae superioris, the latter supplying the medial and inferior recti and the inferior oblique. The branch to the inferior oblique transfers parasympathetic fibres to the ciliary ganglion.

The oculomotor nerve arises from *a nuclear complex*, located ventrally in the periaqueductal grey matter at the level of the superior colliculus, and flanked by the medial longitudinal fasciculi and tectobulbar tracts (*Fig.* 6.17). This nuclear complex has two components:

1. The **general somatic efferent** component is a series of sub-nuclei, described by Warwick (1953) in the monkey (*Fig.* 6.18). These are paired except for a *caudal central nucleus* which supplies both levatores palpebrae superiores. Three lateral nuclei innervate the inferior rectus, inferior oblique and medial rectus of the same side. The superior rectus receives only crossed fibres, its nucleus sited contralaterally in a caudal and medial position. There is no such precise knowledge of localization in humans but it is presumed to be similar.

2. The **parasympathetic** (general visceral efferent) component is known as the *Edinger-Westphal nucleus*. It is dorsal to the somatic nuclei and its neurons relay in the ciliary ganglion, whence short ciliary nerves supply the sphincter pupillae and ciliaris oculi.

Control of ocular movements

Many ocular movements are involuntary, some are initiated voluntarily and continued automatically, and some are purely voluntary. Such movements

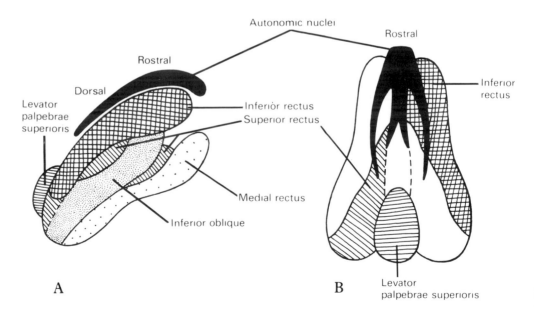

Fig. 6.18 Representation of the right extra-ocular muscles in the oculomotor nucleus of the monkey. (A) Right lateral aspect. (B) Dorsal aspect. (From Warwick R. (1953) *J. Comp. Neurol.* **98**, 480, reproduced by kind permission of the author and publisher.)

are all conjugate, with convergence for close vision (see accommodation and pupillary reflexes, p. 142).

1. **Compensatory ocular movements** maintain a constant retinal (foveal) image despite head and body movement; the mechanism is an action during walking, when the head moves up and down with each stride. This is provided by the vestibular apparatus, augmented by proprioceptive information from the neck muscles. (The role of the cerebellum both in equilibration and in muscular coordination is described in the next chapter.)

2. **Pursuit eye movements** and **automatic scanning** allow vision to 'lock on' to a moving object. A similar mechanism operates in looking out from a moving train: subconsciously, the eyes fix transiently on a succession of passing objects; this may induce a temporary 'railway nystagmus'. Miner's nystagmus is due to persistent subconscious attempts to fix on objects, even in darkness. Locational information passes from the primary visual cortex (Brodmann area 17) to the visual association cortex (Brodmann areas 18, 19); impulses descend to superior colliculi and thence by tectobulbar tracts to 'gaze control centres' (*see* below).

3. **Voluntary scanning** is the ability to examine an area in the visual field and to locate particular features. The frontal eye field of the cortex (Brodmann area 8) coordinates these movements (*see* Applied anatomy). Head movements often accompany those of the eyes. Reading is complex, being an acquired skill and dependent on cortical analysis of language. During learning, the eyes scan by voluntary effort, but when the ability is fully developed, scanning becomes automatic.

Via the *medial longitudinal fasciculi* vestibular information ascends to oculogyric nuclei and descends to cervical motor neurons controlling head movement. The fasciculi also provide connexions between individual oculogyric nuclei, necessary for coordination of eye movements, and are linked to the 'centre for lateral gaze' (PPRF). Through the interstitial nucleus (of Cajal), ascending vestibular impulses are integrated with input from the frontal eye field of the cortex and from the superior colliculus.

The *superior colliculi* receive input from diverse sources, cortical, retinal, auditory and spinal. They function both in the voluntary control of eye movements and also in reflex responses to visual and acoustic stimuli. In the *visual grasp reflex* there is orientation of the eyes, head and body towards such stimuli. These responses cease after ablation of the superior colliculi. Experimental stimulation of a superior colliculus may produce conjugate eye movements. A pineal tumour, as it enlarges and compresses the tectum, successively causes paralysis of elevation, depression and horizontal scan. Input from the visual association cortex is required for automatic scanning and from the frontal eye field for voluntary scanning. The tectobulbar tracts appear to be via interneurons; one such route involves the interstitial nucleus.

The 'centre for lateral gaze', located adjacent to the abducent nucleus in the *PPRF* receives input from the vestibular nuclei, cerebellum, superior and inferior colliculi. It is in continuity caudally with the *nucleus prepositus hypoglossi* which has similar links. The cortical control over eye movements is mediated primarily via the superior colliculi which act largely through the PPRF and nucleus prepositus, and are not linked directly to oculogyric nuclei. These three 'control centres', superior colliculus, PPRF and nucleus prepositus, together with the archecerebellum form a highly integrated and precise system in the control of eye movements; its considerable complexity is incompletely understood. 'The oculomotor system is amongst the most mystifying with respect to its central nervous organization' (Graybiel, 1977).

Pupillary reflexes

Pupillary reflexes involve the autonomic (Edinger-Westphal) component of the oculomotor nucleus. In the *light reflex*, the pupils constrict when light is shone on the retina. If one eye only is stimulated, both pupils constrict, the so-called *consensual reflex*. The afferents are optic nerve fibres which pass to both *pretectal nuclei*, crossing in the posterior commissure. Pretectal nuclei project to the Edinger-Westphal nucleus, from which parasympathetic efferents traverse the oculomotor nerves to ciliary ganglia, whence postganglionic fibres in short ciliary nerves innervate the sphincter pupillae muscles. Note that the reflex connexions are entirely subcortical, in contrast to the accommodation reflex.

The *accommodation reflex* effects three ocular adjustments in near vision: pupillary constriction, convergence of the optic axes and increased convexity of the lens. Since this reflex entails image analysis, optic paths to the cortex must be involved. The cortico-collicular path, and connexions between the superior colliculus and the Edinger-Westphal nucleus complete the central route. The efferent path is the same as that of the light reflex for innervation of the sphincter pupillae and ciliaris oculi; convergence requires coordinated action of all the extra-ocular muscles, some contracting, others relaxing.

Change in pupillary size is primarily due to varying influence in the parasympathetic fibres of the oculomotor nerve; the sympathetic is subordinate in this respect. Like other autonomic nuclei, the Edinger-Westphal receives an input from the hypothalamus.

APPLIED ANATOMY

Every ocular movement requires coordinated adjustment in all the extra-ocular muscles: the primary actions of individual muscles are summarized in Starling's diagram (*Fig.* 6.19).

In *oculomotor paralysis* the ophthalmoplegia is severe: the eye is directed down and outwards due to unopposed actions of the lateral rectus and superior oblique. Ptosis (drooping) of the upper lid results from paralysis of the levator palpebrae superioris. The pupil is dilated (parasympathetic denervation), unresponsive to direct and consensual light reflexes, and to accommodation. Since muscular innervations originate in sub-groups, partial lesions at nuclear level may occur. In an *abducent palsy* abduction of the eye is almost completely lost (the two obliques have a slight abductor component) and ultimately the unopposed medial rectus produces internal strabismus. In *trochlear nerve paralysis* diplopia (double vision) occurs when the eye is directed inferomedially, since the superior oblique takes part in 'down and out' movements (and medial rotation).

Following extradural (middle meningeal) haemorrhage, the underlying temporal lobe may be displaced, compressing the oculomotor nerve of that side against the anterior free margin of the tentorium cerebelli. This results in a fixed dilated pupil on the side of the lesion, a sign of great surgical importance.

The *Argyll Robertson pupil* is primarily associated with syphilis of the central nervous system, though it can occur in other conditions. The pupil is small, does not react to light but contracts well in accommodation. As noted, the afferent routes in the light and accommodation reflexes differ, and may be separately damaged. When a *pineal tumour* compresses the pretectal region the light reflex is lost, pressure on the superior colliculi affects the accommodation reflex and vertical eye movements.

If the *frontal eye field* is damaged, as in vascular deprivation, the patient cannot look voluntarily to the opposite side. In epileptic seizures involving this area, with cortical over-activity, the eyes are deflected contralaterally. *Extrapyramidal disorders* may affect eye control: impaired upward gaze often features in Parkinson's disease or Huntington's chorea; in post-encephalitic Parkinsonism, there may be '*oculogyric crises*' with strong upward deflection of the eyes.

A pontine vascular lesion may affect the *centre for lateral gaze* and the abducent nucleus. In multiple sclerosis, demyelination of the medial longitudinal fasciculus produces *internuclear ophthalmoplegia*, often with convergent or divergent squint due to loss of conjugate movements.

The Trigeminal (V) Nerve

The trigeminal nerve is sensory to the face, scalp, mouth, teeth, nasal cavity and air sinuses, and motor to the masticatory muscles. It enters the ventral pons as a large *sensory root* and, anteromedial to this, a smaller *motor root* emerges.

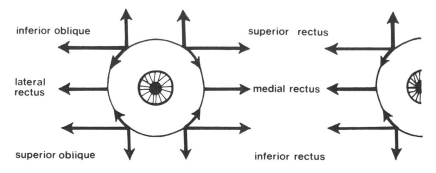

Fig. 6.19 Starling's diagram of the actions of the extrinsic ocular muscles.

Sensory components (general somatic afferent)

Most trigeminal sensory fibres have their unipolar cell bodies in the *trigeminal ganglion*, located in a small recess of dura mater (cavum trigeminale), near the apex of the petrous temporal bone. It differs from a dorsal root ganglion, firstly because there are no visceral afferents, and secondly because proprioceptive fibres pass through it to form a *mesencephalic tract*, whose primary neuron somata are in a uniquely central location in the midbrain. The three divisions, ophthalmic, maxillary and mandibular, converge on the ganglion. The motor root passes laterally under the ganglion to enter the mandibular division, which distributes it. The trigeminal sensory nuclei are joined by the small somatic afferent components carried centrally in the facial, glossopharyngeal and vagus nerves, already described. *Trigeminal sensory nuclei* form a column throughout the brainstem, extending into the first cervical spinal segment (*Fig.* 6.20); there is a rostrocaudal segregation of sensory modalities in this column.

The *mesencephalic nucleus*, mediating proprioception, is a slender column of *unipolar primary neurons* sited laterally in the periaqueductal grey matter

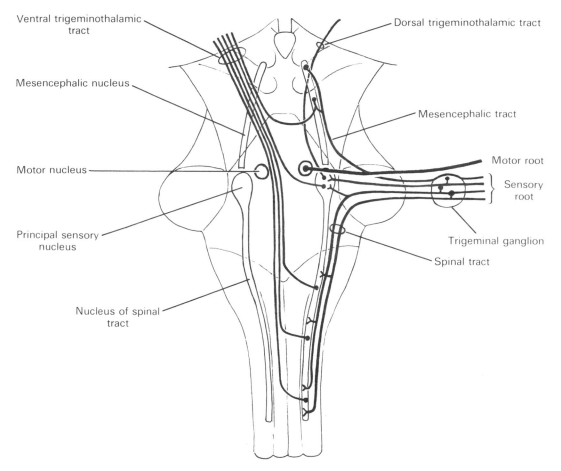

Fig. 6.20 Trigeminal nuclei and their connexions.

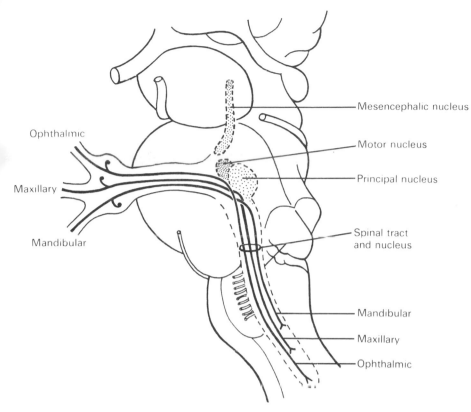

Fig. 6.21 Trigeminal nuclei from lateral aspect. Note that in the spinal nucleus the ophthalmic division is ventral and extends caudally to the cervical region; the mandibular division is dorsal and terminates at mid-medullary level. (After Brodal A. (1981) *Neurological Anatomy*. Oxford, Oxford University Press.)

of the midbrain, reaching caudally to the lateral angle of the fourth ventricle. It is flanked by input fibres, the *mesencephalic tract*. It receives afferents from neuromuscular spindles of the masticatory muscles, from the temporomandibular joint and the teeth. Intense intra-oral proprioception is essential in chewing, controlling the force and accuracy of the bite — how rarely the tongue is bitten, and how aware one is initially of minor structural change due to dental surgery! This nucleus also receives input from proprioceptors in the extra-ocular and facial muscles.

The other sensory fibres have two possible destinations. Some fibres enter the *principal trigeminal nucleus*, which mediates discriminative touch, like the nuclei gracilis and cuneatus. Finely myelinated or non-myelinated fibres descend in the *trigeminal spinal tract*, which enters the *trigeminal spinal nucleus*; this is continuous rostrally with the principal nucleus, and caudally it blends with the substantia gelatinosa and nucleus proprius of the second cervical spinal segment. The rostral part of the spinal nucleus mediates simple touch and pressure sensations; the caudal part is concerned with pain and temperature modalities. Functionally the spinal nucleus resembles the spinal grey horn and it has similar processing mechanisms for modulation of input. Afferents from the three trigeminal divisions rotate, bringing mandibular fibres to a dorsal position in the tract and nucleus, with maxillary fibres central and ophthalmic afferents ventral (*Fig.* 6.21). Moreover, the ophthalmic input extends to cervical level, the maxillary input terminates rostral to this, and the mandibular input does not pass caudal to mid-medullary level. The spinal tract receives input also from the facial, glossopharyngeal and vagus nerves for general somatic sensation in the ear, tongue, pharynx and larynx.

Trigeminal *central projections* are thalamic, cerebellar and nuclear. Fibres from the spinal nucleus reach the *medial ventral posterior (VPM) thalamic nucleus* via the crossed *ventral trigeminothalamic* tract sited immediately dorsal to the contralateral medial lemniscus in the pons (*see Fig.* 5.12). From the principal sensory nucleus most fibres cross, but a few mandibular afferents ascend in a small uncrossed *dorsal trigeminothalamic tract* (*Fig.* 6.20), which ascends through the dorsal pontine tegmentum to lie close to the periaqueductal grey matter in the midbrain: its significance is uncertain (*see Fig.* 5.13). Cortical representation is highly specific and illustrates the functional organization of the cortex into vertical cell units, as experimentally demonstrated in regard to rats' vibrissae: each hair is associated with a single 'barrel' of cells (*see* also p. 227).

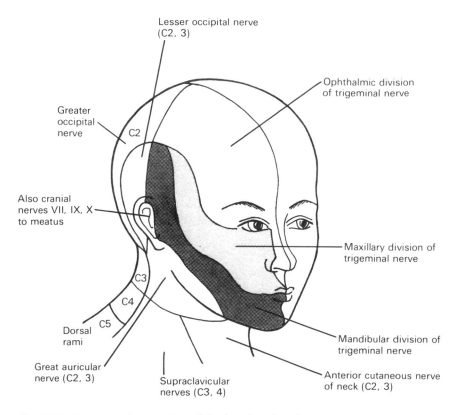

Fig. 6.22 Cutaneous innervation of the head and neck.

The mesencephalic nucleus is connected to the *cerebellum* via its superior peduncle, the spinal nucleus via the inferior peduncle.

Reflex arcs involve the trigeminal, facial and hypoglossal motor nuclei, the nucleus ambiguus and the reticular formation. An example is the corneal reflex: touching the cornea evokes impulses in the ophthalmic nerve, and reflex eyelid closure is effected via the facial nerve. Obviously nuclei controlling mastication, swallowing and phonation must also be co-ordinated. Nasal irritation provokes sneezing, which involves widespread muscular responses. Toothache may inhibit sleep, an effect mediated via the reticular activating system.

Motor component

The *trigeminal motor nucleus* is medial to the principal sensory nucleus. It is branchiomotor to derivatives of the first branchial arch, and is distributed via the mandibular nerve to the muscles of mastication (masseter, temporalis, medial and lateral pterygoids) and to four others (tensor palati, tensor tympani, mylohyoid and the anterior belly of digastric). It receives a bilateral corticonuclear innervation; masticatory muscles act bilaterally (*see* also Applied anatomy).

Course and distribution of the trigeminal nerve
(*Fig. 6.22*)

Note that *although the trigeminal nerve has no intrinsic parasympathetic component at source, all divisions, in their branches are linked to parasympathetic ganglia, and distribute postganglionic fibres.*

The *ophthalmic division* traverses the superior orbital fissure as frontal, lacrimal and nasocilliary branches, supplying sensory fibres to a surface area from the vertex of the scalp to the nasolabial junction, including the conjunctiva. The nasociliary nerve is joined by postganglionic parasympathetic fibres from the *ciliary ganglion* which are derived from the oculomotor nerve and innervate the sphincter pupillae and ciliary muscles.

The *maxillary division* traverses the foramen rotundum, pterygopalatine fossa and infra-orbital canal, emerging on the face. It has meningeal, zygomatic, palatal, alveolar, palpebral, nasal and labial branches. It supplies the skin in the temporal and maxillary regions, upper lip, nasal cavity, hard and soft palate, also the upper teeth and the vault of the pharynx. Through the *pterygopalatine ganglion* it receives postganglionic parasympathetic fibres of the facial nerve; some are distributed in the palatine nerves, others enter the zygomatic branch to reach the lacrimal nerve and innervate the lacrimal gland.

The *mandibular division* is a mixed nerve and contains all the trigeminal motor component. It passes through the foramen ovale, gives off a recurrent meningeal branch and the nerve to the medial pterygoid, then divides into anterior and posterior trunks. The anterior trunk provides a sensory buccal nerve, and three motor branches, the masseteric, deep temporal and lateral pterygoid nerves. The posterior trunk divides into auriculotemporal, lingual and inferior alveolar nerves. The mandibular division supplies the lower teeth, floor of the mouth, anterior two-thirds of tongue (ordinary sensation), the skin over the mandible and part of the auricle. The auriculotemporal nerve is joined by postganglionic parasympathetic fibres from the *otic ganglion* (glossopharyngeal) and distributes these to the parotid gland. The lingual nerve is joined by visceral fibres from the chorda tympani (facial nerve). These are afferent and efferent; the afferent component serves taste in the anterior two-thirds of the tongue; the efferent fibres synapse in the *submandibular ganglion* and are secretomotor to the submandibular and sublingual glands.

APPLIED ANATOMY

Supranuclear lesions. In connexion with the facial nerve it was noted that hemiplegia may include paralysis of the lower facial muscles. Masticatory muscles are little affected, since they have bilateral cortical control. About 15% of such patients have ipsilateral weakness of the masseter (Willoughby and Anderson, 1984).

Infranuclear lesions. *Herpes zoster* has a predilection for the trigeminal ophthalmic division in the elderly; two or three days of severe pain are followed by a vesicular (blistered) rash, which starts in the eyebrow and may involve the entire territory of the trigeminal ophthalmic division, but not beyond: thus only half the nose is affected. Herpes may cause corneal ulceration which can result in corneal opacities. *Trigeminal neuralgia* ('tic douloureux') typically occurs in spasmodic attacks of excruciating pain in one or more of the divisions, without sensory loss. Although usually treated medically, an alternative is 'trigeminal tractotomy', severing connexions with the inferior part of the spinal nucleus which mediates pain, but spares touch sensation and, in particular, retains a corneal reflex.

Occasionally *otitis media* extends to the apex of the petrous temporal bone, affecting the overlying trigeminal ganglion and causing facial pain; it may also involve the abducent nerve, with palsy of the lateral rectus (Gradenigo's syndrome). Nerve lesions sometimes complicate *skull fractures*. An *aneurysm of the internal carotid artery* in the cavernous sinus may compress the ophthalmic and oculogyric nerves.

Syringomyelia may cavitate the central canal in the upper cervical cord and lower medulla. The medullary part of the trigeminal spinal nucleus is compressed progressively in a rostral direction, causing the so-called 'onion skin' phenomenon: initially there is analgesia in the posterior part of the face, but this gradually advances anteriorly in concentric zones towards the 'muzzle area', the last to be affected. This process is informative as to spatial representation in the caudal part of the nucleus.

Cranial nerve summary

Name		Chief Functions	Main Regions Supplied	Components
I	Olfactory	Smell	Olfactory Mucosa	Special sense
II	Optic	Sight	Retina	Brain tract
III	Oculomotor	Eye movement	4 eye muscles and levator palpebrae superioris	Somatomotor. (GSE)
		Pupil constriction Accommodation	Sphincter pupillae and ciliary muscle (via ciliary ganglion & Vi)	Parasympathetic (GVE)
IV	Trochlear	Eye movement	Superior oblique	Somatomotor (GSE)
V	Trigeminal: Vi Ophthalmic	General sensation	Forehead, side of nose, conjunctiva, cornea	Somatic afferent (GSA)
	Vii Maxillary	General sensation	Skin over maxilla, nasal mucosa, mucosa, palate, upper teeth, pharyngeal vault	
	Viii Mandibular	General sensation	Lower teeth, floor of mouth, anterior two-thirds of tongue, skin over mandible	
		Jaw movement	Muscles of mastication (1st arch), also tensor tympani, tensor palati, mylohyoid, digastric (anterior belly)	Branchiomotor (SVE)
VI	Abducent	Eye movement	Lateral rectus	Somatomotor (GSE)
VII	Facial	Facial expression	Muscles of facial expression, hyoid elevators (2nd arch)	Branchiomotor (SVE)
		Salivation	Submandibular and sublingual glands (via submandibular ganglion & Viii)	Parasympathetic (GVE)
		Lacrimation	Lacrimal gland (via pterygopalatine ganglion, Vii, Vi)	
		Taste	Anterior two-thirds of tongue	Gustatory (SVA)
VIII	Vestibulocochlear	Hearing Equilibration	Cochlea. Vestibule	Special sense (SSA)
IX	Glossopharyngeal	Swallowing	Stylopharyngeus (3rd arch)	Branchiomotor (SVE)
		Salivation	Parotid gland (via otic ganglion & Viii)	Parasympathetic (GVE)
		Taste	Posterior one-third of tongue	Gustatory (SVA)
		Common sensation	Posterior one-third of tongue, pharynx	General visceral afferent (GVA)
X	Vagus	Swallowing, Phonation	Pharyngeal muscles. Laryngeal muscles (4 & 6 arches)	Branchiomotor (SVE)
		Visceromotor	Visceral muscles, gut, lungs etc.	Parasympathetic (GVE)
		Visceral sensation	Gut, lungs, heart etc.	General visceral afferent (GVA)
		Taste	Epiglottis	Gustatory (SVA)
		General sensation	External auditory meatus (also from VII and IX)	Somatic afferent (GSA)
XI	Accessory (Spinal)	Head and shoulder movements	Sternomastoid, trapezius	Branchiomotor (SVE)
XII	Hypoglossal	Tongue movements	Tongue muscles	Somatomotor (GSE)

Chapter 7

Cerebellum

General Structure

The cerebellum is in the posterior cranial fossa, beneath the tentorium cerebelli. Centrally it is separated from the pons and medulla by the fourth ventricle. Its surface bears numerous transversely curved fissures between narrow folds, the leaf-like *folia*. Its appearance is thus very different from that of the cerebral cortex. It has two lateral hemispheres, united by a median *vermis* (*Figs*. 7.1–7.3). The *superior vermis* is a slight ridge that extends anteriorly to include the *lingula* on the superior medullary velum. The *inferior vermis* is more clearly demarcated from the hemispheres in the floor of the *vallecula cerebelli:* antero-posteriorly it is divided by fissures into the *nodule, uvula* and *pyramid*. From the nodule, a stalk extends on each side to a tiny lobule, the *flocculus*, and together these form the *flocculonodular lobe*. The *tonsil* is a partly separated lobule which overhangs the inferior vermis; its removal exposes the inferior medullary velum. Raised intracranial pressure may bulge the tonsils downwards into the foramen magnum.

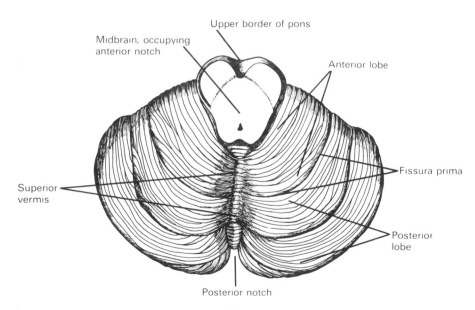

Fig. 7.1 Superior surface of the cerebellum.

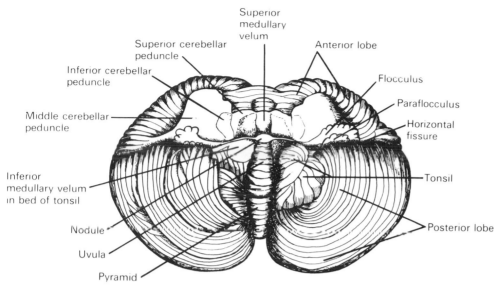

Fig. 7.2 Ventroanterior view of the cerebellum. The right tonsil of the cerebellum has been removed to show the inferior medullary velum.

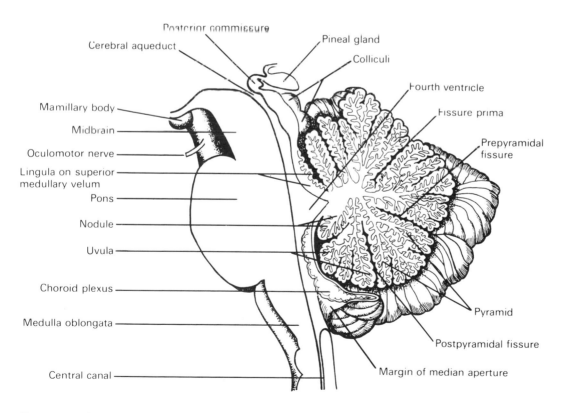

Fig. 7.3 Median sagittal section of the cerebellum and brainstem.

The cerebellum has three main lobes, *anterior, posterior* and *flocculonodular*. On the superior surface a deep *fissura prima* is behind the anterior lobe (*Fig. 7.1*). The remainder of the hemispheres, with the pyramid and uvula, forms the posterior lobe. The flocculonodular lobe has been described. A *horizontal fissure* in the posterior lobe roughly divides the cerebellum into superior and inferior halves: the middle cerebellar peduncles enter this fissure and the flocculi emerge from it.

Deep to the cortex the white medullary core contains individually named *intracerebellar nuclei*, such as the dentate nucleus. There are three paired peduncles. The inferior peduncles ascend from the medulla, the middle enter from the pons, the superior pass from cerebellum to the midbrain.

Structurally and functionally the cerebellum reflects evolutionary history. The *archecerebellum* developed with the vestibular nuclei, is concerned with equilibration, is present in fishes, and in humans is represented by the flocculonodular lobe and lingula. The *paleocerebellum* emerged with terrestrial vertebrates, which required limbs to support the body against gravity; its connexions are therefore predominantly spinal and it is associated with muscle tone, locomotion, posture and other stereotyped movements. It includes the anterior lobe and the uvula and pyramid of the inferior vermis. The *neocerebellum* comprises most of the posterior lobe (except the uvula and pyramid) and is the largest region. It is concerned with the control of non-stereotyped, skilled and learned activities and its size parallels the development of the cerebral hemispheres.

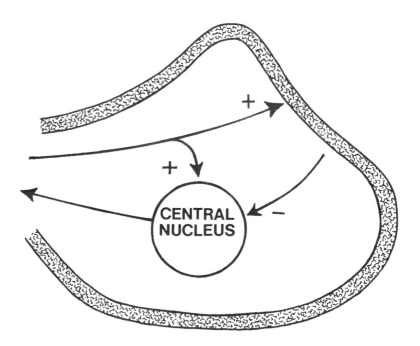

Fig. 7.4 Diagram illustrating excitatory cerebellar input and the inhibitory influence of the cerebellar cortex on the central nuclei.

The detailed structure of the cerebellar cortex is uniform throughout. By contrast, the cytoarchitecture of the cerebral cortex varies according to region. Afferents project to the cerebellar cortex; cortical output is mostly to intracerebellar (central) nuclei, in which efferent fibres originate (*Fig.* 7.4). The influence of the cortex on the nuclei is inhibitory. Collaterals from afferent fibres maintain an excitatory state in each intracerebellar nucleus, and this is controlled by varying inhibition that the nucleus receives from the cortex. As an exception to this general pattern, the vestibular nuclei of the brainstem receive some fibres direct from the cortex.

There are four pairs of nuclei (*Fig.* 7.5) which were given descriptive names long before their functions were known. The *fastigial nucleus* is near the apex of the roof of the fourth ventricle ('fastigium' is the Latin name for the top of a gabled roof). The *globose* (rounded) and *emboliform* (plug-shaped) nuclei are a functional unit. The *dentate nucleus* (toothed in profile) is much larger than the others and particularly prominent in humans.

Nuclear connexions can be summarized as follows:

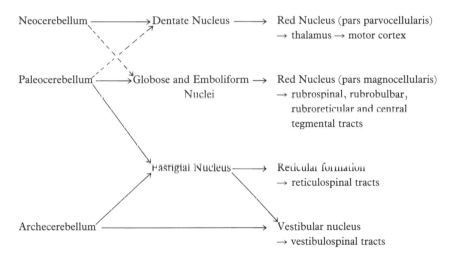

Efferent connexions will be explained later, but note now that the dentate nucleus is particularly associated with the neocerebellum. The globose-emboliform and fastigial nuclei are associated with the paleocerebellum. Primitively the archecerebellum had no central nucleus but some of its efferents relay in the fastigial nucleus. The three parts of the cerebellum are not separate units: there is some overlap and corticonuclear 'exchange' between them.

The Cerebellar Cortex

Most of the cortex is submerged between the folia: only about 15% is visible on the surface. The cortex is trilaminar, with molecular, Purkinje and granular layers (*Figs.* 7.6 and 7.7).

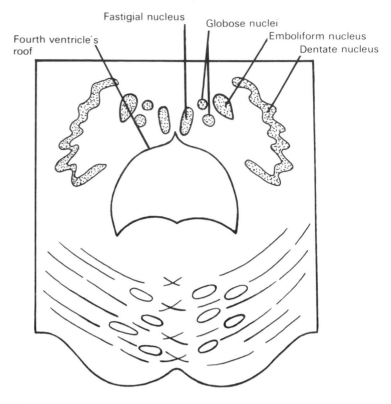

Fig. 7.5 Intracerebellar nuclei in a diagrammatic transverse section.

The *molecular layer* is superficial, contains relatively few cells and consists mainly of fibres: those which run *along* the folia are from the granular cells of the deep layer, while those orientated *across* the folia are Purkinje cell dendrites and associated interneurons. There are two types of interneuron, both inhibitory: the *stellate cells* are in the plane of the Purkinje dendrites; the *basket cells* have a basket-like arborization around the Purkinje cell bodies.

The *Purkinje cells* are very large Golgi Type I neurons whose axons convey cortical output to the intracerebellar nuclei; the axons have recurrent collateral branches. From the archecerebellum some Purkinje axons pass directly to the vestibular nuclei of the brainstem. The large flask-shaped *bodies are arranged in rows along the folia;* relatively few in number, they form a thin layer. Each cell has a profusely branched *dendritic tree orientated transverse to the long axis of its folium;* the primary and secondary branches are smooth, but subsequent ones have numerous dendritic spines.

The wide *granular cell* layer consists of vast numbers (up to 7 million per mm³) of small neurons whose axons ascend into the molecular layer and bifurcate in a T-shaped manner to form *parallel fibres* which run along the folium. Each Purkinje cell's dendritic field includes up to 400 000 synapses with parallel fibres.

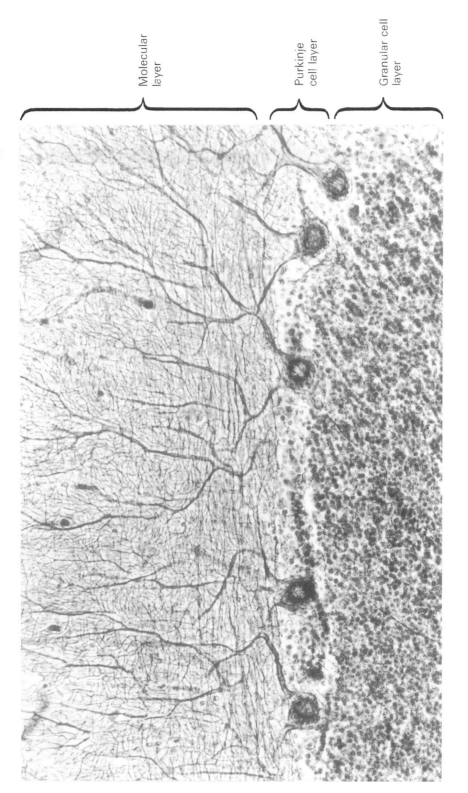

Molecular layer

Purkinje cell layer

Granular cell layer

Fig. 7.6 Photograph of a section through the cerebellar cortex. (Cajal silver stain, × 300.)

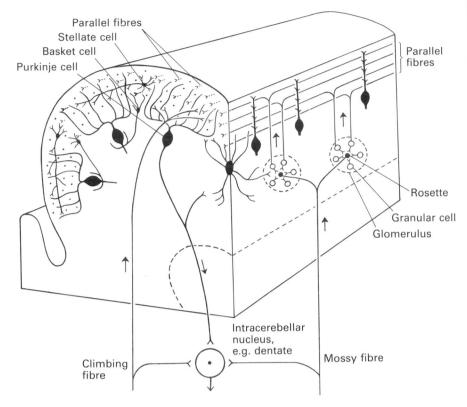

Fig. 7.7 Neuronal organization of the cerebellar cortex. Red: excitatory fibres. Black: inhibitory fibres.

Located superficially in the granular layer there are a few inhibitory *Golgi neurons*. Each of these has a bushy dendritic field which extends into the molecular layer, orientated along and across the folium, serving the territory of about 10 Purkinje cells. Individual Golgi territories approximate to, but do not overlap one another. Their axons are inhibitory to granular cells.

Cerebellar afferents are all excitatory but comprise two very different types of input: **Climbing fibres** provide a *discrete* and *non-divergent input* of pre-integrated information from the contralateral inferior olivary nuclear complex. The inferior olivary nuclei receive ascending (spino-olivary) and descending (central tegmental tract) afferents and project to the whole cerebellar cortex. The principal inferior olivary nuclei project to the neocerebellum, the accessory olivary nuclei, older phylogenetically, are associated with the archecerebellum and paleocerebellum. *Each Purkinje neuron is supplied by a single climbing fibre*, whose branches then twine tendril-like around the smooth areas of its dendritic tree. This highly discrete relationship was originally described histologically by Ramón y Cajal (1911) and later confirmed physiologically by Eccles et al. (1966). A climbing fibre may subdivide a few times to supply up to 10 Purkinje cells only (Eccles 1977).

Mossy fibres comprise all other afferents, diverse in origin and nature, and including those from the pontine nuclei. A *highly divergent input pattern* intermingles these afferents prior to their integration by Purkinje cells. Divergence is brought about as follows: each mossy fibre supplies more than one folium, divides in each folium to reach its anterior and posterior surfaces, divides again in the granular layer, and each terminal forms a bulbous *rosette*, which synapses with about 20 granular cell dendrites. Golgi cell axons have an inhibitory effect at rosettes. The arrangement of the rosette, granular cell dendrites and Golgi cell axons is termed a *glomerulus*. Each granular cell axon bifurcates in the molecular layer into two parallel fibres; these run along the folium and synapse with the dendritic spines of a row of about 400 Purkinje neurons, also with adjacent basket, stellate and Golgi cells. Because of the diffusion of its input to numerous granular cells, one mossy fibre ultimately influences many thousands of Purkinje neurons. As already noted, each Purkinje dendritic field synapses with thousands of parallel fibres and can thus receive, correlate and integrate information from all sources; this is most precisely achieved by selecting only maximally stimulated Purkinje neurons to respond.

The *functional circuitry* is summarized in *Fig*. 7.8. All afferents are excitatory to the cortex and their collaterals are excitatory to the intracerebellar (central) nuclei. Mossy fibre input activates bundles of parallel fibres, creating individual bands of excitation which spread along the molecular layer. When the width of one such a band becomes equal to the width of a Purkinje dendritic field, a row of these neurons fire. Synchronously the flanking stellate and basket cells are stimulated and they inhibit about 10

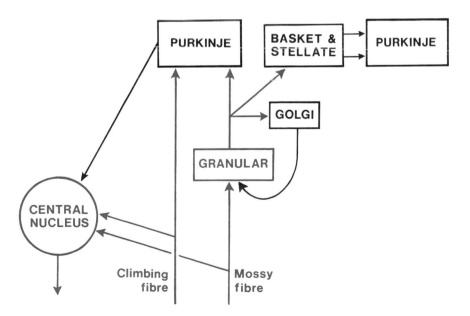

Fig. 7.8 Diagram of the neuronal circuitry in the cerebellum: excitation is indicated in red, inhibition in black. Central nucleus = dentate, globose-emboliform or fastigial.

adjacent rows of Purkinje cells on each side — a selective 'neural sharpening' effect. If the band of excitation becomes too wide, the Golgi cells are activated, these inhibit granular cells and input is reduced. Against this background pattern of activity, the climbing fibres exert specific influences on individual Purkinje neurons. Purkinje axons transmit a constantly changing pattern of inhibition to the central nuclei, a control system sometimes termed 'inhibitory sculpturing'.

Research: learning, memory and motor control

The cerebellum is capable of motor learning and it stores semi-permanent programmes for skilled movements: climbing fibre input from the inferior olive is essential to the development of this. To understand the learning mechanism thought to exist in the cerebellum it is necessary to consider the contrasting *spatial relationships* between the two main forms of input at cortical level. Topographically, the *cerebellar folia, and therefore the cortical parallel fibres, are orientated transverse to the brainstem axis;* the capacity of these fibres (mossy input) alone to excite Purkinje cells is low. The olivary *climbing fibre projections are in para-sagittal strips:* their activation selectively influences the synaptic effectiveness of those parallel fibres which they cut across. The inferior olive has a particular significance in the detection of movement errors: its climbing fibres 'teach' the Purkinje cells which parallel fibre inputs they 'ought' to respond to. This is the instruction-selection theory of cerebellar learning (Eccles, 1977). In addition to long-term teaching effects, the inferior olive has important short-term roles in controlling the dynamic characteristics of movement.

The location and complex nature of cerebellar memory are subjects of current research: for further information *see* Ito (1984), Bloedel et al. (1985), Thompson (1987), Strata (1989).

The parallel fibres, being slender, have a slow conduction rate: a row of regularly spaced Purkinje neurons are excited sequentially at intervals of about a tenth of a millisecond. This may provide a timing mechanism, as required in the control of rapidly alternating voluntary movements. Though this has not been proven experimentally, such skills are lost early in cerebellar disorders. The complex cortical circuitry is still under investigation (Braitenberg, 1967; Ito, 1984).

The paleocerebellum and the globose-emboliform nuclei are concerned with processing spino-cerebellar *feedback*, monitoring movement whilst it is taking place and comparing 'cortical intention' with peripheral performance. The cerebellum not only monitors movement but is also involved in its planning. It receives information from the entire cerebral cortex about the neural activity which underlies and precedes motor action. These 'intention to move' stimuli are conveyed via nuclei pontis and mossy fibres: *the neocerebellum and dentate nucleus are activated before the cerebral primary motor cortex* and are thus able to influence its executive responses. This is a *feed-forward* control mechanism comparable to that used in modern avionics and missile systems. Similar information is being processed concurrently by the corpus striatum.

Cerebellar Peduncles

Detailed components of the three peduncles are:

Superior peduncle:	Efferent	*Dentato-rubro-thalamic tract* Uncinate fasciculus (aberrant fastigiobulbar)
	Afferent	Ventral spinocerebellar tract Rostral spinocerebellar tract Tectocerebellar (from inferior colliculus) Trigeminal (mesencephalic nucleus) Noradrenergic (locus ceruleus)
Middle peduncle:	Afferent only	*Cortico-ponto-cerebellar* Tectocerebellar (from superior colliculus)
Inferior peduncle:	Afferent	*Inferior olivary nuclei* Dorsal spinocerebellar tract Accessory cuneate nucleus Arcuate nuclei Trigeminal (spinal nucleus)
	Afferent and Efferent	*Vestibular* Reticular

The *superior peduncle*, joining the cerebellum to the midbrain, consists mainly of efferent fibres from the dentate nucleus to the contralateral red nucleus and thalamus (*Fig. 7.9*). The *middle peduncle* is the lateral continuation of the transverse fibres of the ventral pons; it is the largest peduncle and contains only afferent fibres. The *inferior peduncle* contains mostly medullary and spinal afferents; connexions with the vestibular nuclei and reticular formation are reciprocal. This peduncle has two parts: a large *restiform body* ascends on the dorsolateral aspect of the medulla; a smaller *juxta-restiform body*, mostly from the vestibular nuclei, joins its medial aspect. As the inferior peduncle enters the cerebellum it turns back between the superior and middle peduncles.

In practice it is essential to recognize that **spinocerebellar connexions are ipsilateral**, and not contralateral as are cerebrospinal connexions.

The locus ceruleus projects unmyelinated noradrenergic fibres to the cortex via the superior cerebellar peduncle: its activity indirectly inhibits Purkinje cell firing. The neurotransmitter organization of the cerebellar cortex is well investigated but complex. For details *see* Nieuwenhuys (1985) or a summary in the latest edition of Gray's Anatomy (Williams et al., 1989)

Afferent Connexions (*Fig. 7.10*)

These may be grouped according to function:

1. **Equilibration.** Vestibulocerebellar fibres are largely from vestibular nuclei, but some are direct, from the eighth nerve to archecerebellum.
2. **Subconscious proprioception.** Most proprioceptive fibres end in the

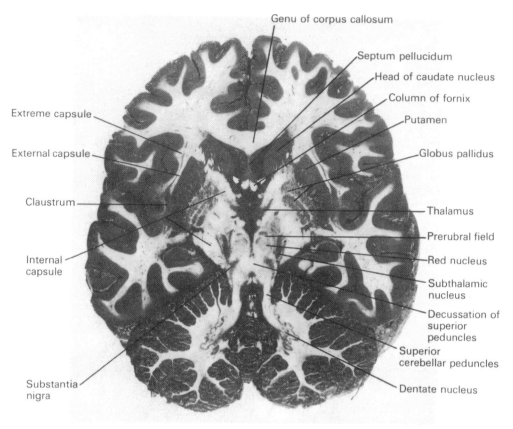

Fig. 7.9 Oblique section through the dentate nuclei and superior cerebellar peduncles. (Mulligan's stain, 0.6 natural size.)

paleocerebellum. There is a dual form of somatotopic representation. In the anterior lobe the projection is ipsilateral: feet anterior, upper limbs posterior; the head is located posteriorly in the superior vermis. There is another body representation, the head anterior and feet posterior, present bilaterally in the posterior lobe adjacent to the inferior vermis.

a. Ipsilateral projections from the spinal cord are via *spinocerebellar*, *cuneocerebellar* and *spino-olivary* paths, and from the face via the *mesencephalic trigeminal nucleus*. Dorsal spinocerebellar and cuneocerebellar tracts convey proprioceptive information from muscle spindles, Golgi tendon organs and cutaneous pressure receptors. Ventral and rostral spinocerebellar tracts convey pre-integrated information about spinal motor activity and reflexes. Ventral spinocerebellar fibres which cross in the cord re-cross at cerebellar level to become ipsilateral in the final projection.

b. *Reticulocerebellar* fibres convey impulses from muscle spindles and from non-specific reticular paths. Also included here is the specific noradrenergic input from the locus ceruleus.

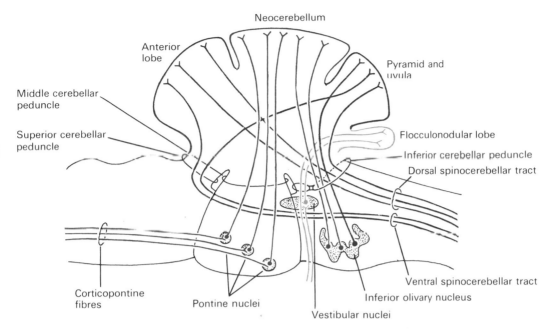

Neocerebellum

Anterior
lobe

Pyramid and
uvula

Middle cerebellar
peduncle

Superior cerebellar
peduncle

Flocculonodular lobe

Inferior cerebellar peduncle

Dorsal spinocerebellar tract

Ventral spinocerebellar tract

Corticopontine
fibres

Pontine nuclei

Inferior olivary nucleus

Vestibular nuclei

Fig. 7.10 Main afferent cerebellar connexions. Blue: neocerebellum. Red: paleo-cerebellum. Green: archecerebellum. There are additional afferents, not shown, from the trigeminal nuclei, the tectum and the reticular formation.

   c. *Tectocerebellar* connexions from the superior and inferior colliculi convey visual and auditory impulses concerned with bodily orientation. The audiovisual centre corresponds to the 'head area' in the superior vermis, immediately anterior to the pre-pyramidal fissure.

3. **Motor control circuits.** The cerebellum coordinates muscle groups, smoothes muscle action, adjusts tone and ensures that the force, direction and extent of movement are appropriate and accurate. It *plans movement* by a feed-forward mechanism in which 'intention to move' signals are relayed through the *cortico-ponto-cerebellar* pathway. Cortico-pontine fibres arise from most regions of the cerebral cortex and descend ipsilaterally to synapse with pontine nuclei; axons from these nuclei cross to form the opposite middle cerebellar peduncle, distributed mostly to the neocerebellum. Cerebellar cortical efferents project to the dentate nuclei, from which the *dentato-rubro-thalamic tract* ascends in the superior peduncle (*Fig.* 7.9) and decussates in the midbrain; some fibres end in the contralateral red nucleus, but most reach the thalamus (ventral lateral nucleus) and relay to the motor cortex, modulating activity in cortico-spinal and corticobulbar tracts. The diffuse origin of the cortico-pontine fibres reflects the fact that the whole of the cerebral cortex is involved in determining and defining motor activity via the pre-programming mechanisms of the cerebellum. *Monitoring* of movement is achieved through spinocerebellar feed-back. In brief, the neocerebellum programmes movement, the paleocerebellum corrects errors.

The inferior olivary nuclei receive descending fibres from the cerebral cortex, red nuclei and the midbrain tegmentum in the *central tegmental tract;* there is also an ascending spino-olivary input. These diverse inputs are correlated in the olive and *olivocerebellar* fibres cross to enter the contralateral inferior peduncle.

Efferent Connexions (*Fig.* 7.11)

1. **Cerebral cortex.** The dentato-rubro-thalamic route to the motor cortex has been described.
2. **Red nucleus.** Round in transverse section, the red nucleus is ovoid rostro-caudally (*Fig.* 7.9). It has a caudal part for descending efferents, relatively minor in humans (pars magnocellularis, of large and small cells); and a phylogenetically more recent rostral region for ascending projections (pars parvocellularis, of small cells). The neocerebellum and dentate nucleus project to the rostral part of the contralateral red nucleus, from thence to the thalamus. The paleocerebellum projects through the globose and emboliform nuclei to the caudal part of the red nucleus, in which descending fibres arise. Some of these enter the *central tegmental tract* and pass to the inferior olive. *Rubrospinal* and *rubrobulbar* tracts cross in the midbrain as the *ventral tegmental decussation; rubroreticular* fibres contribute to the reticulospinal tracts. The rubrospinal tract is large in quadrupeds, much smaller in humans.
3. **Reticular formation.** The main outflow from the paleocerebellum and

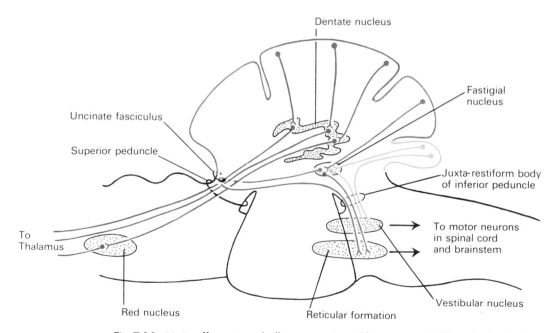

Fig. 7.11 Main efferent cerebellar connexions. Blue: neocerebellum. Red: paleocerebellum. Green: archecerebellum. Rubrospinal connexions are not shown.

fastigial nucleus to the reticular formation is via the ipsilateral inferior peduncle. Because the two fastigial nuclei are in close proximity, some cortical efferents project (incorrectly) to the opposite nucleus; resultant fibres pursue an aberrant course, re-crossing and then hooking over the superior peduncle as the *uncinate fasciculus* en route to reticular and vestibular nuclei. Reticulospinal tracts influence muscle tone via γ motor neurons. Ablation of the fastigial nuclei causes muscle flaccidity.

4. **Vestibular nuclei.** Some efferents from the archecerebellum project directly to the vestibular nuclei, others leave via a fastigial nucleus. Equilibratory control is effected via vestibulospinal tracts and the medial longitudinal fasciculus.

APPLIED ANATOMY

Cerebellar dysfunction may be due to vascular occlusion, neoplastic invasion or demyelinating disease. The clinical signs are ipsilateral if the lesion is unilateral. There are disturbances of equilibration, muscle tone and coordination. The symptoms are most severe when the onset is sudden.

Disturbed equilibrium results in *staggering gait* and a tendency to fall to the side of the lesion if this is unilateral. *Hypotonia* (reduced tone) of muscles is accompanied by weak tendon reflexes.

Ataxia, or incoordination of movement, may take several forms. Tremor, most marked in the upper limb, appears during movement and worsens as the hand reaches its intended goal; hence it is known as *intention tremor*: in contrast to Parkinson's disease it is absent at rest. Inability to gauge the range of a movement, *dysmetria*, results in 'overshoot' (past-pointing) or 'undershoot'. A complex movement is broken down by *decomposition* into a series of simple and often jerky actions, and there is an inability to make rapidly alternating movements such as pronation-supination. Ataxia of vocal muscles produces a *scanning speech* which is jerky, slow and slurred, its sounds too loud or too soft, too long or too short. Cerebellar *nystagmus* is an ataxia of ocular muscles, resulting in horizontal tremor of the eyes, worse on looking to the side of the lesion and usually indicative of involvement of the flocculonodular lobe. The differential diagnosis of nystagmus includes disorders of the vestibular nuclei, eighth nerve or semicircular canals; sometimes it is of congenital origin.

Two main sites are affected, the median vermis and the cerebellar hemispheres. A *vermal lesion* (flocculonodular syndrome) leads to disequilibrium and nystagmus. In children a rapidly growing tumour (medulloblastoma) may affect the vermis, resulting in ataxia of the trunk so severe that the child cannot sit up or hold up its head. Most disorders are neocerebellar: disease of one *cerebellar hemisphere* results in incoordination of skilled movement and hypotonia on the side of the lesion, becoming more severe, with intention tremor and a staggering gait, if either the dentate nucleus or the superior peduncle are involved.

Chapter 8

Diencephalon and internal capsule

The diencephalon is divided into two halves by the slit-like third ventricle and comprises those structures which form the ventricle's floor, walls and roof. These are the hypothalamus, thalamus, subthalamus and epithalamus. The hypothalamic sulcus, extending on each side from interventricular foramen to cerebral aqueduct, is between hypothalamus below and thalamus above (*Fig.* 8.1). The subthalamus is a transitional zone between the midbrain and thalamus-hypothalamus. The epithalamus includes the habenulae and pineal gland in the posterior part of the ventricular roof.

Thalamus

The two thalami form the largest part of the diencephalon, extending anteroposteriorly on each side from interventricular foramen to posterior commissure, and transversely from internal capsule to third ventricle. Each thalamus is an ovoid mass of grey matter; its narrow rounded anterior end is just behind the interventricular foramen, its expanded posterior region forms the *pulvinar*, which overhangs the superior colliculus. The thalami are usually attached across the midline by a narrow *interthalamic connexus* of grey matter. The superior thalamic surface is grooved by the fornix, lateral to which the thalamus forms part of the lateral ventricle's floor (*see Fig.* 8.10). The junction of the superior and medial surfaces is marked by a band of white fibres, the *stria medullaris thalami*.

Thalamic nuclei (*Figs* 8.2 and 8.3)

Thalamic grey matter is partially divided into medial and lateral regions by an oblique sheet of myelinated fibres, the *internal medullary lamina*. Anteriorly this splits to enclose an *anterior nucleus*. The medial region has a large *dorsal medial nucleus* and a small group of *midline nuclei*. The lateral part is divided into dorsal and ventral tiers of nuclei. The caudal part of the dorsal tier forms the *pulvinar*. The medial and lateral *geniculate nuclei* occupy two small swellings, geniculate bodies, on the ventroposterior surface of the pulvinar and these are sometimes collectively termed the metathalamus. The ventral tier is subdivided into *ventral anterior (VA)*, *ventral lateral (VL)* and

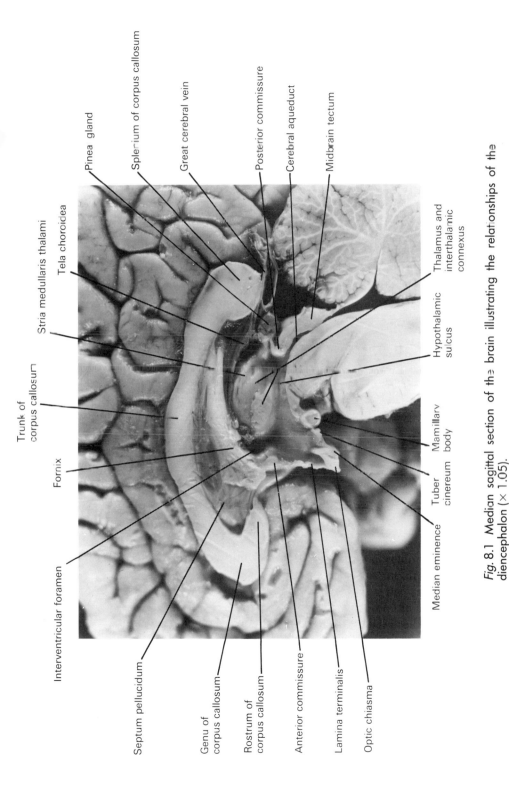

Pinea gland

Splenium of corpus callosum

Great cerebral vein

Posterior commissure

Cerebral aqueduct

Midbrain tectum

Stria medullaris thalami

Tela choroidea

Trunk of corpus callosum

Fornix

Interventricular foramen

Septum pellucidum

Genu of corpus callosum

Rostrum of corpus callosum

Anterior commissure

Lamina terminalis

Optic chiasma

Median eminence

Tuber cinereum

Mamillary body

Hypothalamic sulcus

Thalamus and interthalamic connexus

Fig. 8.1 Median sagittal section of the brain illustrating the relationships of the diencephalon (× 1.05).

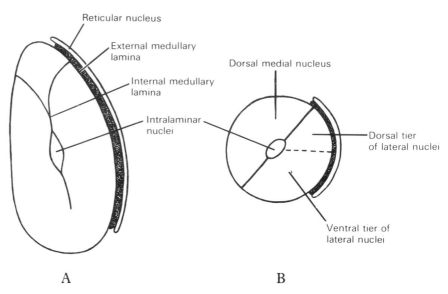

Fig. 8.2 Diagrams of the right thalamus in horizontal section (A) and in coronal section (B).

ventral posterior (VP) nuclei. There are also central *intralaminar nuclei*, the largest being the *centromedian nucleus.* The *reticular nucleus* is a thin curved sheet on the lateral aspect of the thalamus, separated from it by white fibres of the *external medullary lamina.*

Thalamo-cortical connexions are reciprocal: those nuclei which project to the cortex also receive an input from the same cortical area. Thalamic nuclei may be placed in three main functional groups: specific, non-specific and reticular.

Specific nuclei

These receive specific forms of input from certain ascending tracts and project to specific ('primary') cortical areas. They degenerate after ablation of those areas. Functionally they are either sensory (VP and geniculate) or motor (VA and VL).

1. **Ventral posterior nucleus (VP).** This receives ascending somatic sensory fibres. Its lateral division (VPL) receives the medial lemniscus and spinothalamic tracts, its medial division (VPM) receives the trigemino-thalamic input and gustatory fibres from the nucleus solitarius. Thus the head is represented medially, the feet laterally. These nuclei project to the primary sensory area in the postcentral gyrus (*see Fig.* 12.9). There are also connexions with dorsal tier nuclei (integration) and the dorsal medial nucleus (emotional response).

2. **Geniculate nuclei.** The medial geniculate nucleus receives auditory fibres from the inferior colliculus via the inferior brachium, projecting via the

auditory radiation to the primary auditory cortex in the floor of the lateral fissure, and a small amount of outer surface of superior temporal gyrus.

The lateral geniculate nucleus receives the optic tract and projects via the optic radiation to the primary visual cortex in the occipital lobe. The nucleus has a complex six-layered structure and will be considered with the visual system.

3. **Ventral lateral (VL) and ventral anterior (VA) nuclei.** The VL nucleus receives afferents from the cerebellum via the dentato-rubro-thalamic tract and the VA nucleus from the corpus striatum. Both of these nuclei project to the motor cortex (precentral gyrus and premotor area) and contribute to the initiation, organization and control of movement. Motor control mechanisms of the basal ganglia are deranged in Parkinson's

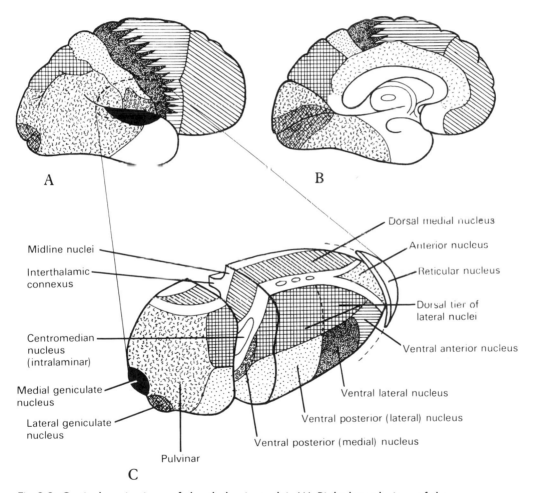

Fig. 8.3 Cortical projections of the thalamic nuclei. (A) Right lateral view of the cerebrum. (B) Median sagittal aspect of the same. (C) Dorsolateral view of the right thalamus showing the arrangement of the nuclei. Equivalent shading patterns indicate the relationships between thalamic nuclei and the cortical areas they influence. (After Williams P.L. *et al.* (1989) *Gray's Anatomy*, 37th edn. Edinburgh, Churchill Livingstone.)

disease: resultant tremor and rigidity can be reduced by surgical destruction of these nuclei.

Non-specific nuclei

These do not receive ascending tracts, but have abundant connexions with other diencephalic nuclei, projecting mostly to cortical 'association areas' in the frontal and parietal lobes and, to a lesser extent, in the occipital and temporal lobes. The cortical association areas are concerned with the correlation and interpretation of information.

1. **Dorsal medial nucleus.** This, the largest sub-nucleus in the medial thalamic region, is highly developed in primates and especially in humans. It receives afferents from other thalamic nuclei and from the hypothalamus. It integrates somatic and visceral afferents and has reciprocal connexions with the prefrontal cortex (frontal association area). It is associated with mood and emotional balance; depending on the nature of current sensory input and previous experience, feelings of euphoria or depression may result. Through its hypothalamic connexions, visceral response to emotion may occur: an unpleasant sight may cause vomiting; tension and apprehension may lead to anorexia or diarrhoea. In psychosomatic disorders, patients have apparently physical illnesses of psychogenic origin. Serious depressive illness has, in the past, been relieved by prefrontal leucotomy, by which the connexions between the dorsal medial nucleus and the prefrontal cortex are severed. The operation may have undesirable side effects such as lethargy and social incompetence; there are more selective forms of surgery but most therapy now relies on antidepressive drugs. Damage to this region of the thalamus results in personality changes which affect intellectual ability, emotional drive, memory and psychological reactions to pain. Similar changes also feature in damage to the prefrontal cortex.

2. **Anterior nucleus.** This receives hypothalamic and limbic afferents from the mamillary body via the *mamillothalamic tract*, and projects through the anterior limb of the internal capsule to the *cingulate gyrus*. It is part of the limbic system, described later, which is concerned with the emotional drives and instinctive behaviour necessary to preservation of the individual and the species. It is also essential in memorization.

3. **Dorsal tier of lateral nuclei.** These receive input from the ventral tier and have reciprocal connexions with the association areas in the parietal, occipital and temporal lobes. They are involved in the analysis and integration of sensory input. The pulvinar receives information from the lateral geniculate nucleus and superior colliculus, and its diffuse cortical projections include Wernicke's area; lesions affect complex forms of visual discrimination. Our understanding of the pulvinar is incomplete but it is of interest that in many animals, though not in humans, there are two visual pathways from retina to cortex: one via the lateral geniculate nucleus is a simple relay and the other via tectum and pulvinar processes information (Sarnat and Netsky, 1974).

Reticular nuclei

1. **The reticular thalamic nucleus.** This is a thin curved sheet of grey matter between the external medullary lamina and the internal capsule. It has diffuse reciprocal connexions with the entire cerebral cortex and all thalamic nuclei via collaterals from corticothalamic and thalamocortical fibres. It modulates thalamic output.

2. **Intralaminar nuclei.** The internal medullary lamina encloses several nuclei, the largest being the *centromedian nucleus (Fig.* 8.3 and *see Fig.* 8.9). These receive afferents from the reticular activating system and from ascending pain pathways. They project to other thalamic nuclei and to the corpus striatum. Experimental stimulation in humans is painful and evokes an 'arousal response', shown by encephalography. They are the thalamic pacemaker of electrocortical activity and profoundly affect levels of consciousness and alertness. They are also involved in awareness of pain at thalamic level: intractable pain can be relieved by their surgical destruction; this also produces somnolence.

3. **Midline nuclei.** In many animals this is an extensive group, located in the wall of the third ventricle and in the thalamic connexus, receiving visceral afferents and connected with the hypothalamus. In humans they are small.

Summary of thalamic functions

Most of the cerebral cortex is influenced by the thalamus. Thalamic nuclei which project to the cortex also receive reciprocal fibres from their cortical areas.

1. *Sensory integration and relay.* All forms of sensory input (except olfactory) converge on the thalamus, where they are correlated into an integrated pattern projected to the cortex.

2. *Motor integration and relay.* The corpus striatum, substantia nigra and cerebellum exert their influence on corticospinal and corticobulbar motor pathways via the thalamus.

3. *Awareness of nociceptive stimuli* occurs in non-discriminative form at thalamic level. In vascular lesions affecting the thalamus, ordinary stimuli may appear excessive and unpleasant; there may be prolonged spasms of spontaneous pain.

4. *Emotional and subjective responses* to sensation. Sensory input is interpreted as agreeable or disagreeable. Connexions with the prefrontal cortex influence mood and personality.

5. *Memory and instinctive behaviour.* The anterior nucleus is part of the limbic system.

6. *Activation and arousal.* The intralaminar nuclei generate much of the low voltage, rapid, desynchronized cortical activity seen in the encephalograms of alert individuals.

APPLIED ANATOMY

Functional and applied aspects of individual thalamic nuclei have already been described. Vascular occlusion may result in a *thalamic syndrome* of combined sensory and emotional symptoms, their severity depending on the extent of the lesion. Sensation from the contralateral side of the body is impaired, its threshold raised, and when perceived it is exaggerated and unpleasant. This may be accompanied by marked emotional instability. Failing blood supply may precipitate spontaneous and intractable pain in the opposite side of the body; surgical destruction of the VP nucleus relieves this but results in hemianaesthesia.

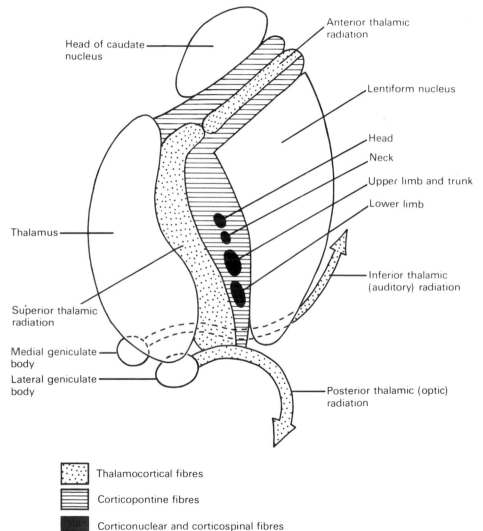

Fig. 8.4 Diagram of the components of the right internal capsule: horizontal section as in *Fig.* 8.5. (After Carpenter M.B. and Sutin J. (1983) *Human Neuroanatomy.* Baltimore, Williams and Wilkins.)

Thalamic radiations and the internal capsule (*Figs* 8.4, 8.5 and *see Fig.* 9.2)

In horizontal section, the internal capsule is a compact aggregation of fibres sited between the thalamus and caudate nucleus medially and the lentiform nucleus laterally. It has a short anterior limb, a genu and a longer posterior limb; retrolentiform and sublentiform parts are respectively behind and below the lentiform nucleus. It consists of motor and sensory cortical projection fibres: these fan out between internal capsule and cortex as the *corona radiata*.

Fibres reciprocally connecting the thalamus and cortex are termed *thalamic radiations*. The *anterior radiation*, in the anterior limb of internal capsule, principally connects the dorsal medial thalamic nucleus with ventral and lateral areas of prefrontal cortex; the anterior thalamic nucleus projects to its

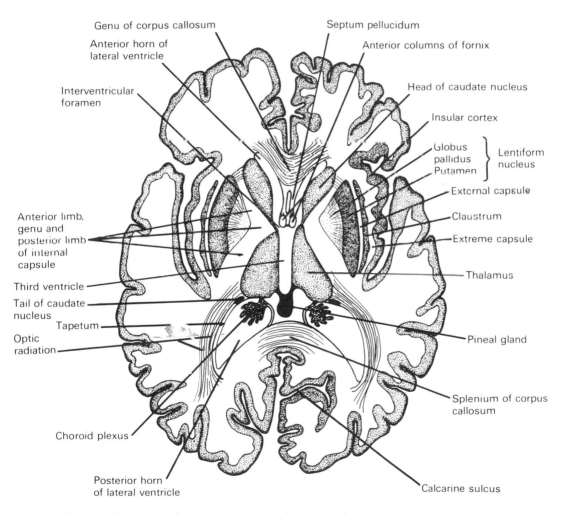

Fig. 8.5 Horizontal section of the cerebrum at the level of the interventricular foramen. (Compare with a photographed section, *Fig.* 9.2.)

medial surface and to the cingulate gyrus. The *superior radiation*, in the posterior limb, connects the VP nucleus with the primary sensory cortex, the VA and VL nuclei with the precentral gyrus and premotor cortex. The *posterior radiation* occupies the retrolentiform part of internal capsule, projecting as the optic radiation from lateral geniculate nucleus to primary visual cortex of the occipital lobe. It also includes fibres between pulvinar and visual association cortex. The *inferior radiation*, in the sublentiform part of internal capsule, is formed by the auditory radiation from medial geniculate nucleus to primary auditory cortex of the superior temporal gyrus. It also contains connexions between pulvinar and auditory association cortex.

Corticofugal fibres descending in the internal capsule are corticopontine, pyramidal (corticospinal, corticonuclear) and extrapyramidal.

Corticopontine fibres have widespread origins in the cerebral cortex. Frontopontine fibres occupy the anterior and posterior limbs of internal capsule, parietopontine and temporopontine its retrolentiform and sublentiform parts. These fibres descend through the basis pedunculi to synapse with ipsilateral pontine nuclei, whose axons aggregate into transverse pontine fibres and cross the midline to form the opposite middle cerebellar peduncle.

Corticonuclear fibres (to motor nuclei of cranial nerves) are just behind the genu of the internal capsule; *corticospinal* fibres are in the posterior half of its posterior limb (for details *see* Kretschmann, 1988).

Extrapyramidal fibres are named according to their destinations: cortico-striate, corticoreticular, corticorubral, corticotectal, cortico-olivary and corti-

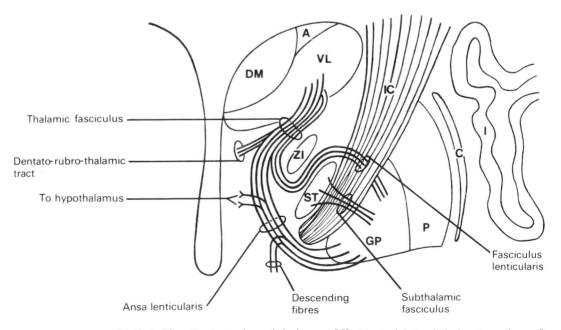

Fig. 8.6 Fibre tracts in the subthalamus. **VL**, Ventral lateral thalamic nucleus; **A**, Anterior thalamic nucleus; **DM**, Dorsal medial thalamic nucleus; **IC**, Internal capsule; **ZI**, Zona incerta, **ST**, Subthalamic nucleus; **GP**, Globus pallidus; **P**, Putamen; **C**, Claustrum; **I**, Insula.

conigral fibres. Most lie near the corticospinal tracts and are affected in lesions of the posterior limb of internal capsule. Corticotectal fibres are in the retrolentiform part. Some corticostriate and corticoreticular fibres are in the external capsule.

Passing transversely through the posterior limb of internal capsule there are fibres from globus pallidus to thalamus (fasciculus lenticularis) and between globus pallidus and subthalamic nucleus (*Fig.* 8.6). The anterior limb is crossed by strata of grey matter which interconnect the head of caudate nucleus with the putamen of lentiform nucleus; inferiorly these nuclei fuse with one another (*see Fig.* 9.3).

APPLIED ANATOMY

The internal capsule receives blood mostly from striate branches of the middle cerebral artery: one large branch prone to rupture is known as the 'artery of cerebral haemorrhage'. The retrolentiform part and ventral region of the posterior limb are supplied by the anterior choroidal artery. Thrombosis or haemorrhage of these vessels results in widespread neurological dysfunction. A lesion in the posterior limb of internal capsule produces an upper motor lesion of the opposite half of the body (hemiplegia), sometimes with partial sensory loss. A vascular lesion in the retrolentiform region causes blindness in the contralateral visual field.

Subthalamus (*Figs.* 8.6–8.9)

The subthalamic region is a transitional zone on each side between midbrain and diencephalon. It lies below and behind the thalamus; the hypothalamus is anteromedial and the internal capsule and globus pallidus ventrolateral to it (*Fig.* 8.6). Ascending tracts such as the medial lemniscus traverse it en route to the thalamus. The red nucleus extends into it: the region between this and the thalamus, the *pre-rubral field*, contains the *thalamic fasciculus* in which fasciculi from globus pallidus to thalamus are joined by the dentato-rubro-thalamic tract.

The *subthalamic nucleus*, shaped like a biconvex lens in coronal section, is adjacent to the medial aspect of the internal capsule, which separates it from the globus pallidus. The subthalamic nucleus and globus pallidus are interconnected by the *subthalamic fasciculus*, which passes transversely through the internal capsule.

The *zona incerta* is a rostral extension of the midbrain reticular formation. It is between the thalamus and the subthalamic nucleus, partly surrounded by tracts of nerve fibres (*Figs* 8.6 and 8.9).

The globus pallidus is the efferent part of the corpus striatum; fibres connecting it to the thalamus traverse this region in two fasciculi. The *fasciculus lenticularis* pierces the internal capsule and arches round the zona incerta, the *ansa lenticularis* curves medially round the ventral border of the internal capsule; these unite as the thalamic fasciculus in the prerubral field

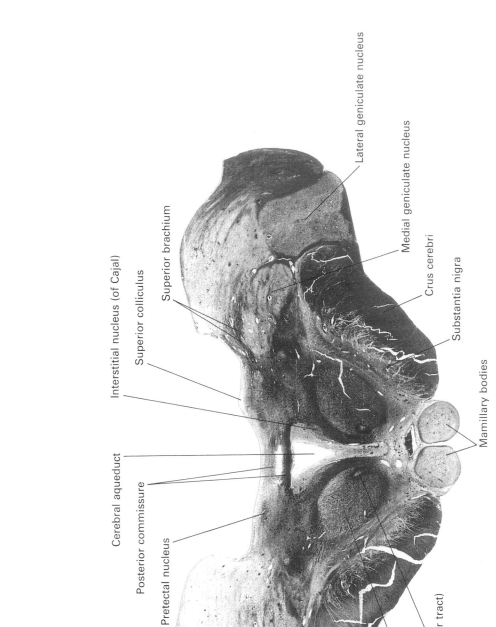

Fig. 8.7 Transverse section at the junction of mesencephalon and diencephalon. (Weigert stain, × 3.)

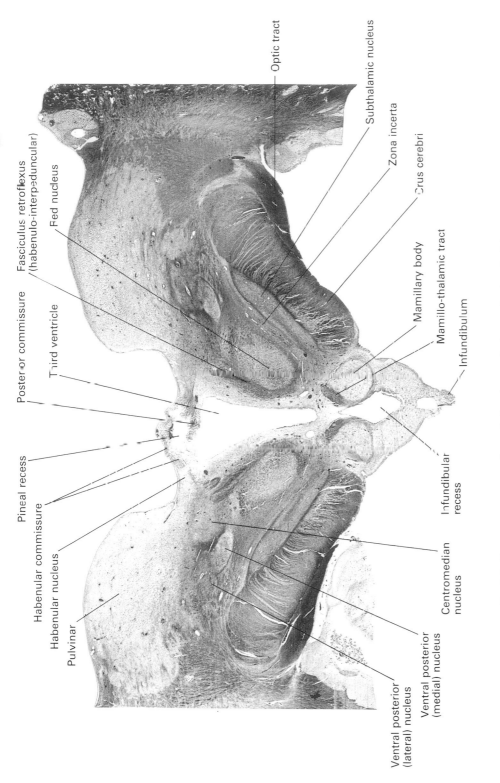

Optic tract

Subthalamic nucleus

Zona incerta

Crus cerebri

Fasciculus retroflexus
(habenulo-interpeduncular)

Red nucleus

Mamillary body

Mamillo-thalamic tract

Posterior commissure

Third ventricle

Infundibulum

Pineal recess

Infundibular recess

Habenular commissure

Habenular nucleus

Pulvinar

Centromedian nucleus

Ventral posterior (medial) nucleus

Ventral posterior (lateral) nucleus

Fig. 8.8 Transverse section through the diencephalon at the level of the infundibulum. (Weigert stain, × 3.)

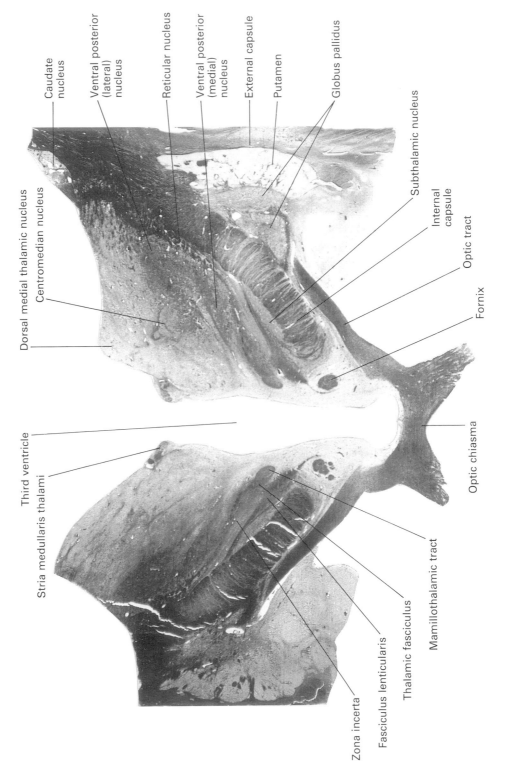

Fig. 8.9 Transverse section through the diencephalon and corpus striatum at the level of the optic chiasma. (Weigert stain, × 2.7.) Compare with Fig. 8.6.

and reach the thalamus. A few fibres descend to the substantia nigra and the midbrain reticular formation.

APPLIED ANATOMY

The subthalamic nucleus is an important extrapyramidal component; it exerts an inhibitory effect on the globus pallidus. Damage to this nucleus, although rare, has dramatic effects. A unilateral lesion induces wild flinging movements (*hemiballismus*) in the contralateral limbs, particularly affecting the shoulder joint, so violent that one patient broke her arm against the side of the cot (Patten, 1977). It may be relieved either medically (chlorpromazine injection) or by stereotactic surgery to the fasciculus lenticularis or globus pallidus.

Epithalamus

The epithalamus includes structures lying posteriorly in the diencephalic roof: the *habenular nuclei, posterior commissure* and *pineal gland (Fig. 8.10).*

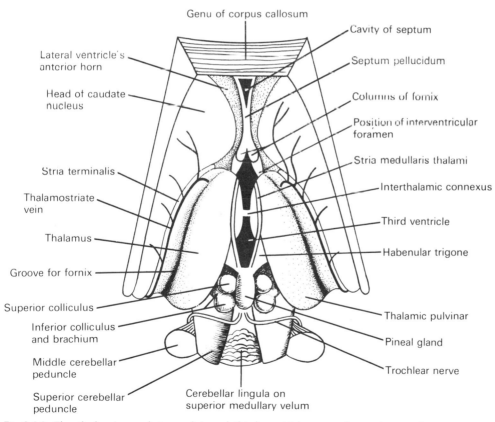

Fig. 8.10 The thalami, caudate nuclei and third ventricle, seen from above after removal of most of the corpus callosum, the body of the fornix and the tela choroidea.

Each *habenular nucleus* lies deep to a *habenular trigone*. Afferents reach it in the *stria medullaris thalami*, whose fibres are applied to the dorsomedial surface of the thalamus (*Fig.* 8.1). These afferents, of diverse origin, are associated with the olfactory or limbic systems, including connexions with the septal area and amygdaloid nucleus (via the stria terminalis) and from the hippocampal formation (via the fornix). These structures are described in Chapter 10. There is also an input from the hypothalamus. Some fibres of the stria medullaris cross the midline as the *habenular commissure* in the upper leaf of the pineal stalk, linking the habenulae. Habenular efferents mostly enter the *fasciculus retroflexus*, which passes to the interpeduncular nucleus. This relays to the midbrain reticular formation and via the *dorsal longitudinal fasciculus* to the autonomic centres of the brainstem controlling salivation, gastrointestinal motility and secretion, a pathway by which olfaction and emotion effect visceral responses. There are habenular efferents to the pineal gland which influence its secretion. Experimental ablation of the habenulae affects metabolism, endocrine and thermal regulation.

The *posterior commissure* (*Figs* 8.1, 8.7, 8.11), in the lower leaf of the pineal stalk, is a composite connexion between the medial longitudinal fasciculi, interstitial nuclei, superior colliculi, pretectal nuclei and posterior thalamic nuclei.

The *pineal gland* is a midline structure overhanging the superior colliculi and below the splenium of the corpus callosum, from which it is separated by the great cerebral vein (*Fig.* 8.1). It is attached to the diencephalon by a *stalk*, which is invaded by the *pineal recess* of the third ventricle; the lower leaf of the stalk is attached to the posterior commissure, the upper leaf contains the habenular commissure. Pinealocytes and neuroglial cells form the gland; pineal secretion passes into the blood and cerebrospinal fluid. For many years the pineal gland attracted little research interest, but this rapidly changed about 25 years ago due to two significant discoveries. Firstly the

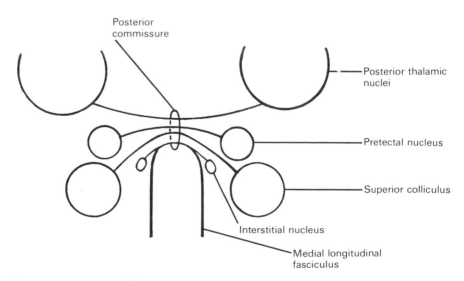

Fig. 8.11 Diagram of the composition of the posterior commissure.

pineal was found to produce a number of metabolically active substances, such as *melatonin* and *serotonin*. Secondly, when the pineal was removed, animals could not detect seasonal changes in day-length and consequently failed to breed at the correct time of year. The level of pineal secretion fluctuates daily and is maximal during darkness. In fish and amphibia the pineal gland is subcutaneous and contains photoreceptors. Mammalian pinealocytes, derived phylogenetically from these receptors, have become secretory cells but remain indirectly photo-responsive. The effect of light in mammals is via the hypothalamus, which receives an input from the retina and influences the pineal through the superior cervical ganglion. Other afferents reach the gland from the habenulae. The pineal is involved, together with the hypothalamus, in the synchronization of circadian rhythms. It has recently been shown that melatonin injections can alleviate jet lag and tiredness after long haul air travel (Petrie et al., 1989).

The pineal exerts a modulating effect, mostly inhibitory, on the hypothalamus and adenohypophysis. There is thus a dual functional relationship between pineal and hypothalamus, each having an effect on the other.

APPLIED ANATOMY

Research has shown that the pineal is an endocrine gland with important regulatory effects on hypothalamus, adenohypophysis and neurohypophysis; through these also on the thyroid, parathyroids, endocrine pancreas, adrenals and gonads. Its secretion is *anti-gonadotrophic:* thus pineal destruction in immature individuals leads to precocious puberty; conversely, a secreting pineal tumour delays its onset. This effect is via the hypothalamus and adenohypophysis. An expanding pineal tumour may compress the pretectal region and superior colliculi, producing fixed, dilated pupils and paralysis of upward gaze. After puberty, calcareous aggregations known as 'brain sand', formerly thought to indicate degeneration but now known to be a by-product of secretory activity, accumulate in the gland and provide a useful midline marker in radiograms.

Hypothalamus

Topography and structure

The hypothalamus forms the lower part of the lateral wall and floor of the third ventricle (*Fig.* 8.1). The hypothalamic sulcus, between the interventricular foramen and the aqueduct, marks its dorsal boundary. It extends posteriorly from the lamina terminalis to the caudal border of the mamillary bodies, blending there into the midbrain tegmentum; the subthalamus lies posterolaterally. Between the optic chiasma and mamillary bodies there is a convex area of grey matter on the ventral surface, the *tuber cinereum*. The pituitary gland is attached by a stalk (infundibulum) to a *median eminence* immediately behind the optic chiasma. Each half of the hypothalamus is described as consisting of medial and lateral zones; a column of the fornix passes between these to reach a mamillary body.

Medial zone (Fig. 8.12A)

This contains many neurons, arranged in anterior, tuberal and posterior nuclear groups. The anterior region includes the *suprachiasmatic, pre-optic, anterior*, and *paraventricular* nuclei, and part of the *supra-optic* nucleus. Axons from the supra-optic and paraventricular nuclei extend to the neurohypophysis as a *supraoptico-hypophyseal tract:* hormone precursors, formed within

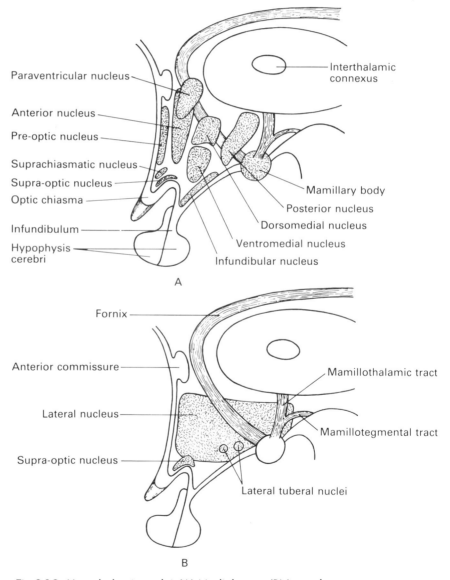

Fig. 8.12 Hypothalamic nuclei. (A) Medial zone. (B) Lateral zone.

the nuclei, are transported along this tract to the neurohypophysis. This anterior region also exerts control over the parasympathetic system (pre-optic and anterior nuclei). The tuberal region comprises *dorsomedial*, *ventromedial* and *infundibular* nuclei. It has metabolic functions and includes a 'satiety centre'. The *tubero-hypophyseal tract* carries 'releasing factors' to the median eminence, transported thence to the adenohypophysis in a *portal system;* each factor effects release (or inhibition) of a particular hormone. The posterior group includes the *mamillary nuclei* and a *posterior* nucleus; a sympathetic control 'centre' is located posteriorly in the hypothalamus (posterior and lateral nuclei).

Lateral zone (Fig. 8.12B)

This has more fibres and fewer neurons than the medial zone. It is traversed by the *medial forebrain bundle* which interconnects the septal area, hypothal-amus and midbrain tegmentum. The *lateral nucleus* consists of diffuse, sparsely arranged neurons, and includes hunger and thirst 'centres'. The *lateral tuberal* nuclei are groups of cells deep to the tuber cinereum. The *supra-optic nucleus* overlies the beginning of the optic tract and the lateral part of the optic chiasma.

Afferent connexions

1. **Visceral and somatic afferents.** General visceral afferents arrive from the vagal sensory nucleus, gustatory afferents from the nucleus solitarius, and somatic afferents from the nipples and genitalia. Retinal afferents, concerned with light intensity, programme a 'biological clock'. There is an input from the olfactory cortex to the medial forebrain bundle.
2. **Limbic system, thalamus and cortex.** The hippocampus, in the floor of the inferior horn of the lateral ventricle is connected by the *fornix* to the mamillary body, with collaterals to other hypothalamic nuclei. The amygdaloid nucleus, in the roof of the inferior horn, has efferents forming the *stria terminalis* which reach the anterior hypothalamic and septal regions. Both these tracts, the fornix and the stria curve round the thalamus (*Figs* 8.1, 8.10, *see Fig*. 10.2). The *medial forebrain bundle* brings afferents from the septal region. The *mamillothalamic tract* connects the hypothalamus to the anterior thalamic nucleus, which has reciprocal links with the cingulate gyrus. These are all part of the limbic system, forming a bording zone (limbus) between the diencephalon and telencephalon.

    The prefrontal cortex transmits emotional, affective information through the dorsal medial thalamic nucleus to the hypothalamus via a periventricular system of fibres on the medial surface of the thalamus.
3. **Pineal gland:** a reciprocal relationship (*see* p.178).
4. **Direct physical and chemical receptors.** Circulating blood is constantly monitored by hypothalamic cells that function as thermoreceptors, osmo-receptors or chemoreceptors.

Efferent connexions

The hypothalamus influences three main regions: autonomic, thalamic-limbic and hypophyseal (pituitary).

1. **Autonomic control.** From the nuclei in the medial zone, periventricular fibres join the *dorsal longitudinal fasciculus* in the periaqueductal grey matter (*see Figs* 5.11–5.16) which passes to autonomic nuclei in the brainstem (salivatory, lacrimal and dorsal vagal motor nuclei) and to spinal autonomic nuclei (vasomotor, sudomotor). From the mamillary body the *mamillotegmental tract* (*Fig.* 8.12) arches caudally to the midbrain tegmentum, projecting to autonomic centres via the reticular formation. Some laterally placed efferents reach the midbrain tegmentum via the *medial forebrain bundle*. Hypothalamic visceral efferents were once considered to be entirely polysynaptic, but some axons have now been traced through from the hypothalamus to the medulla and spinal cord.

2. **Thalamus and limbic system.** The mamillothalamic tract projects to the anterior thalamic nucleus and is connected through this to the cingulate gyrus, as part of the limbic system, whose function may be summarized as the preservation of the individual and the species. Other connexions between hypothalamus and limbic system, already described, contain both afferent and efferent fibres. Connexions between the hypothalamus, dorsal medial thalamic nucleus and prefrontal cortex are also reciprocal.

3. **Hypophysis cerebri**

   a. *Neurohypophysis.* The supra-optic and paraventricular nuclei project to the posterior lobe of the hypophysis as the *supraoptico-hypophyseal tract* (*Fig.* 8.13A); their cells secrete precursors of oxytocin and vasopressin, transported as granules (Herring bodies) by axoplasmic flow along the tract for release into the capillaries of the neurohypophysis. *Oxytocin* causes contraction of uterine muscle and mammary myo-epithelial cells, effects demonstrable after parturition when a baby is put to the breast. *Vasopressin (antidiuretic hormone)*, a vasoconstrictor, has an important antidiuretic effect on the renal collecting ducts. Osmoreceptors and a 'thirst centre' are near the supra-optic nucleus; destruction here results in diabetes insipidus, in which the volume of urine is excessive. Individual nuclei were considered specialized for the production of a single hormone, but it is now known that both hormones are produced in each nucleus. The neurohypophysis has a rich arterial supply from several superior hypophyseal branches and a single inferior hypophyseal branch of the internal carotid artery as the latter traverses the cavernous sinus.

   b. *Adenohypophysis.* The *tubero-infundibular tract* (*Fig.* 8.13B) ends in the median eminence and infundibulum. 'Releasing factors', formed in the tuberal and infundibular nuclei, are carried to the adenohypophysis in a *hypophyseal portal system*. Superior hypophyseal branches of the internal carotid artery form a complex capillary plexus in the median eminence; from this plexus portal veins descend to the adenohypophysis where they open into sinusoids between secretory cells. The adenohypophysis receives its blood supply mostly from

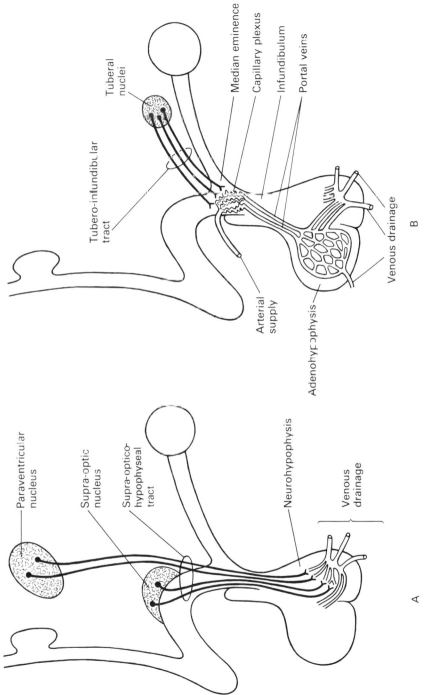

Paraventricular nucleus

Supra-optic nucleus

Supra-optico-hypophyseal tract

Neurohypophysis

Venous drainage

A

Tuberal nuclei

Median eminence

Capillary plexus

Infundibulum

Portal veins

Tubero-infundibular tract

Arterial supply

Adenohypophysis

Venous drainage

B

Fig. 8.13 Hypothalamo-hypophyseal control mechanisms. (A) Supraoptico-hypophyseal tract to neurohypophysis. (B) Hypophyseal portal system to adenohypophysis.

these portal vessels, not from arteries. Venous drainage of the adeno-hypophysis into local venous sinuses is limited, much of it leaves via neurohypophyseal veins. Releasing factors are each specific to cortico-trophin, luteinizing hormone, follicular stimulating hormone, thyro-trophin or somatotrophin. They may promote synthesis as well as release; they **inhibit** the release of prolactin and melanocyte stimulating hormone.

Tanycytes, a variety of astrocyte, interposed between ependymal cells in the floor of the third ventricle, are able to transfer hormones between the cerebrospinal fluid and portal system. The direction of flow in the cells is probably determined by their neural control which is, at present, imperfectly understood. Some neurohypophyseal hormones may pass to the median eminence via reversed flow in communicating capillaries and be secreted by tanycytes into the third ventricle.

Summary of hypothalamic functions

1. *Autonomic control*. Stimulation of the sympathetic or parasympathetic hypothalamic 'centres' affects the cardiovascular, respiratory and alimentary systems. The anterior hypothalamus responds to hyperthermia by causing vasodilatation, sweating and lowered metabolism, while its posterior region responds to hypothermia by causing vasoconstriction, shivering and increased thyroid activity. This thermostatic control is less efficient in the very young and the very old. Circulating bacterial pyrogens stimulate hypothalamic chemoreceptors to produce a febrile response.
2. *Endocrine control*. Hypothalamic centres are sensitive to the feedback effect of circulatory hormonal levels. A castrated animal commonly becomes obese and lazy. Hormone replacement therapy (HRT) is said to minimize autonomic, psychological and physical side effects of the female menopause, which may include flushes, depression and osteoporosis. Neural paths converging on the hypothalamus also influence hormonal release. Some hypophyseal hormones directly affect their target tissues, others, such as adrenocorticotrophic hormone, act through an endocrine intermediary (*Fig.* 8.14).
3. *Food and water intake*. Stimulation of the lateral hypothalamus promotes eating; ablation may lead to death from starvation. Conversely, stimulation of the medial tuberal region causes anorexia. Thus a lateral *'hunger centre'* is functionally balanced against a medial *'satiety centre'*. A *'thirst centre'* in the lateral region regulates fluid intake, influencing renal secretion by regulating the production of antidiuretic hormone.
4. *Emotional expression*. The hypothalamus, informed by the limbic system, prefrontal cortex and other central nervous regions, mediates autonomic emotional responses such as blushing, pallor, sweating, dryness of the mouth, increased gastrointestinal motility, raised blood pressure and raised pulse rate.
5. *Sexual behaviour and reproduction*. Adenohypophyseal gonadotrophin governs aspects of reproductive physiology. The limbic system mediates

complex patterns of associated sexual behaviour such as identification of mate, home-building and care of offspring.

6. *Biological clocks.* There is a cyclical pattern, or *circadian rhythm*, in many tissues and functions. These are influenced by the hypothalamus, itself affected by diurnal rhythms. Based on 24 hours of light and darkness are cyclical patterns in body temperature, waking and sleeping, adrenocortical activity, renal secretion, plasma constituents, and eosinophil count. The most obvious example, the sleeping pattern, may be much disturbed by hypothalamic lesions. The pacemaker, activated by visual input, appears to be in the suprachiasmatic nucleus of the hypothalamus, which in turn affects pineal secretion. As already noted, melatonin influences this phenomenon of diurnal body rhythms.

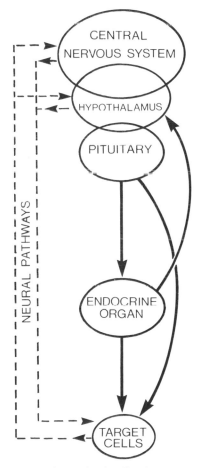

Fig. 8.14 Endocrine control and feedback; neuro-endocrine relationships. Examples of influences on target cells: autonomic and endocrine (e.g. thyroid) effects on the cardiovascular system; blood volume sensors (visceral afferent) and osmoreceptors — anti diuretic hormone release increases renal resorption; nipple stimulation (somatic afferent) in suckling — oxytocin release causes uterine and mammary muscle contraction post partum; lowered body temperature precipitates shivering (somatic efferent). Circulating hormone levels have feedback effects on the hypothalamus, inhibiting or increasing further production and release.

APPLIED ANATOMY

The functional importance of the hypothalamus is disproportionate to its small size. Clinical features of its dysfunction may follow trauma, inflammation, neoplastic compression or ischaemia. *Diabetes insipidus*, developing spontaneously or after head injury, involves impaired secretion of antidiuretic hormone; the urine volume is very large, its specific gravity low; absence of glycosuria differentiates it from diabetes mellitus. Defective temperature regulation, resulting in *hyperthermia* or *hypothermia*, may follow head injury or local surgery. Traumatic anteroposterior displacement of the cerebral hemispheres distorts this region; following severe concussion there may be *somnolence* and '*cerebral irritation*' in which the patient curls up in bed, knees and arms flexed, verbally and physically resenting any interference. Similar '*sham rage*' can be evoked by experimental hypothalamic stimulation. *Fröhlich's syndrome* (dystrophia-adiposo-genitalis), which includes stunted growth, obesity and genital hypoplasia, may occur in children as a result of either a pituitary tumour or hypothalamic dysfunction. *Psychological response to altered endocrine balance* includes premenstrual tension, postpuerperal psychosis and menopausal emotional lability.

Pituitary tumours

Benign tumours (adenomas) arise from specific cell types. Symptoms reflect increased hormone secretion from tumour cells and reduced secretion from other hypophyseal cells which are being compressed; there may also be pressure on adjacent structures, particularly the optic chiasma. Initially fibres from the lower nasal quadrants of the retina are affected and this produces bilateral upper quadrantic visual field defects; untreated it progresses to bitemporal hemianopia (*see Fig.* 11.6). A large tumour may compress the third, fourth and fifth cranial nerves and even the hypothalamus itself.

Tumours of chromophobe cells are non-secretory and produce hypopituitarism by local compression. An adenoma of somatotroph cells secretes excess growth hormone, resulting in *gigantism* in a juvenile and *acromegaly* (enlarged hands, feet and head) in an adult. The discovery of prolactin in 1970 greatly increased our understanding of pituitary tumours (Grossman and Besser, 1985). A *prolactinoma* is often small but even a 2 mm tumour can secrete enough prolactin to cause amenorrhoea in women, impotence and loss of libido in men (inhibition of gonadotrophin) and may provoke lactation in either sex (normally hypothalamic dopamine inhibits prolactin release). Prolactinoma symptoms can be controlled by a synthetic dopamine receptor agonist named bromocriptine. In *Cushing's disease* a relatively uncommon adrenocorticotrophic hormone-producing adenoma causes overactivity of the adrenal cortex.

Pituitary adenomas can be removed by microsurgery through the sphenoidal air sinus. They may also be treated by expertly directed radiotherapy. If adrenocorticotrophic or thyrotrophic cells have been damaged, appropriate hormone replacement therapy is required.

Chapter 9

Corpus striatum

Deep to the cortex in each cerebral hemisphere are masses of grey matter, collectively termed *basal ganglia*. The largest is the *corpus striatum*, topographically divided into a *caudate nucleus* and a *lentiform nucleus*, the lentiform nucleus consisting of an outer *putamen* and inner *globus pallidus* (*Figs* 9.1 and 9.2). Between putamen and the insular cortex is a thin grey sheet, the *claustrum*, of uncertain significance in humans. These masses form a motor complex which functionally includes the *substantia nigra* and the *subthalamic nucleus*. The amygdaloid nucleus has similar developmental origins but is functionally separate, associated with the olfactory and limbic systems.

The major functional division of the corpus striatum is phylogenetic. The globus pallidus is relatively ancient and is termed the *paleostriatum*, or *pallidum*. The *neostriatum*, or *striatum* emerged in reptiles and comprises the caudate nucleus and putamen: originally these were one structure which became partially split by the development of internal capsule fibres (*see Fig.* 1.6). The striatum is largely afferent, the pallidum efferent. These features may be summarized as follows:

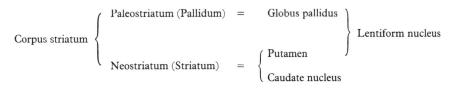

Topography

The *caudate nucleus* has an elongated curved tail (cauda) and is related throughout to the lateral ventricle. It has a large *head* bulging into the lateral wall of the anterior horn of the ventricle (*Fig.* 9.2). The anterior limb of the internal capsule partially separates the caudate head from the putamen of the lentiform nucleus, but numerous strands of grey matter connect them across the internal capsule; inferiorly the two structures are fused (*Fig.* 9.3). This fusion lies immediately above the anterior perforated substance through which the striate branches of the middle and anterior cerebral arteries penetrate to supply the corpus striatum and internal capsule. Near the interventricular foramen the head tapers rapidly into a narrow *body* in the lateral part of the ventricular floor, and a relatively slender *tail* curves down and then forwards in the roof of the inferior horn, with the amygdaloid nucleus located near its tip. A bundle of fibres, the *stria terminalis*, leaves the amygdaloid nucleus and runs along the medial edge of the caudate tail and body. In the floor of the central part of the ventricle, the stria terminalis and a *thalamostriate vein* lie between the caudate nucleus and the thalamus (*see* Figs 8.10, 9.5). The vein receives blood from the thalamus, corpus striatum and internal capsule.

The *lentiform nucleus* appears biconvex in some sections, cuneiform in others. Its lateral surface is gently convex and separated from the claustrum by the *external capsule*. Between the claustrum and insula is the *extreme*

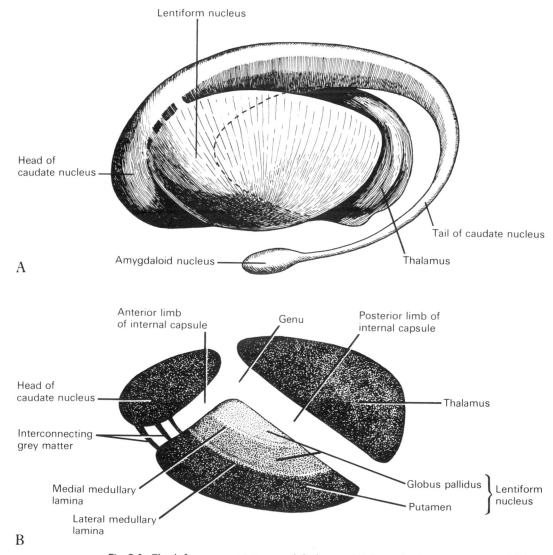

Fig. 9.1 The left corpus striatum and thalamus, (A) from the lateral aspect and (B) in horizontal section.

capsule (*see Figs* 9.2 and 9.4). In transverse sections, the medial surface of the lentiform nucleus is angulated at the genu of the internal capsule, partly separated by the capsule's anterior limb from the caudate head and from the thalamus by its posterior limb. The inferior surface of the lentiform nucleus is deeply grooved by the anterior commissure (interconnecting the temporal lobes) and lies close to the anterior perforated substance. Anteriorly the nucleus is above structures in the roof of the inferior horn of the lateral ventricle; posteriorly it is above the sublentiform part of the internal capsule (auditory radiation).

The amygdaloid nucleus is situated above and in front of the tip of the inferior horn, below the lentiform nucleus.

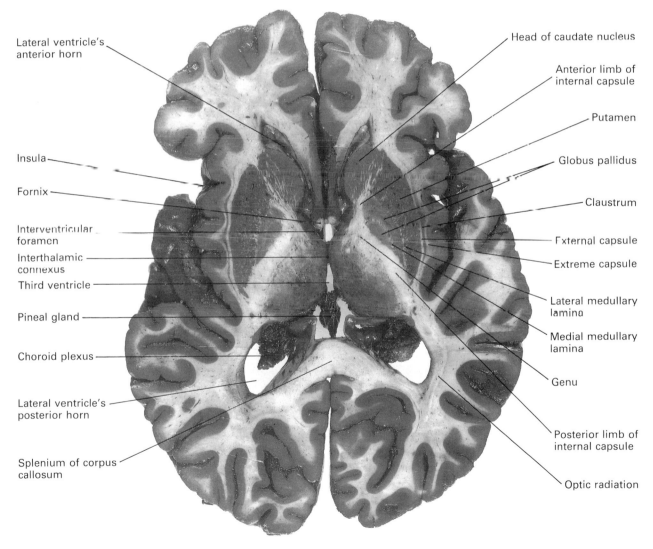

Fig. 9.2 Horizontal section of the cerebrum at the level of the interventricular foramina. (Mulligan's stain, 0.8 natural size.)

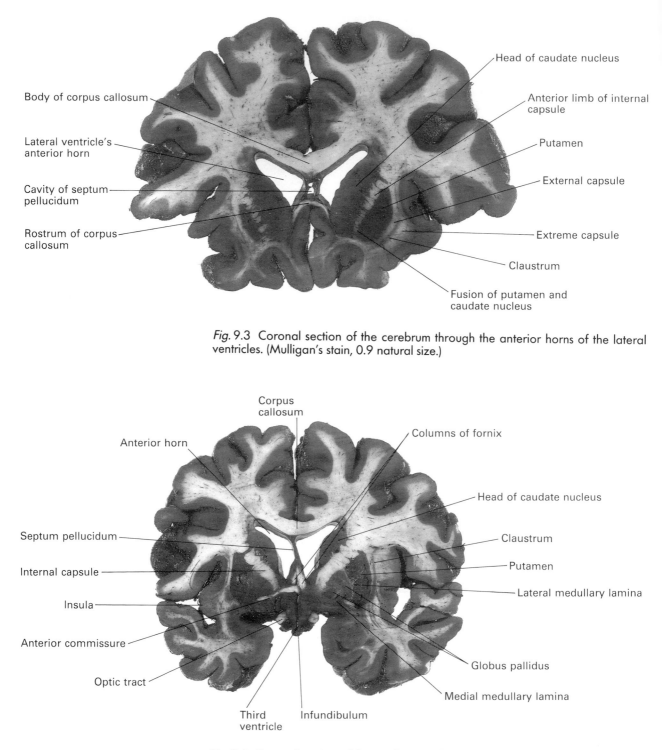

Body of corpus callosum

Lateral ventricle's anterior horn

Cavity of septum pellucidum

Rostrum of corpus callosum

Head of caudate nucleus

Anterior limb of internal capsule

Putamen

External capsule

Extreme capsule

Claustrum

Fusion of putamen and caudate nucleus

Fig. 9.3 Coronal section of the cerebrum through the anterior horns of the lateral ventricles. (Mulligan's stain, 0.9 natural size.)

Corpus callosum

Anterior horn

Columns of fornix

Septum pellucidum

Internal capsule

Insula

Anterior commissure

Optic tract

Head of caudate nucleus

Claustrum

Putamen

Lateral medullary lamina

Globus pallidus

Medial medullary lamina

Third ventricle

Infundibulum

Fig. 9.4 Coronal section of the cerebrum at the level of the infundibulum. (Mulligan's stain, 0.7 natural size.)

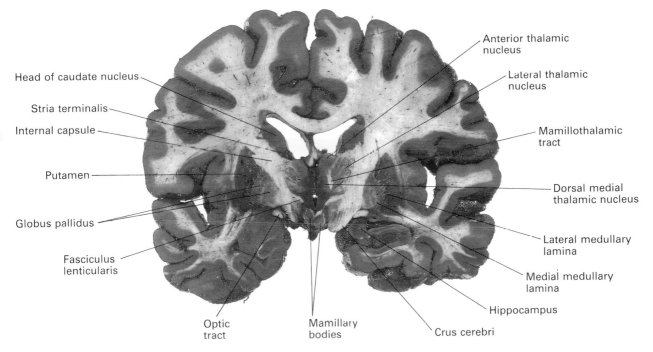

Head of caudate nucleus

Stria terminalis

Internal capsule

Putamen

Globus pallidus

Fasciculus
lenticularis

Optic
tract

Mamillary
bodies

Crus cerebri

Anterior thalamic
nucleus

Lateral thalamic
nucleus

Mamillothalamic
tract

Dorsal medial
thalamic nucleus

Lateral medullary
lamina

Medial medullary
lamina

Hippocampus

Fig. 9.5 Coronal section of the cerebrum at the level of the mamillary bodies.
(Mulligan's stain, 0.8 natural size.)

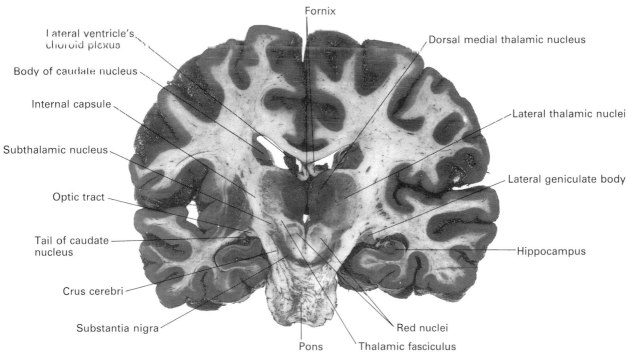

Lateral ventricle's
choroid plexus

Body of caudate nucleus

Internal capsule

Subthalamic nucleus

Optic tract

Tail of caudate
nucleus

Crus cerebri

Substantia nigra

Pons

Fornix

Dorsal medial thalamic nucleus

Lateral thalamic nuclei

Lateral geniculate body

Hippocampus

Red nuclei

Thalamic fasciculus

Fig. 9.6 Coronal section of the cerebrum through the thalami, crura cerebri and
pons. (Mulligan's stain, 0.8 natural size.)

In section the lentiform nucleus displays a dark external zone, the putamen, and a lighter internal part, the globus pallidus. The putamen is densely cellular and identical in structure to the caudate nucleus. The globus pallidus is traversed by many myelinated fasciculi, giving it a pale colour. There is a thin lateral medullary lamina of white fibres between the putamen and globus pallidus; a medial medullary lamina divides the globus pallidus into medial and lateral segments (*Figs* 9.2 and 9.5).

Striatal Connexions

The *striatum* (caudate nucleus and putamen) is the receptive region of the corpus striatum; most of its output is to the globus pallidus (the pallidum). Some efferents also reach the substantia nigra. A knowledge of the relevant neurotransmitters is vital to an understanding of basal ganglia disease; their pathways are illustrated in *Fig.* 9.7 and described in Chapter 15. (*See* also Marsden, 1982; Nieuwenhuys, 1985.)

Striatal afferent fibres

Afferents are received from the *cerebral cortex, substantia nigra* and *thalamus*. *Corticostriate* fibres are profuse and arise from most parts of the cerebral cortex, particularly the somatomotor region, and have a topographical arrangement. Thus the 'facial region' of the primary motor cortex projects to the ventral putamen, and the 'leg area' to its dorsal part. These fibres enter the striatum via the internal and external capsules; they are not collaterals of the corticospinal and corticobulbar fibres but arise from a layer of small pyramidal cells in the external half of cortical lamina V. *Nigrostriate* fibres utilize dopamine as a neurotransmitter and exert a constant tonic inhibition: in Parkinson's disease, characterized by tremor and muscular rigidity, this influence is lacking and the striatum is overactive. *Thalamo-striate* fibres mostly start in the centromedian nucleus, and also in smaller intralaminar nuclei and the dorsal medial nucleus. *Brainstem afferents* from the raphe nuclei of the midbrain transport serotonin (5–HT) to the striatum and exert an inhibitory modulation here. (Nuclei of the raphe have been mentioned in relation to a descending pain control pathway.)

Striatal efferent fibres

Most striatal efferents are *striatopallidal*, myelinated fibres passing to the globus pallidus. *Striatonigral* fibres mostly carry inhibitory γ-aminobutyric acid (GABA) neurotransmitter to the substantia nigra, but a few are excitatory and use substance P. It is clinically significant that, although there are reciprocal connexions between striatum and substantia nigra, their main neurotransmitters are different.

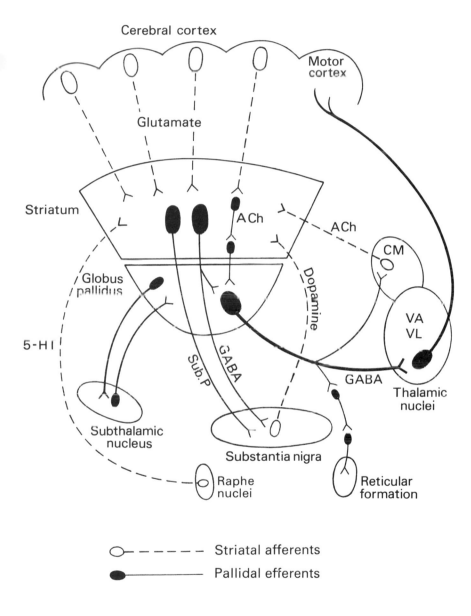

Fig. 9.7 Neurotransmitter anatomy of basal ganglia. ACh = acetylcholine; GABA = γ-aminobutyric acid; Sub.P = substance P; 5-HT = 5-hydroxytryptamine (serotonin); CM = centromedian thalamic nucleus; VA = ventral anterior thalamic nucleus; VL = ventral lateral thalamic nucleus. (Adapted from Marsden C.D. (1982) Lancet **ii**, 1141–1147.)

Pallidal Connexions

As the main efferent component of the corpus striatum, the globus pallidus receives most of the striatal output; it also has reciprocal connexions with the subthalamic nucleus.

Pallidal efferents

Outflow from the globus pallidus is mainly to the thalamus. As previously noted, this is via two fasciculi; the *ansa lenticularis* looping round the posterior limb of the internal capsule and the *fasciculus lenticularis* traversing the internal capsule (*see Figs* 8.6 and 9.5). These fasciculi enter the region between the red nucleus and the thalamus (prerubral field) to meet the dentato-rubro-thalamic tract and unite as the *thalamic fasciculus* (*see Figs* 7.9 and 9.6). This leads to thalamic ventral anterior (VA) and ventral lateral (VL) nuclei, which project to the motor and premotor cortex. The corpus striatum and cerebellum influence descending pathways via this thalamocortical projection.

In the absence of movement the corpus striatum exerts an inhibitory influence on the thalamus. Before a motor command signal is issued by the motor cortex, there is widespread activity in the cerebral cortex and this is projected to the corpus striatum and cerebellum for processing. Such corticostriate input preceding movement reduces existing pallido-thalamic inhibition: thalamic activation of the motor cortex results. Synchronously, as a result of input from cerebral cortex to cerebellum, there is dentato-thalamic excitation. Thus the VA and VL thalamic nuclei assist in regulating the commands of the motor cortex. A decision to undertake a voluntary movement is cortically mediated; the means whereby it is organized is largely subcortical. In summary, there is a neurological distinction between *what* is to be done (cortical) and *how* it is to be done (basal ganglia and cerebellum).

The *subthalamic fasciculus* passes through the internal capsule from globus pallidus to subthalamic nucleus (*Figs* 8.6 and 8.9) and also conveys fibres from the subthalamic nucleus to the globus pallidus. *Pallidonigral* efferents pass to the substantia nigra. A small group of *pallidotegmental* fibres reaches the reticular formation of the lower midbrain and contribute to the central tegmental tract, but there is no direct projection beyond this to the brainstem or the spinal cord as is seen in lower vertebrates.

Functions of the Basal Ganglia

In sub-mammalian vertebrates, the thalamus and corpus striatum are sensory and motor integrating and control centres, combined in the performance of stereotyped activity. In later evolution, the activities of the corpus striatum become subordinate to and coordinated with, those of the cerebral cortex. It remains essential to the control of muscle tone and the qualitative organization of movement. The executive functions of the motor cortex require a substratum of available motor programmes, which are mostly developed in childhood. The basal ganglia have a major role in this organization: thus a disorder such as Parkinsonism commonly features poverty of movement, difficulty in initiating, controlling and terminating it. The corpus striatum, substantia nigra and subthalamic nucleus are functionally interdependent. Disease in any part of this nuclear complex upsets total function, and the symptoms reflect general derangement, commonly termed 'extrapyramidal disorder'. Dysfunction of one component may result in over-activity in another part of the complex ('release phenomenon').

APPLIED ANATOMY

Diseases of the basal ganglia (extrapyramidal disorders) cause changes in muscle tone and the occurrence of abnormal involuntary movements which are collectively termed '*dyskinesia*'. The latter take various forms: *tremors; athetosis* — uncontrolled writhing movements of the distal parts of limbs, particularly the hands and forearms; *chorea* — rapid, jerky, purposeless movements, often accompanied by grimacing and twitching of the facial muscles; *ballismus* — violent flailing limb movements at shoulder or hip.

Parkinson's disease is characterized by tremor, rigidity and slowness of movement. The hands tremble continuously even when at rest, unlike the intention tremor of cerebellar disease which occurs during movement. Muscular rigidity, with slowness and general poverty of movement, results in a shuffling gait, stooped posture, slow speech and mask-like, emotionless face. The condition follows degeneration of dopamine-producing neurons in the substantia nigra and their nigrostriate axons, with a consequent absence of dopamine in the striatum (melanin, normally present in the substantia nigra, is a by-product of dopamine metabolism). The rigidity, but not the tremor, is alleviated by administration of L–dopa which, unlike dopamine, crosses the blood–brain barrier. Tremor is probably resultant upon rhythmic overaction in the cholinergic interneurons of the striatum; it is slightly relieved by anticholinergic drugs. Rigidity can be reduced by stereotactic surgery, placing a small destructive lesion in the VA and VL thalamic nuclei; this diminishes the thalamo-cortical effects of abnormal striatal discharges.

Athetosis follows cerebral injury during birth, or congenital maldevelopment; it is accompanied by spasticity. Degeneration is usually found in the neostriatum and the adjacent cortex.

Huntington's chorea is a hereditary disorder which appears in adult life and progresses to dementia. It is associated with degeneration of striatonigral GABA neurons, and intrastriatal cholinergic neurons. The loss of GABA-mediated control of the substantia nigra allows its dopaminergic neurons to inhibit striatal activity excessively. The cerebral cortex becomes thin and the striatum grossly atrophic. *Sydenham's chorea*, a disease of children, is associated with rheumatic fever; patients usually recover. Small haemorrhagic lesions in the corpus striatum have been described in fatal cases.

Hemiballismus consists of violent, jerky, flinging movements of limbs contralateral to a damaged subthalamic nucleus, usually the result of vascular occlusion. This disorder has been produced experimentally in monkeys by localized destruction in the subthalamic nucleus. It is much more difficult to mimic other disorders of the basal ganglia by experimental methods.

Research: neural transplantation

Striatal implants of dopamine-containing neurons of fetal origin are effective in controlling experimentally induced Parkinsonism in rats: fetal material is used because this is less likely to be rejected by the host. Early enthusiasm for transplanting human fetal cells into the caudate/putamen in human Parkinsonism has given way to caution (Williams, 1990). But there have been a few spectacular successes and a neurosurgeon in Mexico City claims that '60% have shown appreciable signs of functional recovery' (Madrazo, 1990). Carefully controlled small trials in advanced cases of the disease are continuing; increased understanding of how these grafted cells function and of the complex variables in technique will probably make this a useful form of treatment over the next decade. Autograft implantation of dopamine cells from patients' own adrenal glands is also being evaluated.

In Sweden, Professor Björklund has produced experimental lesions of the caudate/putamen in rats which result in morphological and biochemical changes resembling Huntington's disease. These can be ameliorated by grafts of fetal striatal tissue into the lesioned striatum. Grafted neurons receive afferents from the normal striatum and establish synaptic connexions with the globus pallidus and, to a lesser extent, with substantia nigra (Björklund et al., 1987).

Chapter 10

Olfactory and limbic systems

In most vertebrates the olfactory sense is of primary importance, and the olfactory part of the brain, or *rhinencephalon*, is relatively large. In such *macrosmatic* animals it is related not only to searching for food, but also to mating, identification of offspring, danger, defence and offence. A *vomero-nasal organ* (of Jacobson), present on each side of the anterior part of the nasal septum in all orders of mammals except the Cetacea, contains pheromone receptors essential for location of mate and initiation of the reproductive process (*see* Wysocki, 1979). Humans are *microsmatic*, with a much reduced olfaction and no functional vomeronasal system: the rhinencephalon is relatively small and is overshadowed by the great development of the cerebral hemispheres. The olfactory cortex occupies a small area; the wider emotional and behavioural reactions, originally associated with the rhinencephalon, are mediated by the limbic system.

Olfactory Pathways

The olfactory epithelium in humans occupies only about one square inch in the nasal roof. It contains *neurosensory cells*, bipolar neurons whose peripheral processes have ciliated receptors that are sensitive to odiferous substances dissolved or suspended in the overlying mucus. Superficially located and easily damaged by infection, these neurons have a limited natural life span and are constantly being replaced by differentiation of epithelial stem cells: new axons grow centrally, a unique form of regeneration into the central nervous system. Their non-myelinated axons form about 20 bundles of *olfactory nerves* on each side which traverse the cribriform plate of the ethmoid bone and pierce dura mater to terminate in the olfactory bulb, where they converge on *synaptic glomeruli*. There is further convergence to secondary sensory neurons, either *mitral cells* (shaped like a mitre) or smaller *tufted cells*, whose axons form the *olfactory tract*. There are also some efferent (centrifugal) fibres in the tract and inhibitory interneurons in the bulb which are involved in editing information. The *anterior olfactory nucleus*, a small aggregation of neurons at the junction of the bulb and tract, has axons which cross to the opposite bulb in the anterior cerebral commissure. Posteriorly the olfactory tract divides into *medial* and *lateral olfactory striae* at the anterior perforated substance (*Fig.* 10.1). The medial stria, of minor significance in man, carries a few fibres to the anterior perforated substance and anterior commissure. The lateral stria leads to the *primary olfactory cortex* which occupies the uncus and anterior end of the parahippocampal gyrus. This projects to the *olfactory association (entorhinal) cortex*, which adjoins it posteriorly, also to the amygdaloid nucleus (dorsomedial part), hypothalamus and thalamus (dorsal medial nucleus).

The *diagonal stria* (of Broca) passes between the amygdaloid nucleus and the septal area, forming a caudal boundary to the anterior perforated substance. The *septal area* is located anterior to the lamina terminalis and inferior to the rostrum of corpus callosum.

Autonomic responses to olfaction, such as salivation and gastric secretion, are mediated by two pathways from the septal area and hypothalamus to the brainstem. The main projection is via the *medial forebrain bundle* which traverses the lateral part of the hypothalamus and enters the midbrain tegmentum. The other route is less direct, via the slender *stria medullaris thalami* which crosses the medial surface of the thalamus to reach the habenular nucleus (*see Fig.* 8.10), relays there to the interpeduncular nucleus of the midbrain and then forms the *dorsal longitudinal fasciculus*. This slender, unmyelinated fasciculus is located ventrolaterally in the periaqueductal grey matter, and descends on each side in the floor of the fourth ventricle (*see Figs* 5.11–5.15). Descending hypothalamic and limbic efferents also utilize these pathways.

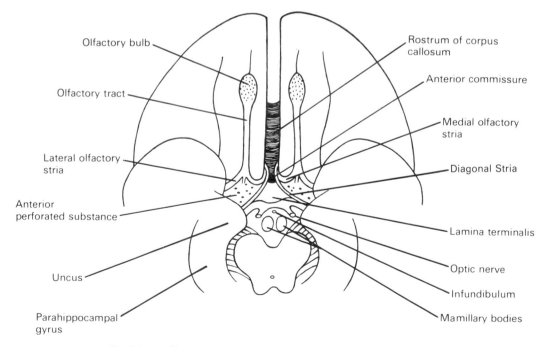

Fig. 10.1 Olfactory structures on the ventral surface of the brain. (The optic nerves have been retracted posteriorly.)

APPLIED ANATOMY

Head injuries which involve anteroposterior movement of the brain may tear the olfactory nerves and cause permanent *anosmia*. Such a patient frequently complains of loss of taste, since much of our interpretation of taste is related to olfactory stimuli. If a cribriform plate is fractured, cerebrospinal fluid may leak into the nose, and bacteria may enter, causing meningitis. *Uncinate fits* occur when epilepsy involves the temporal lobe: the 'aura' before an attack takes the form of olfactory hallucinations.

The Limbic System

The limbic system is so named because it occupies a bordering zone (limbus) between the diencephalon and telencephalon; functionally it is intermediate between the emotive and cognitive aspects of consciousness. Sensory input from the thalamus and hypothalamus is processed here in regard to those emotional and behavioural reactions which relate to the preservation of the individual and the species. The limbic system has an important role in memorization.

The major limbic components (*Fig. 10.2*) are the *septal area*, *cingulate* and

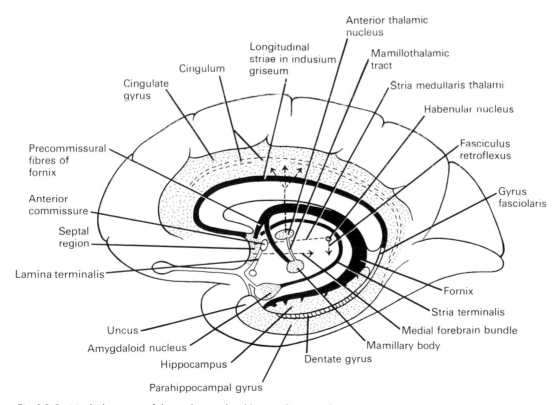

Fig. 10.2 Medial aspect of the right cerebral hemisphere to show structures included in the limbic system (stippled) and their tracts (black).

parahippocampal gyri, *hippocampal formation*, *amygdaloid nucleus*, *mamillary bodies* and *anterior thalamic nucleus*. Sparse grey matter on the upper surface of the corpus callosum, the *indusium griseum*, and in the septum pellucidum have developmental and phylogenetic significance (*see Fig.* 1.8).

Limbic pathways include the *fornix, mamillothalamic tract, cingulum, stria terminalis* and *medial* and *lateral longitudinal striae*. Output to the brainstem is via the *medial forebrain bundle, stria medullaris thalami* and *mamillotegmental tract*.

Many of these structures have a curvature determined by progressive development of the cerebral hemispheres, first posteriorly, then anteroinferiorly around the diencephalon. The hippocampus, a relatively ancient structure (archecortex), is located dorsally in reptiles and early mammals, curving over the anterior (olfactory) commissure from the septal area, a pattern also seen in the early stages of development of the human brain (*see Fig.* 1.8). With the development of the cerebral hemispheres (neocortex) and corpus callosum, the hippocampus has been displaced downwards into the temporal lobe and rolled medially. The indusium griseum and longitudinal striae indicate the track of this displacement and provide a vestigial connexion in humans between the hippocampus and the septal area.

Hippocampal formation

This comprises the *hippocampus, dentate gyrus* and *subiculum*. The subiculum

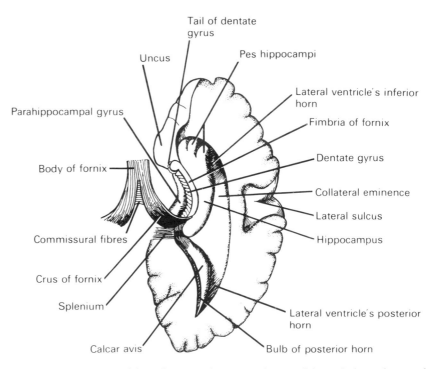

Fig. 10.3 A dissection of the inferior and posterior horns of the right lateral ventricle.

is a transitional zone between the three-layered hippocampal archecortex and the six-layered neocortex of the parahippocampal gyrus.

The hippocampus (*Fig.* 10.3) is an area of cortex rolled into the floor of the inferior horn of the lateral ventricle and continuous through the subiculum with the parahippocampal gyrus. The name 'hippocampus', meaning 'sea horse', is derived from its appearance in coronal section (*Fig.* 10.4). Its anterior extremity forms a paw-like *pes hippocampi*. On its ventricular surface is a layer of white matter, the *alveus*, whose fibres converge medially to a longitudinal band, the *fimbria of the fornix*. The choroid fissure and choroid plexus are above the fimbria. Posteriorly the hippocampus ends beneath the splenium of the corpus callosum.

The *dentate gyrus*, a serrated band of grey matter between the fimbria and subiculum, is overhung by the fimbria and is best viewed from the medial aspect. Anteriorly the dentate gyrus blends with the uncus; posteriorly it continues through the slender *gyrus fasciolaris* into the *indusium griseum*, the vestigial grey matter on the upper surface of the corpus callosum. The *medial* and *lateral longitudinal striae*, two narrow fasciculi embedded in the indusium griseum on each side, extend forwards to the septal area (*Fig.* 10.5).

The hippocampus has three neuronal layers termed molecular, pyramidal

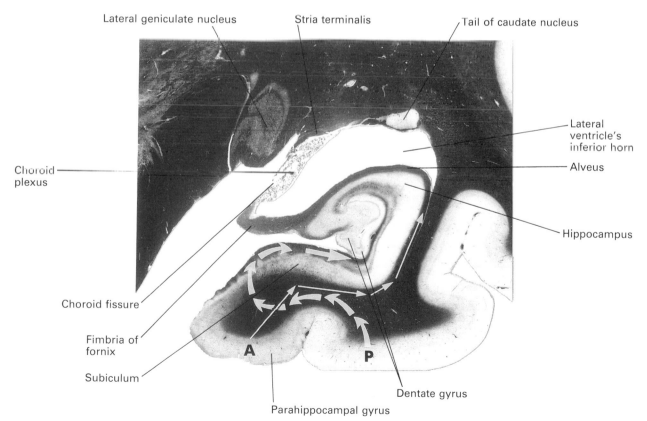

Fig. 10.4 Coronal section through the hippocampal formation. (Lithium haematoxylin and darrow red stain, × 4). **A**, alvear path. **P**, perforant path.

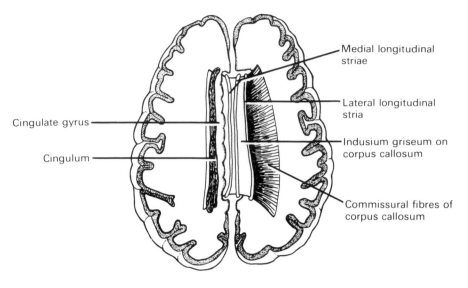

Medial longitudinal striae

Lateral longitudinal stria

Indusium griseum on corpus callosum

Commissural fibres of corpus callosum

Cingulate gyrus

Cingulum

Fig. 10.5 Superior aspect of the corpus callosum. The cerebral hemispheres have been sectioned above the cingulate gyri, the left cingulate gyrus dissected to reveal the cingulum and the right cingulate gyrus removed and some callosal fibres shown.

and polymorphous; axons of pyramidal neurons pass through the polymorphous layer and alveus into the fornix. The dentate gyrus is also trilaminar, but its middle layer is of granular cells.

Connexions of the hippocampal formation (*Figs* 10.2 and 10.6)

The input to the hippocampal formation from the parahippocampal gyrus is via two routes: the 'alvear' path enters the hippocampus from its ventricular surface (beneath the alveus), the 'perforant path' passes through the subiculum to reach the dentate gyrus. All efferents from the dentate gyrus pass to the hippocampus.

The fornix is the efferent tract of the hippocampus. Posteriorly the fimbriae form two *crura* which curve over the thalami and unite above in the *body* of the fornix; here a *hippocampal commissure* between the crura interconnects the two hippocampi (*Fig.* 10.3). The body of the fornix is closely related above to the corpus callosum and is separated below from the thalami by the choroid fissures. Anteriorly, the body of the fornix divides into two *columns* which arch down towards the anterior commissure, and form the anterior boundary of the interventricular foramen on each side. The columns of the fornix traverse the hypothalamus and end in the *mamillary bodies*. Each mamillo-thalamic tract has reciprocal connexions with its *anterior thalamic nucleus*, and this projects to the ipsilateral cingulate gyrus. Within the gyrus, a bundle of myelinated fibres, the *cingulum*, curves posteroinferiorly into the *parahippocampal gyrus*, and thus to the hippocampus. This path is named the 'Papez circuit'(*Fig.* 10.6), after the neuroanatomist who described it in 1937

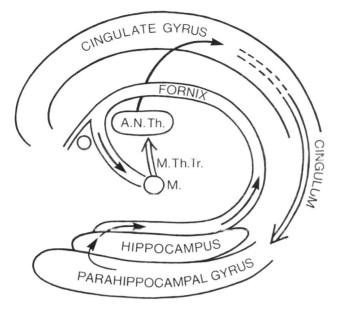

Fig. 10.6 The Papez Circuit. A.N.Th., anterior thalamic nucleus. M.Th.Tr., mamillo-thalamic tract. M, mamillary body.

as being significant in emotional behaviour: more recently it has been found to be essential for the process of memorization.

The anterior column of the fornix gives off a *precommissural fasciculus* to the septal area; the postcommissural fibres pass not only to the mamillary body but also directly into the medial forebrain bundle. Another connexion between hippocampus and septal area is via the fibres of the *longitudinal striae* above the corpus callosum.

Amygdaloid nucleus

This almond-shaped mass is anterior to and above the tip of the lateral ventricle's inferior horn. As already noted, its dorsomedial part has olfactory connexions. Its larger, ventrolateral part is included in the limbic system and has complex cortical, thalamic and hypothalamic afferents. *Its limbic efferent tract is the stria terminalis*, which runs posteriorly in the roof of the inferior horn, medial to the tail of the caudate nucleus, and curves into the floor of the body of the lateral ventricle, where it lies between the caudate nucleus and the thalamus. It projects to the septal area, anterior hypothalamus and dorsal medial thalamic nucleus, affecting emotional behaviour.

Limbic projections to the brainstem

There are three paths (*see also* p. 182) by which the limbic system influences autonomic centres in the brainstem:

1. *Medial forebrain bundle*, from the septal area and hypothalamus.
2. *Stria medullaris thalami:* afferents are from the septal area, hypothalamus, stria terminalis and fornix; it crosses the medial surface of thalamus to the habenular nucleus, from thence via the fasciculus retroflexus to the interpeduncular nucleus and dorsal longitudinal fasciculus. There is also a direct input from the hypothalamus to this fasciculus.
3. *Mamillotegmental tract*, from mamillary body to midbrain tegmentum.

Functions of the limbic system

The limbic system has close reciprocal links with the hypothalamus, thalamus and cortex and it functions as part of an integrated complex. Phylogenetically ancient, it is concerned with the *preservation of the individual and the species*. Individual responses to a challenging situation may involve offensive or defensive reactions, anger, fear, acceleration of heart and respiration. Species preservation includes sexual responses, mating and the care of offspring.

The limbic system participates in a *memory retention* mechanism. Lesions of the hippocampus or any interruption of the Papez circuit will depress memorization of recent events, although long-established memories are unaffected. Localized lesions of the hippocampus can sometimes be demonstrated by magnetic resonance imaging (Press et al., 1989). As noted previously, the anterior and dorsal medial thalamic nuclei are involved in memorization. The nature of long-term memory storage is imperfectly understood.

There are so-called 'pleasure centres' in the limbic system. Thus, if a human septal area is stimulated by an electrode under local anaesthesia, the patient becomes much less inhibited and even euphoric. Less significantly, there are also 'aversion centres'. The balance of activity in these centres represents reward or punishment and is a neural substrate in *motivation* and in the *emotional equilibrium* between euphoria and depression. The anterior and dorsal medial thalamic nuclei are involved in this (p.168). The local concentration of monoamine neurotransmitters is sometimes abnormal in psychological disorders and, as described below, this can be improved therapeutically.

APPLIED ANATOMY

Bilateral removal of anterior parts of the temporal lobes, either experimentally or in the treatment of severe epilepsy originating here, results in the *Klüver-Bucy syndrome*, which is characterized by increased appetite, loss of recent memories, docility and hypersexuality, the latter often bizarre.

Experimental stimulation of the *amygdaloid nuclei* produces excitability, fear and rage; repeated stimulation may establish long-term aggressive attitudes. Stereotactic surgical lesions have been used clinically to reduce pathological aggression in extreme cases. Normally there are very high levels of opiate here, presumably released as required in response to stress.

Following *Wernicke's encephalopathy*, a vitamin deficiency associated with alcoholism, there is a permanent memory loss; haemorrhage into and atrophy of the mamillary bodies may be found post mortem.

Temporal lobe epilepsy has been mentioned in connexion with olfactory hallucinations. Other symptoms such as altered awareness of surroundings, bizarre behaviour, temporary amnesia and unusual visceral sensations may be due to limbic dysfunction.

The medial forebrain bundle also includes the ascending fibres of a *mesolimbic pathway*. This conveys dopamine from the ventral tegmentum of the midbrain, noradrenaline from the locus ceruleus and serotonin from the raphe nuclei. Excessive dopamine activity here appears to be a feature of *schizophrenia* and this can be treated by drugs which block dopamine receptors; unfortunately such therapy may also affect nigrostriate tracts and produce side effects which resemble Parkinson's disease. Post mortem reports of brains from schizophrenic patients have shown a gross asymmetry of dopamine content in the two amygdalae, the left amygdala having an abnormally high concentration (Reynolds, 1983; MacKay, 1984).

One of the early antihypertensive drugs, reserpine, was found to cause severe *depression:* it lowers the concentration of noradrenaline and serotonin in the limbic system. Monoamine oxidase inhibitors have the opposite effect and can be used to treat depression. The tricyclic antidepressants such as imipramine inhibit the re-uptake of amines from the synaptic cleft to the presynaptic terminal.

Chapter 11

Visual system

The optic nerve and retina develop from an outgrowth of the forebrain vesicle. Near the skin this outgrowth invaginates as a bilaminar optic cup, one layer becoming the black pigmented retinal epithelium, the other forming the neural layers of the retina. These two basic laminae are closely apposed, but may separate in the clinical condition, 'detached retina'.

The Retina

From within outwards (i.e. from vitreous to choroid) the retina consists of *nerve fibres, ganglion cells, bipolar cells, photoreceptors* and *pigment epithelium*, with supportive neuroglial cells (*Fig.* 11.1). The nerve fibres converge to the *optic disc*, slightly medial to the posterior ocular pole, pierce the sclera, become myelinated and form the optic nerve. The optic disc, insensitive to light, is termed the 'blind spot'. The central retinal artery and vein also traverse the disc. Immediately lateral to the disc and in line with the visual axis is the oval, slightly yellow *macula lutea*, which has a central depression, the *fovea centralis*, where visual acuity is maximal; there are no nerve fibres or blood vessels in front of it. In purposeful vision the eyes are directed so that the retinal image is on the macula.

The *pigment epithelium* contains melanin which absorbs light and prevents backscatter. Its external aspect is firmly attached to the choroid; its internal surface is infolded between individual photoreceptors. The *photoreceptors*, rods and cones, have an external light-sensitive segment containing photopigments, a cell body and a synaptic base. They transduce light into electrical energy. *Rods* are more numerous than cones, contain the pigment rhodopsin (visual purple), and are most sensitive in conditions of low illumination, for example at night. The fovea is 'night-blind' because it contains no rods. *Cones* are more discriminative of detail and are sensitive to colour; each cone contains one of three pigments sensitive to blue, green or red light. Cones predominate in the macula and diminish rapidly away from it; only cones are present in the central fovea.

In the retina (*Fig.* 11.1) there is direct neuronal transmission from photoreceptors via bipolar cells to ganglion cells whose axons form the optic nerve; there is also modulation and integration of input through a laterally interacting system of interneurons — horizontal and amacrine cells.

Horizontal cell dendrites synapse between photoreceptors and bipolar cells; they increase contrast by lateral inhibition. *Amacrine cells* modulate transmission between bipolar and ganglion cells; they are very responsive to changes in light intensity. It has recently been suggested that rod bipolars do not synapse directly on ganglion cells but only via amacrine cells (Daw, et al., 1990).

Input is either convergent (rods) or relatively non-convergent and more discriminative (cones). Large numbers of rods synapse with one bipolar cell, many of which converge to one ganglion cell. This summation contributes to sensitivity of the rod system in poor lighting, but limits discrimination. There is little such convergence among cones, and foveal cones have a 1:1:1 ratio with their bipolar and ganglion cells, thus ensuring high resolution. Retinal nerve fibres are non-myelinated, an optical advantage since myelin is highly refractile.

The physiology of vision is complex: a brief summary is given here. *Bipolar neurons* are of two functional types, responding positively either to light or dark photoreceptor-exposure. Ganglion cells also have differing responses. Each *ganglion cell* receives input via bipolar neurons from a circular field of photoreceptors. Some ganglion cells are termed 'on centre' because they are excited by light at the centre of the field; they are inhibited by light at its periphery. Others are termed 'off centre' because they respond positively to peripheral and negatively to central field illumination (Kuffler, 1973). The implication is that the ganglion cells detect contrasts, as in borders and shapes, rather than general illumination levels. This 'centre-surround antagonism' also applies to the processing of complementary

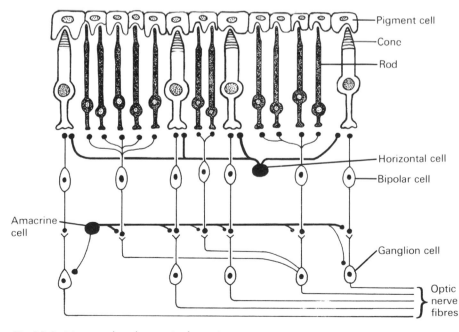

Fig. 11.1 Neuronal pathways in the retina.

colours. Thus if a ganglion cell is only excited by a spot of red light in the centre of its field, it will be inhibited by surrounding green illumination. Such cells are termed 'spectrally opponent'; others are non-opponent and any wavelength can produce on/off responses. Colour analysis is only completed at cortical level but its correlation begins in the retina. Some ganglion cells are sensitive to movement in their fields.

Visual Pathway

The two *optic nerves* extend from the eyes to the optic chiasma, each nerve containing about one million axons, myelinated by oligodendrocytes, and surrounded by pia mater, arachnoid mater and dura mater. Pia mater invests the nerve and is separated from the arachnoid by the subarachnoid space. The central retinal vessels traverse this space, and if the cerebrospinal fluid pressure is abnormally raised, the vein is compressed, with resultant oedema of the optic disc (papilloedema). The dural sleeve fuses with the ocular sclera. At the optic chiasma, fibres derived from the nasal half of each retina cross. Some crossed fibres loop forward slightly into the contralateral optic nerve before entering the optic tract; some loop backwards into the ipsilateral tract before crossing (*see Fig.* 11.6). Each *optic tract* extends from the chiasma to the lateral geniculate body, where most of its fibres end. A few fibres leave each optic tract to descend in a *superior brachium* to the ipsilateral superior colliculus and both pretectal nuclei. A strong retinocollicular stimulus can induce reflex head and eye movements, as towards a flash of light; the pretectal nuclei serve the pupillary light reflex. The *optic radiation* (geniculo-calcarine tract) is in the retrolentiform part of the internal capsule. Fibres

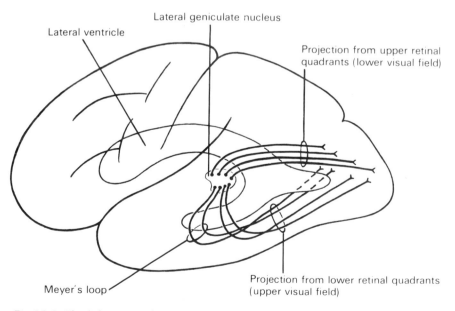

Fig. 11.2 The left optic radiation viewed from the lateral aspect.

passing to the primary visual cortex above the calcarine sulcus fan out round the lateral ventricle's posterior horn; fibres passing to the visual cortex below the sulcus loop down into the temporal lobe, lateral to the ventricle's inferior horn (Meyer's loop) (*Fig.* 11.2). The optic radiation also includes fibres projecting *from* the occipital cortex to the lateral geniculate nucleus and superior colliculus (*see* below).

The *primary visual cortex* (area 17 of Brodmann) is located in the walls and depths of the calcarine sulcus. It is also known as the striate cortex, because section reveals a horizontal *visual stria* (of Gennari) in its grey matter (*see Fig.* 12.5) The *visual association cortex* (areas 18, 19) occupies the rest of the occipital lobe; it processes information received from area 17 and is concerned with complex aspects of visual perception. It has an input from the thalamic pulvinar and is the source of corticocollicular fibres mediating the pupillary accommodation reflex, visual grasp reflex and automatic scanning (*see* p.141). The adjoining postero-inferior surface of the temporal lobe (area 20) is involved in visual pattern recognition and storage of visual memories. Remembering the position of an object in space is one of the functions of the superior parietal lobule (area 7).

Image Projection and Processing

Light from the left half of the visual field impinges on the right halves of the two retinae, which project to the right visual cortex. The cornea and lens produce a retinal image which is inverted and reversed (left to right), and this pattern is transferred to the visual cortex. As illustrated in *Fig.* 11.3, a sequential cortical projection requires decussation of the optic nerves. In the panoramic vision of sub-mammalian vertebrates there is total decussation. In human binocular vision half the fibres decussate: the resultant fusion of images viewed from a slightly different angle by each eye produces stereoscopic perception of depth and distance.

There is very accurate point-to-point projection from the retina, in the visual pathway, to the visual cortex. *Fig.* 11.4 shows that the lower retinal quadrants are represented in the outer half of the ipsilateral geniculate nucleus and project to the visual cortex below the calcarine sulcus. The upper retinal quadrants project to the medial half of their lateral geniculate nucleus and to the visual cortex above the sulcus. There is a disproportionately large macular representation in the geniculate nuclei and in the posterior third of the primary visual cortices. This accords with the macula's functional importance; the number of fibres from the macular ganglion cells is large because of the discrete, non-convergent projection from its photoreceptors.

Each *lateral geniculate nucleus* has six layers of neurons, numbered 1–6 from the ventral to the dorsal surface. Crossed optic fibres terminate in layers 1, 4 and 6, uncrossed optic fibres in layers 2, 3 and 5. It is not simply a relay station: in each lamina there is further integration of visual input by interneurons, but there is little exchange between laminae.

Axons from the lateral geniculate nucleus terminate in the visual stria of

Gennari (*see Fig.* 12.5), which is in layer IV (*see* Chapter 12) of the *primary visual cortex*. Binocular integration is effected in layers II and III and from thence efferents pass to the visual association cortex. 'Solitary cells' (of Meynert) in layer V of areas 17, 18 and 19 project to the superior colliculus. Layer VI has feedback links to the lateral geniculate nucleus which modulate input.

As input is processed through neurons in the retina, lateral geniculate nuclei, primary visual and association cortex, it is built into increasingly complex forms whereby progressively sophisticated perception is achieved. Thus area 17 elicits the orientation of an image, area 18 is concerned with stereoscopic vision, area 19 with colour and movement, area 20 (postero-

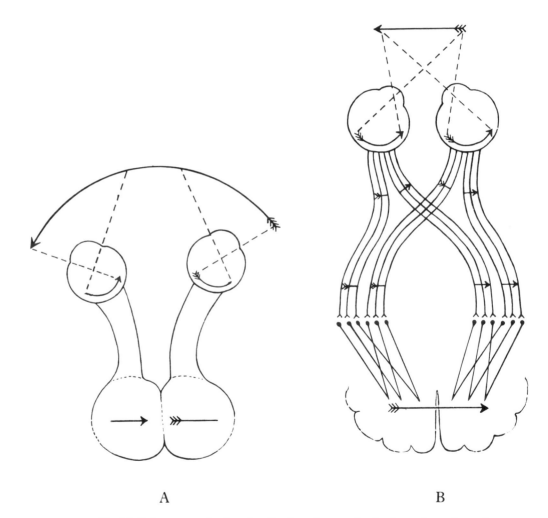

A   B

Fig. 11.3 Image projection in visual pathways. In the hypothetical condition (A), with no decussation of optic nerves, central projection of the image would be illogical. In (B) half the optic nerve fibres decussate; image projection is sequentially reconstructed in pathways to visual cortex. (After Sarnat H.B. and Netsky M.G. (1974) *Evolution of the Nervous System*. Oxford, Oxford University Press.)

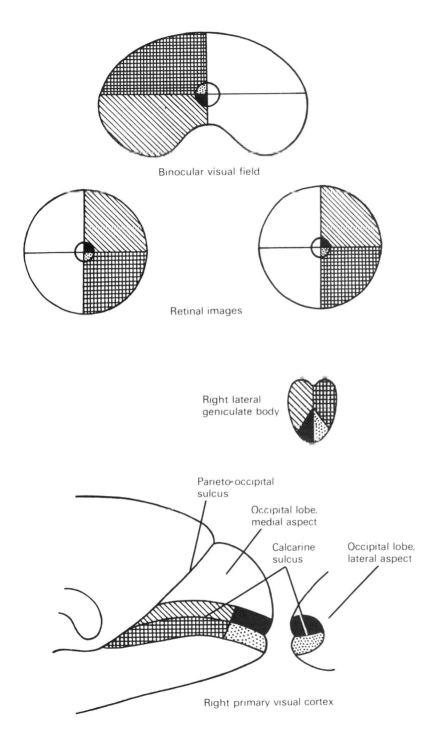

Binocular visual field

Retinal images

Right lateral
geniculate body

Parieto-occipital
sulcus

Occipital lobe,
medial aspect

Calcarine
sulcus

Occipital lobe,
lateral aspect

Right primary visual cortex

Fig. 11.4 Representation of the visual fields in the retinae, right lateral geniculate nucleus and visual cortex.

inferior surface of temporal lobe) with identification and recognition, area 7 (superior parietal lobule) with the spatial position of objects. Pupillary reflexes and the control of eye movements are described on p.141–2.

Research: cortical columnar organization, callosal connexions

Hubel and Wiesel (1974) showed that visual cortical neurons are organized into narrow columns, extending from the cortical surface to the central white matter. Whereas geniculate cells respond to spots of light shone on the retina, these cortical neurons react to lines and edges; each column reacts to only one orientation of an image. They are hence termed *orientation columns*. Adjacent columns represent angular shifts of about 10°. They are grouped into larger *ocular dominance columns* each of which receives an input from only one eye (*Fig.* 11.5). The visual cortex contains alternating right and left ocular dominance columns, about 1 mm wide in humans, each containing a series of orientation columns covering a 180° pattern of linear excitation in the visual field. This regular arrangement of the cortical ocular dominance columns is only partially developed at birth; full development depends on subsequent binocular excitation. Deprivation of input from one eye in the neonatal period results in irreversible cortical change, an imbalance in the size of left-right columns and permanent loss of normal binocular vision. This is an example of *neuronal plasticity*, in which cells of the stimulated column expand connexions into the adjacent quiescent area (Hubel et al., 1977). It has obvious practical implications in the management of the newborn.

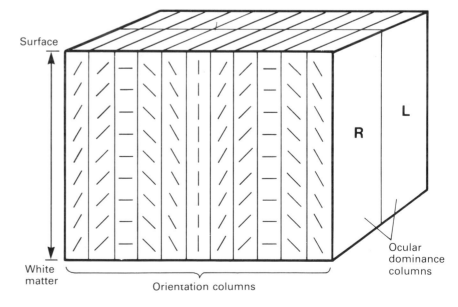

Fig. 11.5 Simplified diagram of ocular dominance and orientation columns in the primary visual cortex. The actual shift between orientation columns is about 10°.

Recent investigations have shown that commissural fibres of corpus callosum to occipital lobes are restricted to narrow boundary zones between the visual cortical areas 17, 18 and 19. Moreover, these callosal connexions link only the cortical representations of the vertical meridian of each retina — a narrow vertical strip between right and left halves. It is reported that the ganglion cells of each meridian have axons that bifurcate to enter both optic tracts (Choudhury et al., 1965; Garey et al., 1968; Zeki et al., 1970; Fisken et al., 1975).

APPLIED ANATOMY

Visual defects may be mapped in detail by using an instrument called a perimeter. Gross defects can be detected by the confrontation method. The subject faces the examiner, eye to eye, and the latter moves an object, midway between him or herself and the subject, from the periphery towards the visual field and from differing directions. In each test the subject states when the object enters his or her visual field, and the examiner compares this rough estimate of the field with his or her own perceptions.

Lesions of the visual pathway are illustrated in *Fig.* 11.6. Defects are

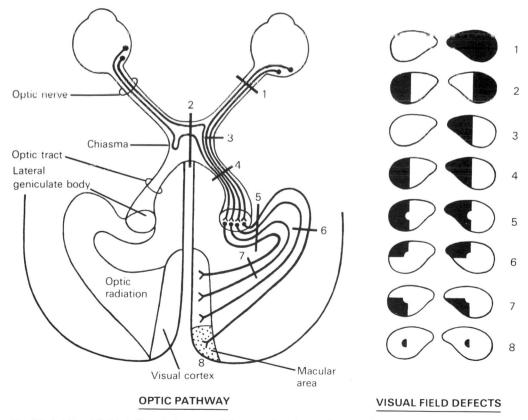

OPTIC PATHWAY **VISUAL FIELD DEFECTS**

Fig. 11.6 Visual field defects in lesions of the visual pathway (*see* text).

described in terms of the loss of visual fields. Loss of half a visual field of one or both eyes is *hemianopia*. Damage of one optic nerve (1) results in monocular blindness. A pituitary tumour may compress decussating fibres in the optic chiasma (2), causing bitemporal hemianopia. Pressure at the lateral edge of the optic chiasma (3) results in ipsilateral nasal hemianopia; if this is due to aneurysm of the internal carotid artery in the cavernous sinus, there may also be a paralysis of eye muscles (ophthalmoplegia) due to compression of nearby cranial nerves III, IV and VI. A lesion of the right optic tract (4) produces a left homonymous hemianopia — loss of the same half of the visual field of both eyes. A complete lesion of the optic radiation (5) has a similar effect but, because the radiation fans out, partial or *quadrantic* defects are more common (6, 7). In field defects due to thrombosis of the posterior cerebral artery there is often 'macular sparing', sometimes assumed to be due to a branch of the middle cerebral artery reaching the macular area of the primary visual cortex (5, 6, 7). Damage of the cerebral occipital pole, usually due to trauma, may destroy the macular area, producing a *central scotoma* (8). Sometimes a genetic disorder causes a primary degeneration of the macula: the resultant loss of central visual acuity is a severe disability.

Chapter 12

Cerebral cortex

Cytology and Cytoarchitecture

The external cerebral surface is a grey mantle (pallium) of neurons and
neuroglia; its total area of more than two square feet is folded into gyri and
sulci. Cortical thickness, greater over gyri, less in sulci, varies from 4.5 mm
in the primary motor area to 1.5 mm in the primary visual area. It reaches
almost maximum extent by the age of twelve years; its synaptic complexity
continues to increase and this changes throughout life. Some impression of
its intricacy is gained by considering the vast number of neurons (estimates
vary between 14 000 million and 2 600 million), and then noting that a single
pyramidal neuron may take part in 60 000 synapses within the cortex.

Primitively the cortex served olfaction; such rhinencephalic derivatives
archecortex (hippocampus, dentate gyrus) and *paleocortex* (olfactory) — are
three-layered. The six-layered *neocortex* started to emerge in reptiles, became
truly evident in mammals and reached its evolutionary summit in humans,
comprising 90% of the human cortex. The cingulate gyrus has a *mesocortex*,
intermediate histologically and functionally as part of the limbic system.

Cortical neurons

Golgi Type I neurons, with long axons, are either *pyramidal* or *fusiform*.
Golgi Type II neurons, with short axons, are either *stellate* (granular),
horizontal neurons (of Cajal) or *Martinotti* neurons (with ascending axons)
(*Fig.* 12.1).

Pyramidal neurons have cell bodies which vary in height from 10 μm to
120 μm; the latter *giant pyramidal cells* (of Betz) occur only in the primary
motor cortex. The pyramidal cell apex and an apical dendrite are directed
towards the cortical surface, basal dendrites spread laterally, and all have
dendritic spines; the axon emerges from the cell base and has recurrent
collateral branches. Pyramidal axons enter the white matter as *projection
fibres* (to spinal cord, brainstem, basal ganglia and diencephalon), as *commissural fibres* (inter-hemispheric) and as *association fibres* (intra-hemispheric).
Some small, superficially placed, pyramidal cells have short axons passing
only to deeper cortical laminae. Large and medium somata are in lamina V,
medium and small cells in laminae III and II.

Fusiform neurons are similar to pyramidal cells but their somata are spindle-

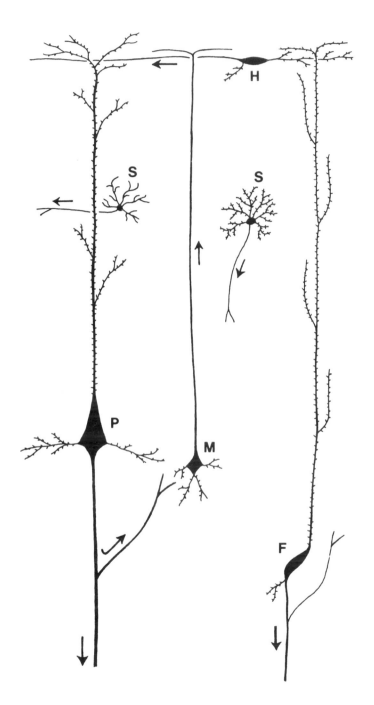

Fig. 12.1 Cortical neurons. **H**, horizontal neuron (of Cajal); **S**, stellate neuron; **P**, pyramidal neuron; **M**, Martinotti neuron; **F**, fusiform neuron.

shaped and in lamina VI; a long apical dendrite is directed towards lamina I, there are short basal dendrites, their axons form projection fibres.

Stellate neurons (granular cells) are concentrated in laminae II and IV, but are present throughout the cortex, except in lamina I. Each has a small, 8–10 μm star-shaped somata, with a short axon and many dendrites.

Neurons of Martinotti, polygonal cell bodies with short dendrites, have axons directed *towards* and often into lamina I, giving off collaterals en route. The somata occur in all laminae, except I.

Horizontal neurons (of Cajal) have small, fusiform somata, a dendrite at each pole and a longer axon, all parallel to the surface and restricted to lamina I. Obvious in the newborn, they are sparse in adults.

Laminar structure of the neocortex (*Figs* 12.2 and 12.3)

Regional cortical variations will be described later; the general pattern and functional attributes of the six-layered neocortex are:

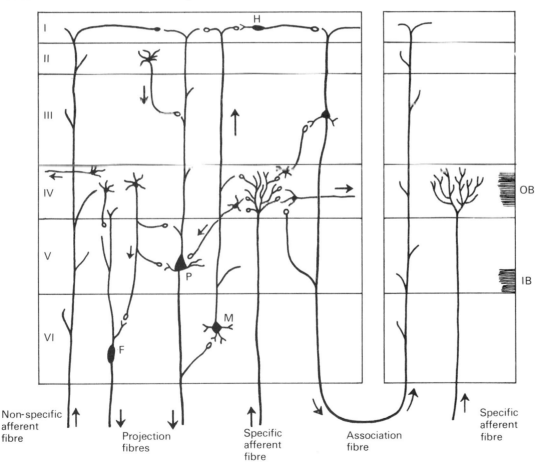

Fig. 12.2 A simplified diagram of intracortical circuits. **OB, IB**, outer and inner bands of Baillarger; **H,P,M,F** as in *Fig.* 12.1; laminae of the cortex are numbered I–VI.

I.   *Molecular lamina*. The most superficial lamina, this is a *synaptic field* with few cells and many fine nerve fibres, including dendrites of pyramidal and fusiform neurons and axons of Martinotti neurons.

II. *External granular lamina*. Involved with *intracortical circuits* are large numbers of stellate and small pyramidal neurons with dendrites entering lamina I and axons directed to deeper laminae.

III. *External pyramidal lamina*. Concerned with *association* and *commissural* efferents and afferents, this contains medium-sized pyramidal cells superficially and larger ones more deeply, mingled with stellate and Martinotti neurons.

IV. *Internal granular lamina*. Receptive of *specific thalamic afferents* (e.g. from geniculate or ventrel posterior nuclei), this contains numerous somata of stellate neurons. In contrast to non-specific thalamic and reticular afferents to association cortex, which diffuse through all layers, specific afferents have localized bushy terminals (*Fig. 12.2*): these form the *outer band of Baillarger*, most marked in the primary visual area, hence the name 'striate cortex' (*see Fig. 12.5*).

V.   *Inner pyramidal lamina*. This is a *major source of projection fibre efferents*, corticospinal, corticobulbar, extrapyramidal (e.g. corticostriate), corticopontine and corticothalamic. It is characterized by the presence of medium and large pyramidal neurons; in the primary motor area, giant Betz cells contribute 3% of pyramidal tract fibres. Axon collaterals form the *inner band of Baillarger* in the deep part of this lamina (*Fig. 12.4*). Stellate and Martinotti neurons also occur.

VI. *Multiform lamina*. This is also an *efferent* lamina with neurons of various forms, many fusiform, forming projection fibres. Martinotti neurons are often numerous. This lamina mingles with the white matter, being pervaded by fibre bundles entering or leaving the cortex (*Fig. 12.3A*).

It has been discovered that substantial numbers of projection fibres, destined for sub-cortical centres, have collateral branches which form callosal connexions with the opposite hemisphere (Szentágothai, 1987).

In identifying these laminae, first identify the outer and inner bands of Baillarger in the middle of lamina IV and the deep part of lamina V respectively; second observe that laminae I and II are relatively narrow, lamina III very wide. Vertical intracortical fibres include dendrites and axons of pyramidal neurons and the axons of Martinotti neurons.

Cortical classification

Homotypical cortex (Greek *homos* = the same as): characterizes 'association areas' (*see* functional localization). The structure of all association areas is very similar and six cortical layers are evident. There are minor regional variations: thus the visual association cortex includes some pyramidal-type 'solitary cells' (of Meynert), the origin of corticocollicular fibres.

Heterotypical cortex (Greek *heteros* = different): the primary sensory and motor cortices differ structurally from one another; the former is described as granular, the latter as agranular. A six-layered pattern is obscured by the blending of laminae II–V, with a predominance here of either stellate (sensory) or pyramidal (motor) neurons (*see Fig.* 12.3B) The primary visual and auditory areas and the anterior part of the postcentral gyrus (Brodmann area 3) have a *granular cortex* with many stellate but few pyramidal neurons

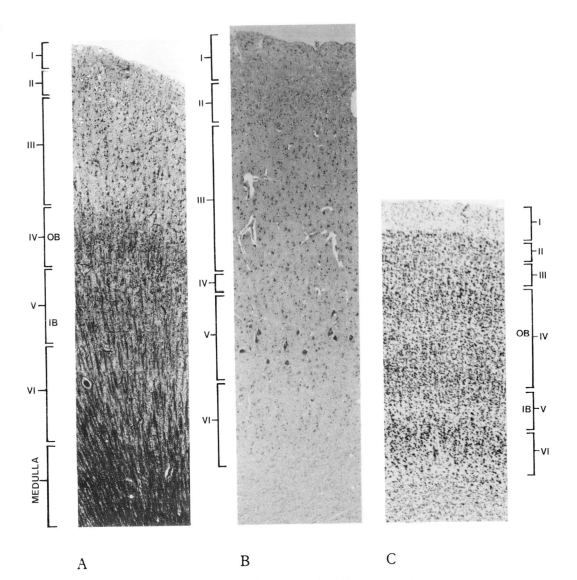

A   B   C

Fig. 12.3 Sections showing cortical structure, homotypical and heterotypical. Some dissimilarities are due to different staining methods. In the homotypical prefrontal cortex (A) myelinated fibres and cells are stained (lithium haematoxylin and darrow red). In the heterotypical motor cortex (B) and visual cortex (C) only the cells are stained (by cresyl violet and toluidine blue respectively). Note the width of layer IV in the visual cortex. Identify the inner (**IB**) and outer (**OB**) bands of Baillarger. Laminae of the cortex are numbered I–VI. (× *c*.32, photographs by J.A. Findlay.)

in laminae II–IV (*see Fig.* 12.3C). The primary motor and premotor areas have an *agranular cortex:* pyramidal neurons spread through layers II–V.

Allocortex, of three layers, includes arche- and paleocortex; it is described in Chapter 10.

Brodmann (1909) classified the cortical areas in a cytoarchitectural map, based on a study of sub-human primate brains; fifty-seven areas were numbered. Though still widely used, such a division, with functional attributes, is over-precise. Even a basic division into 'motor' and 'sensory' areas is too rigid; for example some corticospinal fibres originate from the parietal 'sensory' cortex.

Functional columnar organization

Neuronal circuits of the cortex are arranged in vertical columns, most evident in sensory areas. The neurons in each column have a common receptive field, respond to and process the same stimuli. A column has its own pattern of afferent, efferent and internuncial fibres. The human cortex

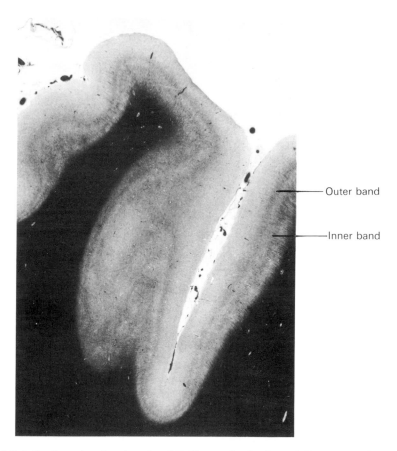

— Outer band

— Inner band

Fig. 12.4 Section showing bands of Baillarger in the frontal (homotypical) cortex. (Lithium haematoxylin and darrow red stain, × 6.)

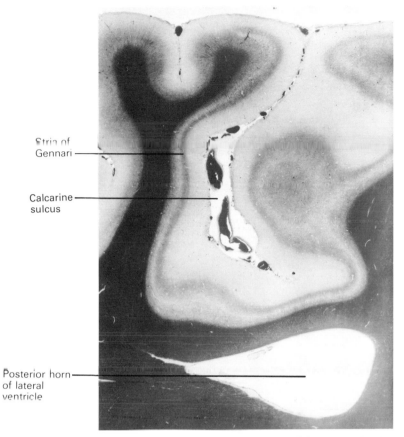

Stria of
Gennari

Calcarine
sulcus

Posterior horn
of lateral
ventricle

Fig. 12.5 A section of primary visual cortex. Note the stria of Gennari in both walls
of the calcarine sulcus. The lateral ventricle's posterior horn has also been sectioned.
(Lithium haematoxylin and darrow red stain, × 5.)

excels in its multitudinous stellate neurons, which form complex vertical interlaminar circuits and also link adjacent columns. Columnar organization is clearly demonstrable in the primary visual cortex where input from right and left eyes alternates in ocular dominance columns (*see Fig.* 11.5). A column is about 0.5 mm wide and its height is the cortical thickness; each is further subdivided into orientation columns.

Cerebral White Matter

This is a compact mass of vast numbers of association, commissural and projection fibres and associated neuroglia.

Association fibres (*Fig.* 12.6)

These are intra-hemispheric, interconnecting cortical areas within one hemi-

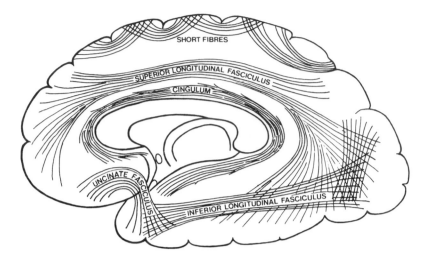

Fig. 12.6 The principal association fibres in the cerebrum.

sphere. They vary in length: *short association fibres* link adjacent gyri; *long association fibres* connect different lobes. The *cingulum*, in the cingulate gyrus, is a limbic association bundle between the septal area and the parahippocampal gyrus. The *uncinate fasciculus* extends from the motor speech area and the frontal lobe's orbital surface, and hooks round the lateral fissure to reach the temporal pole cortex. The extensive *superior longitudinal fasciculus* connects the frontal and occipital poles, curves into the temporal lobe, receiving and giving off fibres en route. The *fronto-occipital fasciculus* pursues a similar course but is more deeply placed, separated from the superior longitudinal fasciculus by the corona radiata. The *inferior longitudinal fasciculus* connects the visual association area with the temporal lobe.

Commissural fibres

These are inter-hemispheric, joining corresponding sites of the two hemispheres. Neocortical commissures are in the *corpus callosum* and the much smaller *anterior commissure*. Others are *habenular* (between the habenular nuclei), *hippocampal* (between the crura of the fornix) and the *posterior commissure* (between the superior colliculi and the pretectal regions).

The *corpus callosum* is a massive, arched, interhemispheric bridge flooring the midline longitudinal fissure and roofing both lateral ventricles. It has a thin superficial grey mantle, the *indusium griseum*, embedded in which are white fibres of the *medial* and *lateral longitudinal striae*. The anterior cerebral vessels run in its pia mater. It is overhung by the median *falx cerebri* and overlapped on each side by the cingulate gyri. It is described as having a rostrum, genu, trunk and splenium (*see Figs* 8.1 and 12.7). The curved anterior *genu* extends as a thin *rostrum* to the lamina terminalis. The *trunk*, the main body, ends posteriorly as a thickened *splenium* which overhangs the

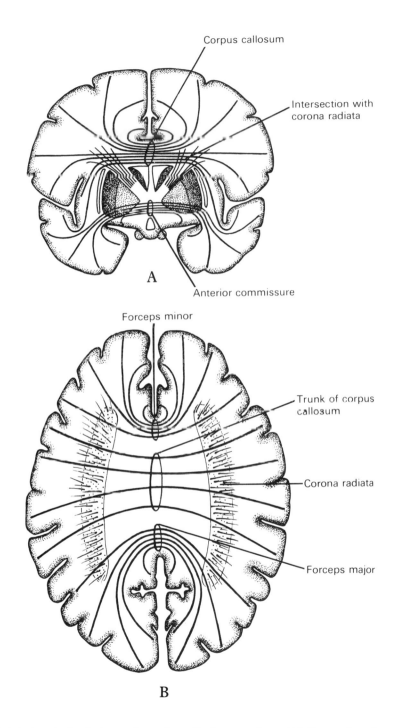

Fig. 12.7 Interhemispheric (commissural) cortical connexions. (A) Coronal section through the anterior commissure and corpus callosum. (B) Transverse section through the corpus callosum.

thalamic pulvinars, pineal gland and midbrain tectum. The *septum pellucidum* is a thin median sheet of white and grey matter comprising two laminae separated anteriorly by a small central cavity (*see Figs* 9.3 and 14.6). It is covered by ependyma and continuous with deep aspects of the rostrum, genu and anterior part of the trunk of corpus callosum; posteriorly the trunk fuses with the body of fornix (*see Fig.* 9.6). A *transverse fissure*, containing the tela choroidea of the third ventricle, posterior choroidal arteries and great cerebral vein, is inferior to the splenium. Callosal fibres traverse the medullary centres of the hemispheres to reach the cortex. Fibres of the rostrum interconnect the orbital surfaces of the frontal lobes. Fibres in the genu radiate forwards as the *forceps minor* to the medial and lateral surfaces of the frontal lobes. Fibres in the callosal trunk pass laterally to extensive areas of the cortex, intersecting the corona radiata en route. Fibres from the splenium curving posteriorly into the occipital lobes form the *forceps major* which bulges into the medial ventricular wall as the *bulb of the posterior horn* (*see Fig.* 10.3). Those fibres which arch over the posterior horn's roof and lateral wall, and over the lateral wall of the inferior horn, constitute the *tapetum*, a thin white lamina between ependyma and optic radiation (*see Fig.* 8.5).

The *anterior commissure* is an oval bundle which crosses in the upper part of the lamina terminalis, immediately in front of the columns of the fornix. Laterally it divides into two fasciculi, unequal in size. The anterior fibres pass from the anterior olfactory nucleus of one side to the olfactory bulb of the other and in humans they are few in number. Posterior fibres form a large bundle that deeply grooves the inferior aspects of the lentiform nuclei en route to anterior regions of the temporal lobes, including the parahippocampal gyri.

Commissural fibres are essential for the interhemispheric transfer of information for bilateral responses and in learning processes. Commissural fibres between occipital lobes, significant in stereoscopy, are limited to narrow boundary zones between the visual cortical areas (p. 213). There are no commissural connexions between cortical areas representing the hands, or between those for the feet. Severance of the corpus callosum in young monkeys causes a 'split brain' effect: trained to perform a task with one forepaw, they are unable to replicate the act with the other paw. Section of the optic chiasma and splenium prevents the interchange of visual information between hemispheres. In treating disabling epilepsy it is sometimes necessary to divide the corpus callosum. Not only the brain, but also the the mind is then divided: two 'individuals' in one body may produce bizarre effects. One hand may tie the dressing-gown cord, the other hand unties it. Only one side of the brain is literate, so the left hand may try to close a book which is is being read and held in the right hand, or slap the face when watching a television programme.

Projection fibres

Corticofugal fibres project to the spinal cord, brainstem and diencephalon as corticospinal, corticobulbar, extrapyramidal (corticostriate, corticorubral, cortico-olivary, corticoreticular, corticonigral), corticopontine, corticothalamic and hypothalamic connexions. *Corticopetal* fibres relay from thalamus to cortex, except for olfactory input. Almost all efferent fibres traverse the internal capsule; some corticostriate fibres enter the external capsule; thalamocortical fibres *ascend into* the internal capsule. Between internal capsule and cortex fibres fan out as the *corona radiata*.

Functional Localization

As already noted, the cerebral cortex is not divided into exclusively somatomotor and somatosensory regions. The pre- and postcentral areas are both sensorimotor, the former predominantly motor, the latter mostly sensory. There are supplementary somatomotor and somatosensory areas. The *relative* significance of these functional attributes can be expressed in an abbreviated form as follows: precentral somatomotor = Ms I, supplementary somatomotor = Ms II; primary somatosensory = Sm I, supplementary somatosensory = Sm II. There are also visual and auditory primary sensory areas. Almost all the cortex supplies corticopontine fibres (from pyramidal neurons in the outer part of lamina V), which relay to the cerebellum.

The cortex can be regarded as consisting of two main types, 'primary' motor and sensory areas (mostly heterotypical in structure) and association areas (homotypical); but this is merely a convenient simplification of its complexities. The association areas have increased relatively throughout evolution to reach their summit in humans (86% of the human cortex, 11% in the rat). Much of our understanding of such areas derives from clinical investigation of localized cortical injury. The diverse functions of the association areas include the interpretation of sensory input in relation to experience, qualitative analysis, the correlation of differing modalities (e.g. visual and auditory), complex behavioural responses and all 'thought'.

Parietal lobe

The *primary somatosensory area*, Sm I, occupies the *postcentral gyrus*, extending to the medial surface of the *posterior part of the paracentral lobule (Fig.* 12.8); it receives input from the ventral posterior thalamic nucleus. Histologically there are three narrow strips of cortex (Brodmann areas 3, 1, 2); area 3, in the posterior wall of the central sulcus, has a granular heterotypical structure and responds to tactile stimuli; areas 1 and 2 have a homotypical structure and react to deep stimuli and joint movement. Nociceptive (pain or thermal) sensation reaches consciousness at thalamic level, but its qualitative and spatial evaluation is cortical. Gustatory impulses are received in the junctional region of the postcentral gyrus and insula.

The area of cortex concerned with a body region is related to its functional skill and innervation density rather than to size; cortical areas representing the mouth, face, eye and hand are disproportionately large (*Fig.* 12.9). The

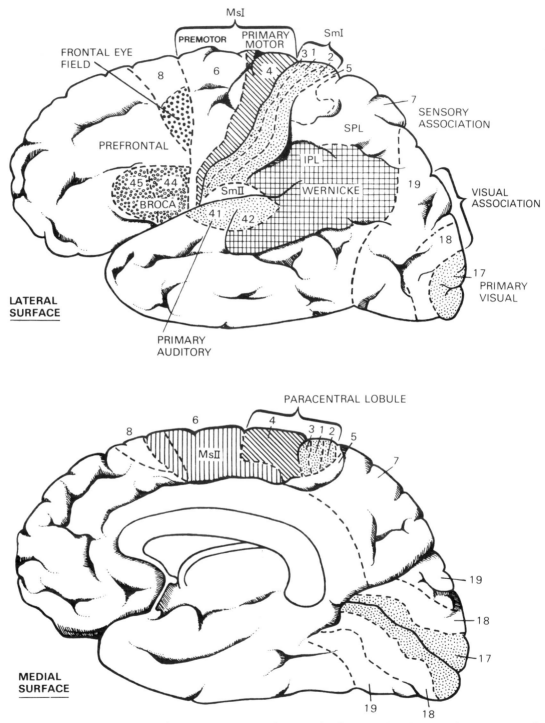

Fig. 12.8 The cerebral cortex showing the functional and cytoarchitectural (Brodmann) areas (1–45). **SPL**, superior parietal lobule; **IPL**, inferior parietal lobule; **Ms I**, precentral somatomotor; **Ms II**, supplementary somatomotor; **Sm I**, primary somatosensory; **Sm II**, supplementary somatosensory.

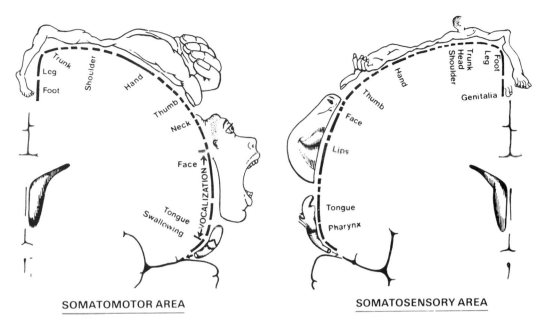

Fig. 12.9 Motor and sensory homunculi showing proportional somatotopic representation in the cortex. (After Penfield W. and Rasmussen T. (1950) *The Cerebral Cortex of Man*. New York, Macmillan.)

body image is inverted: the pharynx, tongue and jaws are inferolateral, followed by the face, hand, arm and trunk; the lower limb, anal and genital regions are superomedial and extend into the paracentral lobule. Most somatic input is contralateral, although some from the oral region is ipsilateral and the pharynx, larynx and perineum project bilaterally.

Localization is very discrete, for example each vibrissa of the rodent muzzle is represented by an aggregation, or 'barrel unit', of neurons in lamina IV. A tangential section in the plane of this cortical lamina reveals that the arrangement of units (barrelfield) corresponds precisely to the pattern of the whisker pad. It is noteworthy that although whisker pads are present on the muzzle when a mouse is born, cortical barrel units only start to develop three days later: peripheral stimulation has caused neurons to migrate into an organized cortical map. There is a critical post-natal period (day 1–6) during which deprivation of stimulation or destruction of hair follicle receptors prevents normal organization of this region of sensory cortex (Jeanmonod et al., 1981). Similar neuronal plasticity has been noted in the development of the visual cortex (p. 212), the critical period here in monkeys and cats extends from two weeks to four months after birth. The cortical effects of such sensory deprivation are most severe if they are prolonged and occur early in a critical phase, becoming less marked if applied later to a more mature system.

The *supplementary somatosensory area*, Sm II, is in the superior lip of the lateral fissure, with the face anterior and the lower limb posterior. It has connexions with Sm I and the thalamus, some being bilateral. Its functional significance is uncertain.

Somatosensory association area

The *superior parietal lobule* (areas 5, 7) has reciprocal connexions with Sm I and with the dorsal tier of lateral thalamic nuclei. It is concerned in discriminative aspects of sensation, such as the qualities of shape, roughness, size and texture, and also in remembering the positions of objects in space. It is responsible for a general awareness of the contralateral body image and the location of its parts. A lesion here may cause an inability to identify familiar objects manually (tactile agnosia). An afflicted individual may appear unaware of the side of the body opposite to the lesion, neglecting to wash or shave it.

The *inferior parietal lobule* (areas 39, 40) functions with the posterosuperior part of the temporal lobe; the combined region, *Wernicke's area*, is concerned with the interpretation of language through visual and auditory input. Sensory and motor 'speech areas' exist only in one hemisphere, in the left hemisphere of right-handed individuals, and this is the 'dominant hemisphere'. Damage results in word-blindness, *alexia*, and an inability to copy, *agraphia*, both being forms of *sensory aphasia*, the inability to understand written and spoken language.

Occipital lobe

The *primary visual area* (area 17) is in the upper and lower lips and depths of the calcarine sulcus, extending to the occipital pole and occasionally slightly beyond to the lateral surface. Input is from the lateral geniculate nucleus via the optic radiation (geniculo-calcarine tract). Histological features of the striate cortex have been described above; its columnar organization is described in Chapter 11. The orientation of lines and borders is detected here. The left visual field projects to the right visual cortex; the superior retinal quadrants (lower visual field) project to the upper wall of the calcarine sulcus, inferior quadrants (upper field) to the lower wall; the macula has extensive representation, occupying approximately the posterior third of the primary visual area.

The *visual association area* (areas 18, 19) occupies most of the remaining occipital cortex. It receives input from area 17 and has reciprocal connexions with the pulvinar. It is concerned with the further abstraction and analysis of visual information. Area 18 is necessary for stereoscopic vision, area 19 is concerned with eye movements and colour recognition; for recognition of complex patterns it is linked with the adjoining area 20 (posteroinferior temporal surface). As a centre for automatic scanning, its solitary cells (of Meynert) form a cortico-collicular connexion which, via the superior colliculus, coordinates involuntary eye movements, as in following moving objects. This area is linked with the 'frontal eye field' which activates voluntary scanning (*see* Control of eye movements, p. 140).

Temporal lobe

The human temporal neocortex is highly evolved; during development, part of it is submerged in the lateral fissure: two *transverse temporal gyri* (of Heschl) form its floor, bounded medially by the *insula*. The inferomedial margin, derived from the more primitive allocortex, is in-rolled as the *hippocampal formation* in the floor of the lateral ventricle's inferior horn. The temporal lobe has diverse attributes such as linguistic interpretation, auditory, vestibular and visceral functions; its anterior pole ('psychical cortex') and hippocampal formation are involved in memory and behaviour. Connexions with the limbic system extend the functions of the temporal lobe beyond its physical boundaries.

The *primary auditory area* (areas 41, 42) is mostly in the two transverse temporal gyri (of Heschl), extending slightly to the outer surface of the superior temporal gyrus. Area 41 is heterotypical granular cortex; area 42 is homotypical and is mainly an auditory association area. Input from the medial geniculate nucleus is via the auditory radiation, which also includes some efferent fibres which descend to medial geniculate nucleus and inferior colliculus, concerned with selectivity and neural sharpening. A tonotopic cortical representation has been described, with low frequencies anterior and high frequencies posterior. Since auditory input is bilateral, a unilateral cortical lesion causes some deafness in both ears; if the damaged area is in the dominant hemisphere, comprehension of language is affected. The *auditory association* area is posteroinferior to the primary cortex; in the dominant hemisphere it functions with the inferior parietal lobule as Wernicke's area, essential to linguistic comprehension.

Vestibular representation is imperfectly defined; it is contralateral and adjoins the 'face area' of Sm I. The *insula*, deeply submerged in the lateral fissure, is surrounded by a circular sulcus and overlapped by parts of the frontal, parietal and temporal lobes, termed the *opercula;* stimulation in humans evokes visceromotor and sensory effects such as nausea, salivation, gastrointestinal movements and alterations in blood pressure.

The *anterior part of the temporal lobe* ('psychical cortex') is described in Chapter 10. If it is removed bilaterally, together with the hippocampal formations, the abnormal behaviour of the Klüver-Bucy syndrome results. Stimulation may evoke visual or auditory memories of past events, tumours may cause visual or auditory hallucinations. Lesions of the uncus may be associated with olfactory and gustatory hallucinations known as 'uncinate fits'.

Complex visual *pattern recognition* is located in the posteroinferior part of the temporal lobe (area 20), adjoining the visual association cortex. In particular, a localized lesion here produces the rare condition of *prosopagnosia*, inability to recognise familiar faces.

Frontal lobe

The frontal cortex is divisible into a somatomotor *precentral region*, anterior to the central sulcus, and a larger *prefrontal association cortex*.

The precentral region or *first somatomotor area*, Ms I, includes the *precentral gyrus* (area 4) and the *premotor area* (area 6); the latter occupies the posterior parts of superior, middle and inferior frontal gyri. Both are agranular heterotypical cortex with numerous pyramidal neurons, but they differ physiologically; it is hence customary to designate areas 4 and 6 as 'primary motor' and 'premotor' respectively. A great deal of interacting information underlies all 'executive' responses by the motor cortex: the corpus striatum and cerebellum process input from widespread areas of cortex and project to Ms I via the ventral anterior and ventral lateral thalamic nuclei prior to motor activation. Though it is the major source of corticospinal and corticobulbar fibres, some of these originate in the somatosensory areas posterior to the central sulcus. The frontal eye field and motor speech area are immediately anterior to the premotor area.

The *primary motor area* (area 4) is in the anterior wall of the central sulcus and adjacent precentral gyrus, extending to the anterior part of the paracentral lobule on the medial surface, an area wider above than below (*Fig.* 12.8). Giant pyramidal cells (of Betz), up to 120 μm in diameter, are most numerous in its superomedial part: only about 3% of the pyramidal fibres originate in them, the majority being derived from medium-sized pyramidal neurons. Approximately 30% of pyramidal fibres (corticospinal and corticobulbar) come from area 4, 30% from area 6, the remainder from the parietal lobe. Somatotopic representation in area 4 is in the form of an inverted homunculus (*Fig.* 12.9) in which the size of bodily regions is related to motor skill rather than to muscle bulk: thus the face, tongue, larynx and hand are disproportionately large, the trunk and lower extremities small. Appropriate electrical stimulation usually produces simple contraction of contralateral muscle groups. Skilled movements require intricate synaptic interactions which cannot be experimentally evoked. Bilateral movements occur in the masticatory, laryngeal, pharyngeal, upper facial and extra-ocular muscles. There are also 'centres' for the control of micturition and defaecation in the superomedial parts of the frontal lobes. Ablation of area 4 in primates initially results in flaccid paralysis, then partial recovery with impairment of skill, particularly in fine digital movements and in the distal limb muscles. Excessive stimulation produces 'pattern convulsions' similar to Jacksonian epilepsy, spreading from a focus in orderly progression throughout the body.

The *premotor area* (area 6), anterior to the primary motor area, is wider above than below and extends onto the medial surface. It is closely associated with area 4 in the planning and control of movement. The cortical origins of extrapyramidal fibres (corticostriate, corticoreticular, corticorubral, cortico-olivary) are diffuse, but many arise from this area. To produce movements experimentally, stronger stimulation is required here than in area 4 and resultant movement patterns are more generalized and often postural, such as rotation of head and trunk, flexion or extension of limbs. Lesions produce weakness of axial and proximal limb muscles, affecting posture and gait.

The *supplementary motor area*, Ms II, is on the medial surface of the frontal lobe, anterior to the paracentral lobule (area 6, part of 8). In monkeys the body is represented horizontally, with the head anterior. Reports of experimental studies on Ms II have varied. Stimulation produces movements which are mostly bilateral and postural in nature; bilateral lesions markedly affect motor function and also cause loss of speech. Its significance in humans is unclear.

The *frontal eye field*, situated posteriorly in the middle frontal gyrus, occupies the lower part of area 8 and adjacent parts of areas 6 and 9. Stimulation causes contralateral conjugate ocular deviation. It is the 'centre for voluntary scanning', for consciously-directed eye movements, as in searching visual fields for particular features.

The *motor speech area of Broca* (areas 44, 45) is situated posteriorly in the inferior frontal gyrus of the dominant hemisphere, on the left side in right-handed individuals, the same side as Wernicke's area. Dominance of one hemisphere is genetically determined; right or left handedness may be influenced by educational and other factors. Lesions in this area result in *motor aphasia:* although language is understood, it cannot be expressed in speech or writing.

The *prefrontal area* includes those parts of the frontal lobe not yet described. It has reciprocal connexions with dorsal medial and anterior thalamic nuclei through the anterior thalamic radiation, and with the hypothalamus; frontopontine fibres project to the cerebellum via the nuclei pontis. Association fibres connect with the parietal, occipital and temporal lobes. Commissural fibres of the forceps minor and the genu of corpus callosum (to medial and lateral surfaces) and from the rostrum (to orbital surfaces) unite corresponding areas of prefrontal cortex of both sides. Until the discovery of specific anti-depressant drugs, prefrontal leucotomy was sometimes performed, bilaterally severing the connexions between thalamus and the orbito-frontal cortex. The post-operative sequelae illustrate some functions of this area, for example relieved depression, altered affective tone and reduced emotional content of pain. Extensive bilateral frontal lobe injuries have a detrimental effect not only on emotional balance, but on behaviour and intellect, resulting in a profound change of personality. The prefrontal cortex is concerned with depth of emotion, with social, moral and ethical awareness, and with the ability to concentrate, to elaborate ideas and to solve problems; it is also concerned with planning, foresight, judgement, the correlation and evaluation of information and the choice of appropriate responses.

General Considerations

Cerebral dominance

In manual dexterity and linguistic skill the left hemisphere is genetically dominant in right-handed individuals; the human brain appears unique in this respect. Left-handedness is a less definite phenomenon and is not necessarily related to cerebral dominance. Imperfectly developed dominance may be associated with difficulties in reading, writing, drawing and spatial analysis. The dominant hemisphere is concerned with language, speech, mathematical and analytical functions. The non-dominant hemisphere processes spatial, geometrical and pictorial information; though almost 'illiterate', it is necessary for musical appreciation and expression. The myelination and function of the corpus callosum are incomplete until two or three years after birth, during which time both hemispheres process linguistic information. Young children sustaining damage to a dominant left hemisphere can become skilfully left-handed and can learn to speak, read and write, utilizing the early neural plasticity which is lost as age progresses. (For further reviews of neural plasticity *see* Stein et al., 1974; Cotman, 1978; Milgram et al., 1987; Petit and Ivy, 1988.)

Sleep

Sleep was regarded as a purely passive state, a nocturnal depression of the reticular activating system due to fatigue. It is now known to be an active and complex process with two contrasting and alternating intrinsic rhythms, separately identifiable by encephalography and controlled from brainstem centres by specific neurotransmitters.

Slow wave sleep is characterized by synchronized high voltage, low frequency, encephalographic waves. Most muscles relax, but postural adjustments occur. There is parasympathetic dominance: the heart rate and blood pressure decrease, respiration is slow and regular and gastrointestinal movements are increased.

Paradoxical sleep, occurring at intervals during the night, is associated with ocular movements, and is named 'paradoxical' because encephalography shows desynchronized, low voltage, fast waves, like those seen in the waking state. Sympathetic activity evokes a raised heart rate and blood pressure, respiration is rapid and irregular and gastrointestinal movements are decreased. Muscle tone is depressed, apart from characteristic bursts of rapid eye movements; hence the alternative name 'REM sleep'. The ocular movements are triggered by phasic electrical activity in the pontine reticular formation, lateral geniculate nuclei and occipital cortex, known as ponto-geniculo-occipital (PGO) spikes; these are probably initiated by ascending impulses from the medial and inferior vestibular nuclei.

The *pontine raphe nuclei* contain serotonin and are involved in slow wave sleep; those in the caudal pons act as a priming mechanism for paradoxical sleep. Damage to the nuclei of the raphe is said to produce total insomnia. The *locus ceruleus*, near the periaqueductal grey matter, contains noradrenaline (norepinephrine) and is active in paradoxical sleep; there is also evidence that acetylcholine is involved in this process. These complex interrelationships are incompletely understood.

Memory

It is necessary to distinguish between input, storage and retrieval of information. The hippocampal formations have a particular role in memory input; lesions of the limbic system may impair this. The anterior parts of the temporal lobe appear to be concerned not only with input but also with storage: electrical stimulation may result in recall of previous experience. Learning requires a storage of information. Experimental ablation of any area of the cortex slows the rate of learning in proportion to the area lost; certain regions have additional specific contributions, for example the visual and auditory regions. Even mild but diffuse cortical compression, as by chronic subdural haematoma, leads to impaired learning and memory.

The extent of dendritic fields and complexity of intracortical circuits increase in response to sustained and varied input; conversely, inactivity causes thinning of the cortex. There is continual synaptic turnover and remodelling (Jones, 1988). Blindness leads to atrophy of the visual cortex, and neonatal monocular deprivation permanently affects ocular dominance (*see* p. 212). The plasticity of the central nervous system is most active in youth. 'Old dogs cannot learn new tricks', but experience and the resultant ability to evaluate increases with age. Old age generally entails defective memory for recent events, recall of distant events being unaffected; this is a normal phenomenon, differing from 'senile dementia' (Alzheimer's disease), in which there is generalized cerebral atrophy, often with a profound change in personality. The reverberating circuits which encode short-term memory may be disrupted by deep anaesthesia or trauma, leaving long-term memory unaffected; this implies a more permanent physical change for the latter, probably based on selective facilitation of presynaptic terminals. The prefrontal cortex is necessary for the motivation and concentration required in complex learning processes.

APPLIED ANATOMY

Functional correlations of cortical areas have been mentioned in this chapter. Damage to these may result from a cerebrovascular accident, such as haemorrhage, thrombosis or embolism, or from cerebral tumours, other forms of intracranial compression, or in head injuries (*see* also p. 286). Localizing symptoms are summarized here.

Motor cortex. Damage to the *precentral area* produces spastic paralysis of the contralateral limbs; normally extrapyramidal fibres from this area inhibit muscle tone. If one *frontal eye field* is affected, the eyes 'look to the side of the lesion'. Destruction of the *motor speech area* results in expressive (motor) aphasia or an inability to speak, linguistic comprehension being unaffected.

An unusual example of neural plasticity is demonstrated in a middle-aged patient who, as a young child, had the right cerebral hemisphere removed because of severe epilepsy; although he has little useful movement of the left hand, he can walk almost normally. In such cases, areas of the developing central nervous system may assume some of the functions of missing components; this capacity is lost after early childhood.

Sensory cortex. Lesions of the *primary somatosensory area* result in contralateral loss of sensory discrimination, although crude awareness, particularly of nociceptive stimuli, is retained at thalamic level. Dysfunction of the *somatosensory association areas* leads to tactile agnosia, that is inability to appreciate three-dimensional shape (astereognosis), size, weight or texture when identifying familiar objects by touch; there is also a lack of awareness of the body's contralateral side. The non-dominant parietal lobe has a more general capacity for pictorial and spatial analysis; lesions may result in an inability to arrange the sequential components of complex movements, a form of apraxia. Sensory aphasia, the inability to recognize spoken or written words, follows damage to *Wernicke's area* in the dominant hemisphere. Lesions of the *primary visual area* cause contralateral visual field loss proportional to the extent of the damage. Defects of the *visual association areas* impair visual recognition; local damage to the postero-inferior surface of the temporal lobe produces prosopagnosia, an inability to remember faces. A lesion in the lateral fissure may affect the *primary auditory area* causing partial bilateral deafness, the vestibular area causing vertigo, and the insula causing visceral effects such as nausea, salivation and altered blood pressure. The personality may be severely affected by bilateral damage to the *prefrontal cortex* or the *temporal lobes*.

Research

Fetal neurons may survive when implanted experimentally into senile rat brains; cells containing acetylcholine appear to improve memory, dopamine cells improve balance. Experiments also suggest a possibility that Alzheimer's disease may be ameliorated by non-fetal cell transplantation: fibroblasts, modified by genetic engineering to produce 'nerve growth factor' and injected into rat brains appear to halt degeneration. Neuron transplantation in Parkinson's disease and Huntington's disease is reviewed on page 196.

Chapter 13

Meninges, cerebrospinal fluid and cerebral ventricles

Three continuous membranes or *meninges*, the dura mater, arachnoid mater and pia mater, surround the brain and spinal cord. Their intracranial arrangement differs from that in the vertebral canal and will be described separately.

Intracranial Meninges

Dura mater

This is often regarded as bilaminar, with an external *endosteal layer* of periosteum, continuous through cranial foramina and sutures with the pericranium, and an internal *meningeal layer*, a strong fibrous membrane continuous with the vertebral dura mater at the foramen magnum. The meningeal dura mater and endosteum are adherent except where *dural venous sinuses* intervene. Meningeal dura mater ensheathes the cranial nerves in their osseous foramina, fusing externally with their epineurium; the sheaths of the optic nerves fuse with the ocular sclera.

The meningeal dura mater is infolded as septa between parts of the brain (*Fig. 13.1*). The sickle-shaped median *falx cerebri*, between the cerebral hemispheres, is narrow anteriorly where it is attached to the ethmoid crista galli and wider posteriorly where it joins the horizontal tentorium cerebelli. Its upper convex margin, attached to endosteum parasagittally as far as the internal occipital protruberance, encloses a *superior sagittal sinus;* its unattached lower concave edge contains an *inferior sagittal sinus*. The *straight sinus*, formed by the junction of inferior sagittal sinus and great cerebral vein, runs in the attachment of the falx cerebri to the tentorium cerebelli.

The *tentorium cerebelli*, roofing the posterior cranial fossa, is between the cerebellum and the cerebral occipital lobes. Its free edge bounds the *tentorial incisure*, traversed by the midbrain. Its peripheral border is attached to the margins of the bony grooves for the *transverse sinuses*, to the superior edges of the petrous temporal bones (where it encloses *superior petrosal sinuses*) and to the posterior clinoid processes of the sphenoid bone. The free edge extends forwards to the anterior clinoid processes, crossing the attached border. The triangular interval between free and attached borders is pierced by oculomotor and trochlear nerves as they enter the lateral wall of the

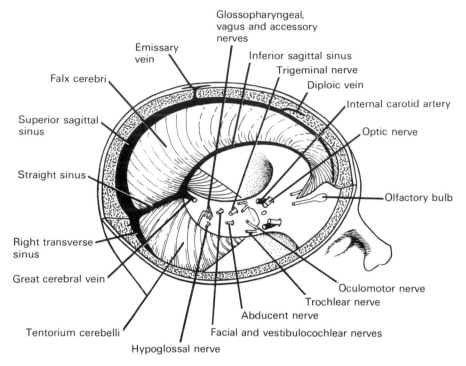

*Fig.*13.1 Cerebral dura mater, its reflexions and dural venous sinuses viewed from the superolateral aspect, the brain having been removed.

cavernous sinus on each side. Near the apices of the petrous temporal bones, the meningeal dura mater is evaginated under each superior petrosal sinus as a *cavum trigeminale*, partially enclosing the trigeminal ganglion.

The smaller *falx cerebelli* extends down from the tentorium cerebelli in the posterior cerebellar notch; at its attachment to the internal occipital crest it encloses an *occipital sinus*. The *diaphragma sellae* roofs the sella turcica and is perforated by the pituitary infundibulum.

The *dural arterial supply* is from numerous branches of the internal carotid, ascending pharyngeal, maxillary, occipital and vertebral arteries. The *middle meningeal artery*, branching from the maxillary artery, traverses the foramen spinosum to lie between the endosteal and meningeal layers of dura mater. Its anterior and posterior branches groove and supply bones of the cranial vault; the meningeal veins lie between the arteries and bone.

The anterior (frontal) branch crosses the pterion, the posterior (parietal) ascends backwards towards the lambda. A fracture of the thin squamous temporal bone may cause a 'middle meningeal haemorrhage' from the artery or vein, producing an *extra-dural haematoma*. The nerve supply to the supratentorial dura is trigeminal, while the infratentorial supply is from the vagus and the upper three cervical nerves.

Dural venous sinuses (*Figs* 13.1, 13.2, *see Figs* 6.15 and 14.6)

The venous sinuses are between the meningeal and endosteal layers of dura mater; they are lined by endothelium, have no valves, and drain to the internal jugular veins. They receive cerebral, diploic and meningeal tributaries and, through skull foramina, communicate via valveless emissary veins with extracranial vessels. Because of the free communication with veins of the face and scalp, cutaneous sepsis may cause infective thrombosis of an intracranial sinus.

The *superior sagittal sinus*, in the attached border of the falx cerebri, extends from the foramen caecum (where it may communicate with nasal veins) to the internal occipital protruberance, continuing there usually into the right transverse sinus at the *confluence of the sinuses*. Here it communicates with the left transverse, occipital and straight sinuses. Large clusters of *arachnoid villi*, concerned in the absorption of cerebrospinal fluid, form *arachnoid granulations* projecting into the *venous lacunae* of the superior

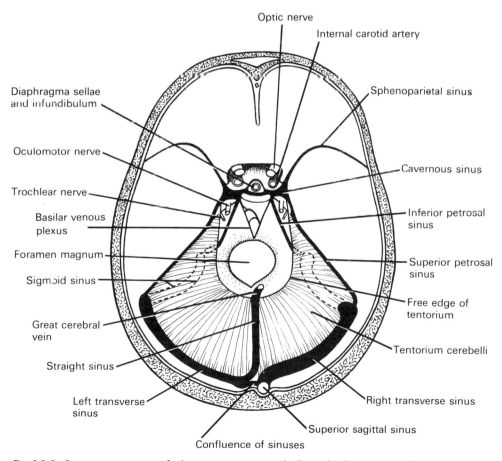

Fig. 13.2 Superior aspect of the tentorium cerebelli with the venous sinuses exposed.

sagittal sinus (*Fig.* 13.3). As these granulations enlarge with age they create parasagittal depressions in the inner surface of the cranial vault. *Superior cerebral veins* ascend to reach the superior sagittal sinus and its lacunae; **they traverse the subdural space** (between dura and arachnoid): traumatic posterior displacement of the brain may tear these veins, causing *subdural haemorrhage*.

The *inferior sagittal sinus*, in the lower border of falx cerebri, receives veins from the falx and medial cerebral surfaces. It joins the great cerebral vein to form the *straight sinus* at the junction of falx cerebri and tentorium cerebelli. At the confluence of sinuses the straight sinus usually turns into the left transverse sinus.

The paired *transverse sinuses*, in the attached margin of the tentorium cerebelli, groove the occipital bone; they become *sigmoid sinuses* on the inner surface of the mastoid temporal bones, continuing as the internal jugular veins at the jugular foramina. A chronic middle ear infection involving mastoid air cells may cause an infective thrombosis in the adjacent sigmoid sinus. Each transverse sinus receives the superior petrosal sinus, the inferior anastomotic vein, inferior cerebral and cerebellar veins. The small *occipital sinus* in the falx cerebelli, between the confluence of sinuses and foramen magnum, communicates there with the sigmoid sinus and the vertebral venous plexus.

Cavernous sinuses (*see Fig.* 6.15) flank each side of the body of sphenoid from superior orbital fissure to the apex of petrous temporal, and are so named because of their internal trabeculation. Each is traversed by an internal carotid artery, its sympathetic plexus and an abducent nerve, covered by endothelium. In the lateral wall of each sinus, between meningeal

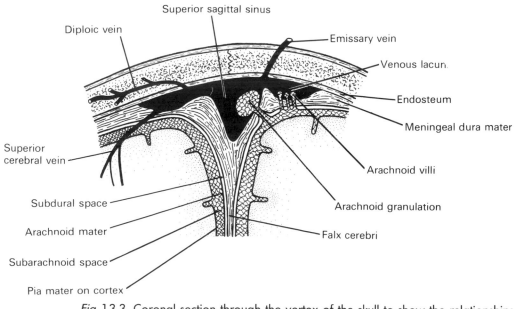

Fig. 13.3 Coronal section through the vertex of the skull to show the relationships of the superior sagittal sinus and the meninges.

dura mater and endothelium, are the oculomotor, trochlear, ophthalmic and maxillary nerves. The two sinuses are interconnected by veins in the diaphragma sellae; anteriorly they communicate with *ophthalmic veins*, and hence with facial veins; facial infection may thus spread to cavernous sinuses, a potentially fatal event prior to the discovery of antibiotics. Each sinus receives input from the *superficial middle cerebral vein* and the *sphenoparietal sinus*, a small channel under the lesser wing of sphenoid. A *basilar venous plexus* crosses the clivus to the foramen magnum, communicating there with the internal vertebral venous plexus. Posteriorly each cavernous sinus drains via a *superior petrosal sinus* to the transverse sinus, and via an *inferior petrosal sinus* through the jugular foramen to the internal jugular's bulb. A number of *emissary veins* connect each cavernous sinus with the pterygoid and pharyngeal venous plexuses through the foramina ovale, spinosum and lacerum.

Arachnoid mater and pia mater

Between the meningeal dura mater and arachnoid mater a cleavage plane, the *subdural space*, is traversed only by cerebral veins en route to the dural venous sinuses. In contrast, the *subarachnoid space*, between the arachnoid mater and pia mater, contains a web of trabeculae (arachnoid = spidery), cerebrospinal fluid, cerebral arteries and veins. Vascular *pia mater* follows the contours of gyri and sulci, closely applied to the cortical surface.

Until recently it was thought that the subarachnoid space continued around blood vessels as they entered the cortex: our present understanding is illustrated in *Fig*. 13.4. Perivascular pial sheaths in the subarachnoid space continue round intracerebral arteries, but not veins. This probably prevents the noradrenergic innervation of intracerebral arteries from affecting brain tissue (Zhang et al., 1990). A *subpial space*, recently described, extends around penetrating blood vessels; its function is imperfectly understood. In the rat there is very rapid transport from the surface of the brain to retropharyngeal lymph nodes, probably via subpial and perivascular spaces (Weller, 1990).

The *arachnoid mater* is a delicate, impermeable, avascular membrane; unlike the pia mater, it bridges sulci and other surface irregularities. The width of the subarachnoid space is therefore variable, narrow over gyri, wider over sulci and cerebral fissures, and wider still at the cerebral base, where it forms subarachnoid cisterns (*Fig*. 13.5). Into the largest, the *cerebellomedullary cistern* (cisterna magna), between the cerebellum and medulla, cerebrospinal fluid escapes from the fourth ventricle via the median and lateral apertures (of Magendie and Luschka). Other cisterns are the *pontine, interpeduncular, chiasmatic* and *superior*. The superior cistern with the subarachnoid spaces flanking the midbrain are termed the *cisterna ambiens* by clinicians: it contains the great cerebral vein and the posterior cerebral and superior cerebellar arteries. (The cisterns and ventricles can be examined radiographically, *see* Applied anatomy.)

The subarachnoid space surrounds each cranial nerve for a short distance at its foramen. Around the optic nerves the space reaches the sclera; the

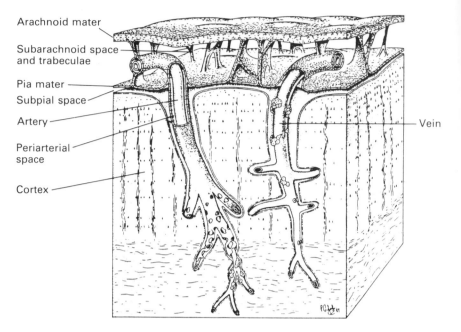

Arachnoid mater

Subarachnoid space
and trabeculae

Pia mater

Subpial space

Artery

Periarterial
space

Cortex

Vein

Fig. 13.4 The relationships of the pia mater to intracerebral arteries and veins. (From Zhang E.T., Inman C.B.E., and Weller R.O. (1990), *J. Anat.*, **170**, 120. Reproduced by kind permission of the authors and publisher.)

central retinal artery and vein cross it, and raised cerebrospinal fluid pressure may compress the vein, causing oedema of the optic disc or *papilloedema*.

Ventricular choroid plexuses develop where the pia mater and ependyma are in contact (*see* below, cerebrospinal fluid).

Spinal Meninges

The *spinal dura mater*, continuous with the intracranial meningeal dura mater, is attached to the edge of the foramen magnum, the bodies of the second and third cervical vertebrae and the posterior longitudinal vertebral ligament. *Arachnoid mater* adheres to the internal aspect of the dura, and both meninges extend to the level of the second sacral vertebra. The dura mater and arachnoid mater are evaginated by the spinal nerve roots, fusing with the epineurium just beyond the dorsal root ganglia (*see Fig.* 4.2). A narrow *extradural (epidural) space*, traversed by nerve roots, also contains a valveless vertebral venous plexus, arteries, fat and lymphatics. A local anaesthetic injected into the space affects nerve roots, in 'epidural anaesthesia'. The *pia mater* closely invests the spinal cord and roots, thickened along its ventral fissure as a midline *linea splendens* and drawn out on each side as a *denticulate ligament* with twenty-one 'teeth' that are attached to the arachnoid and dura mater. The spinal *subarachnoid space* is not trabecular.

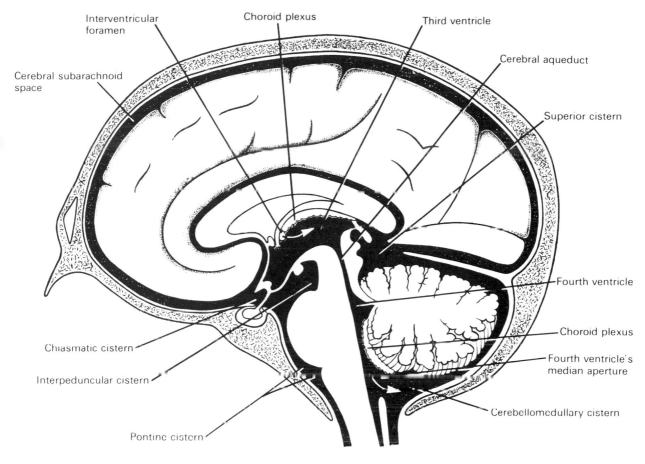

Fig. 13.5 Median sagittal section to show the subarachnoid cisterns. Arrows in the interventricular foramen and in the median aperture of the fourth ventricle indicate the circulation of cerebrospinal fluid.

Distal to the spinal cord, the *lumbar cistern* extends from second lumbar to second sacral vertebrae and contains the cauda equina (lumbosacral nerve roots) and filum terminale. A needle may be inserted safely into the cistern in the third or fourth lumbar interspinous spaces; if strictly median this should not touch the nerve roots.

Cerebrospinal Fluid

Cerebrospinal fluid (CSF) is secreted by choroid plexuses in all the ventricles, but mostly into the lateral ventricles, whose plexuses are the largest. Where the pia mater and its vessels contact ependyma during development, these form a double membrane with vascular fringes, the *tela choroidea* (*see* development, Chapter 1). As the cerebral hemispheres and corpus callosum

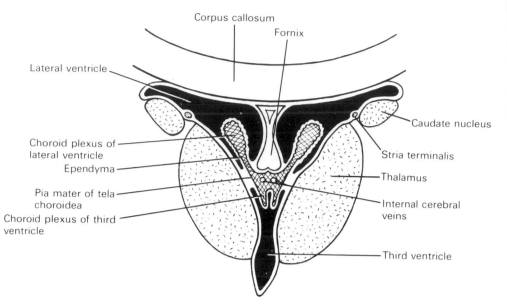

Fig. 13.6 Coronal section posterior to the interventricular foramen showing the choroid plexuses of the third and lateral ventricles.

grow caudally, the tela choroidea becomes trapped between them. Thus the tela enters the *transverse fissure* between the splenium above and tectum of midbrain below, and extends forward between the body of fornix and roof of third ventricle. The arrangement of choroid plexuses in the lateral and third ventricles is shown in *Figs* 13.6 and 13.7, and in the fourth ventricle in *Fig.* 5.5. The tela choroidea roofs the third ventricle, and plexuses in its margins invaginate the ependyma of each lateral ventricle through a *choroid fissure*. Interposed between telencephalon and diencephalon, this fissure is C-shaped, extending on each side posteriorly from the interventricular foramen: in the lateral ventricle's body it is bounded superiorly by fornix, inferiorly by thalamus; in the inferior horn it is between stria terminalis above and fimbria below.

A choroid plexus has a convoluted surface, covered by a single layer of specialized cuboidal epithelium whose cells have a distinct basement membrane and apical microvilli (*Fig.* 13.8). Tight junctions between these cells form a *blood–CSF barrier*. The presence of numerous mitochondria and enzymes such as adenosine triphosphate indicates that CSF is not a mere filtrate; its selective secretion involves energy-dependent active intracellular transport. The underlying stroma contains many capillaries, some fenestrated, supplied by the anterior and posterior choroidal branches of the internal carotid and posterior cerebral arteries respectively.

A brain of 1500 g weighs only 50 g when submerged in CSF. The fluid cushion protects the brain by limiting its displacement during sudden acceleration or deceleration of head movement. Cerebrospinal fluid provides

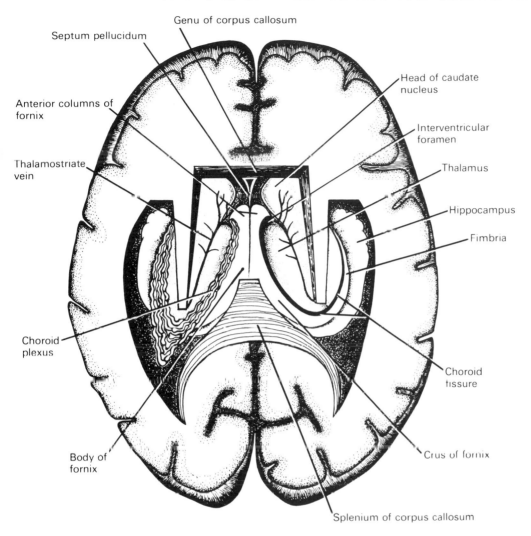

Septum pellucidum

Genu of corpus callosum

Head of caudate
nucleus

Anterior columns of
fornix

Interventricular
foramen

Thalamus

Thalamostriate
vein

Hippocampus

Fimbria

Choroid
plexus

Choroid
fissure

Body of
fornix

Crus of fornix

Splenium of corpus callosum

Fig. 13.7 A dissection of the lateral ventricles viewed from the superior aspect: on the right side the choroid plexus has been removed to reveal the choroid fissure.

the special environment essential for neural tissue: there is no barrier to diffusion between them. It has a much lower protein content than blood plasma (6.5 g protein/100 g plasma; 0.025 g protein/100 g CSF); the glucose content is about half that of blood, the chloride content slightly more in CSF. Normally clear and colourless, with a specific gravity of 1.003–1.008, it has less than 5 lymphocytes/mm³. In bacterial meningitis the fluid is cloudy, with raised protein content and a vastly increased number of cells. Analysis of CSF has diagnostic value in many central nervous diseases.

Cerebrospinal fluid volume averages 140 ml, of which about 30 ml is intraventricular. About 500 ml is secreted daily, passing from lateral

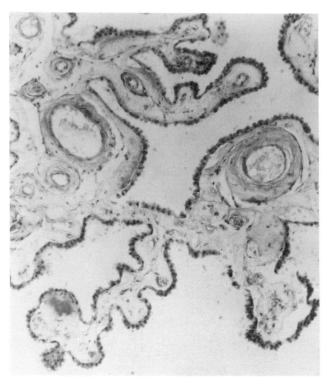

Fig. 13.8 A section of choroid plexus. Note the large capillaries and convoluted epithelium. (Haematoxylin and eosin, × 125.)

ventricles to third ventricle, via the cerebral aqueduct to the fourth ventricle and thence via median and lateral apertures to the subarachnoid space. Some fluid is also derived from neural metabolism and intracerebral capillaries, diffusing through pia mater into the subarachnoid space. Absorption into the venous sinuses is through the arachnoid villi, which act as one-way valves, opened when the CSF pressure exceeds the venous pressure. There is also some absorption via small spinal veins into the vertebral venous system.

The CSF pressure, 80–180 ml of saline, is measured with the patient horizontal, a needle in the lumbar cistern connected to a manometer. The pressure is increased by coughing, straining or sitting up. It is also raised by manual compression of the internal jugular veins, indicating normal communication between the cerebral and spinal subarachnoid spaces (Queckenstedt's sign).

Blood–brain Barrier

Selective filtration is necessary to provide the particular environment required by the central nervous system. The blood–brain and blood–CSF barriers and the free diffusion between brain and CSF are illustrated diagrammatically:

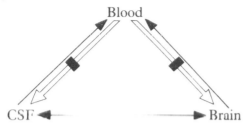

A blood–CSF barrier was noted above in the description of choroid plexuses.

Intravenous vital dyes stain most tissues except the brain. The blood–brain barrier of cerebral capillaries is formed largely by the continuous nature of their endothelial cells which are united by tight junctions. In addition, 85% of the surrounding capillary basal lamina is covered by the 'end feet' of astrocytes (*see Fig.* 2.7) which provide a selective nutritive path to neurons. Intravascular chemicals may enter the brain either because they are lipid-soluble and can cross membranes, or by active transport mechanisms in the endothelium and glia, which contain enzymes controlling the transport of amines, amino acids and sugars. Thus, dopamine cannot pass but L–dopa can; having entered the endothelium it is converted there to dopamine. In Parkinson's disease there is dopamine deficiency, alleviated by the administration of L–dopa.

Some diseases cause a 'breakdown' of the blood–brain barrier. Normally penicillin cannot enter the central nervous system: it has low lipid solubility, is bound to plasma albumin, and the choroid plexus transports it from the CSF to the blood. However, in bacterial meningitis, encephalitis and uraemia, penicillin crosses the barrier. There may also be a local breakdown in brain tumours; radioactive-labelled albumin then enters the tumour tissue selectively, facilitating diagnosis and localization.

Certain small cerebral regions with secretory functions have fenestrated capillaries; these include the pineal gland, neurohypophysis and hypothalamic median eminence. *Tanycytes*, specialized astrocytes interposed between ependymal cells in the third ventricle's floor, are able to transfer hormones in either direction between CSF and the pituitary portal system.

Topography of Cerebral Ventricles

For purposes of revision, ventricular relationships in the cerebrum are described here.

Lateral ventricles (*see Figs* 1.11; 9.2–9.6; 13.7)

These two cavities, lined by ependyma and filled with CSF, are within the cerebral hemispheres. Anteriorly they are separated only by the septum pellucidum and each communicates with the third ventricle via an interventricular foramen (of Monro); posteriorly and inferiorly they diverge. Each comprises a central body, anterior, posterior and inferior horns.

The *anterior horn*, anterior to the interventricular foramen, extends into the frontal lobe. It is triangular in coronal section. The roof and anterior wall are formed by the trunk and genu of corpus callosum. The convex surface of the head of caudate nucleus forms the lateral wall and most of the floor; the callosal rostrum enters the medial part of the floor. The medial wall is the septum pellucidum; a column of the fornix in the septum's postero-inferior border bounds the interventricular foramen.

The *body* extends from interventricular foramen to the level of the splenium. Its roof is the corpus callosum. The medial wall anteriorly is the septum pellucidum with the body of fornix in its inferior margin; posteriorly, behind the septum pellucidum, the corpus callosum and body of fornix are fused. The floor is formed medially by the upper surface of thalamus, laterally by the body of caudate nucleus, with the stria terminalis and thalamostriate vein in the groove between these. The choroid fissure is between fornix and thalamus; the tela choroidea is attached to the under surface of the fornix, covers much of the upper surface of the thalamus and has the choroid plexus in its lateral edge (*see Fig*. 14.6).

The *posterior horn*, variable in size, extends into the occipital lobe. Its roof and lateral walls are formed by tapetal fibres of corpus callosum. Fibres of the forceps major bulge into the medial wall as the bulb of the posterior horn; below this another elevation, the calcar avis, is produced by the deep calcarine sulcus.

The *inferior horn* (*Figs* 10.3 and 10.4) curves downwards round the posterior aspect of thalamus and passes forwards into the temporal lobe to within 2.5 cm of the temporal pole. The tapetum extends over the posterior part of the roof into the lateral wall. The tail of caudate nucleus and the stria terminalis are in the roof, reaching the amygdaloid nucleus at the tip of the horn. Laterally in the floor the deep collateral sulcus produces the collateral eminence. Medially in the floor is the hippocampus, covered by the alveus, fibres of which form the fimbria of the fornix; this continues posteriorly into the crus of the fornix. Between fimbria and stria terminalis the choroid plexus invaginates through the choroid fissure.

The third ventricle (*see Figs* 1.11, 8.1)

The cavity of the diencephalon is a narrow median cleft. It communicates with the lateral ventricles via interventricular foramina and with the fourth ventricle via the cerebral aqueduct.

Its *anterior boundary* is the lamina terminalis, extending from the optic chiasma to the anterior commissure and the rostrum of corpus callosum. On each side, behind the anterior commissure and in front of the interventricular foramen, the columns of the fornix arch down and sink into the lateral walls to reach the mamillary bodies.

Each *lateral wall* is formed by thalamus above, hypothalamus below:

separating these, the hypothalamic sulcus extends between interventricular foramen and cerebral aqueduct. The two thalami are closely approximated and usually linked by a thalamic connexus of grey matter. The lateral wall is limited above by the stria medullaris thalami.

The *floor* is mostly hypothalamic. In rostrocaudal sequence, behind the optic chiasma, are the infundibulum, tuber cinereum, mamillary bodies, subthalamus and midbrain tegmentum. In front of the optic chiasma is an optic recess, behind the chiasma an infundibular recess extends into the infundibulum.

The *posterior boundary* includes the cerebral aqueduct, posterior commissure, a pineal recess into the pineal stalk, habenular commissure and a suprapineal recess.

In the *roof* a thin layer of ependyma stretches between the striae medullares thalami. Blending with this, a double fold of pia mater forms the tela choroidea, from which two slender parasagittal choroid plexuses project into the third ventricle.

APPLIED ANATOMY

The cranium contains the brain, blood and CSF, an increase in the volume of any one of which results in the decrease of another. Compensation is possible within physiological limits, sneezing or straining cause transient venous congestion, but some CSF may be displaced through the foramen magnum.

In *hydrocephalus* the volume of CSF is increased and, before fusion of cranial sutures, a child's skull can greatly enlarge. In *internal hydrocephalus* the ventricular system is obstructed, commonly at the fourth ventricle's foramina, due to basal meningitis, but sometimes due to congenital stenosis of the aqueduct. In *communicating hydrocephalus* the obstruction is outside the brain, for example adhesions between the midbrain and tentorial incisure, or blockage of arachnoid granulations after meningitis. The brain is compressed and the cortex atrophies. In *senile dementia*, cerebral atrophy is accompanied by a compensatory enlargement of the subarachnoid space and ventricles.

Cerebral oedema, due to an impaired blood–brain barrier, may follow head injury, meningitis, cerebral anoxia, uraemia and other toxic conditions, leading to coma. *Raised intracranial pressure* causes papilloedema, slow pulse, raised blood pressure and impaired consciousness.

Radiological investigations

These include the injection of radio-opaque fluid into the internal carotid or vertebral arteries (cerebral *angiography, see Fig.* 14.5), injection of air into the ventricles (*ventriculography, Fig.* 13.9) or into the lumbar cistern (*encephalography*). These methods are now largely replaced by *computerized*

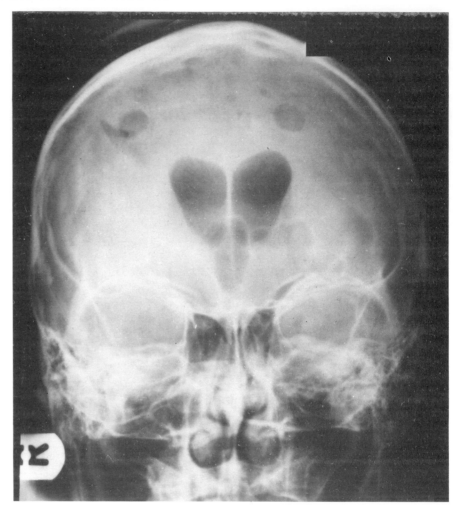

Fig. 13.9 A ventriculogram: air has been injected into the lateral ventricles through holes in the skull. Note the midline septum pellucidum.

tomography (CT scan, *Fig.* 13.10), a radiological technique producing serial cross-sections of the cranial contents and *magnetic resonance imaging* (MRI) (*Fig.* 13.11).

Whereas CT scans are based on tissue density, MRI also reflects biochemical composition. Protons of hydrogen atoms in body tissues act like small bar magnets, their north and south poles normally orientated at random. When an intense magnetic field is applied to the body the protons all line up with this (equilibrium position). A second electromagnetic field transmitted at an angle to the first causes them to flip from this position, returning to 'equilibrium' on its cessation. This 'nuclear magnetic resonance' produces radio signals which, with pulsed excitation, are converted into an MR image. Tissues behave differently according to their composition and biological

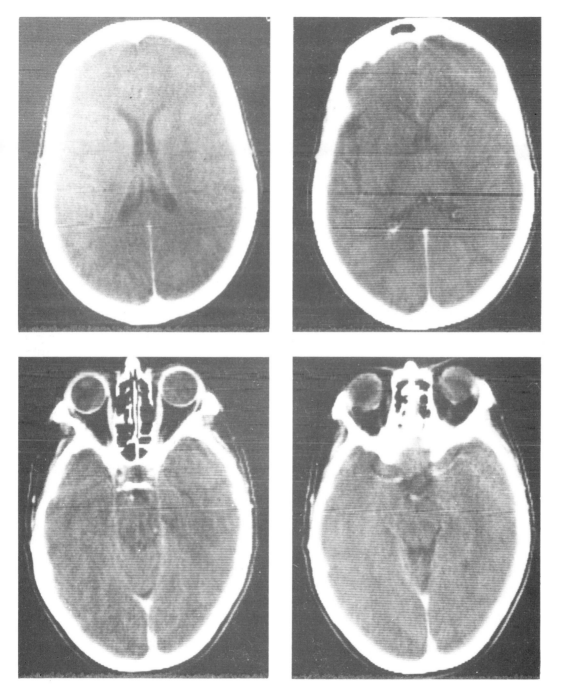

Fig. 13.10 Computerized tomography. These radiographic 'sections' of the brain
are taken at an angle of 25° to the base line of the skull.

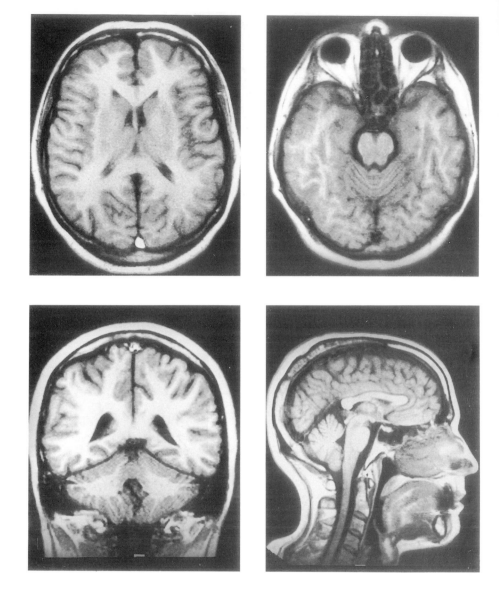

Fig. 13.11 Nuclear magnetic resonance scans. Compared with CT scans these have greater clarity, differentiate between tissues such as grey and white matter and are more versatile, being used in coronal and sagittal as well as transverse planes. (Films supplied by Bristol M.R.I. Centre.)

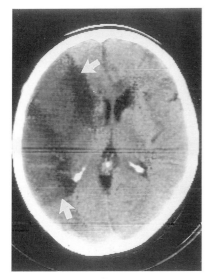

A

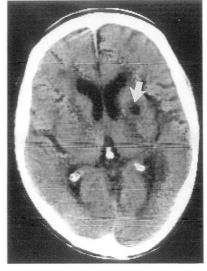

B

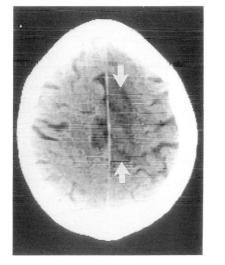

C

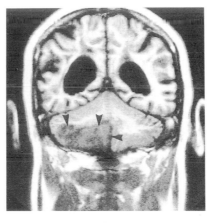

D

Fig. 13.12 Brain scans following arterial thrombosis: infarction is indicated by arrows. (A) Middle cerebral artery thrombosis: grey and white matter are affected (CT). (B) A single striate artery is occluded, producing a very localized infarct of the anterior limb of the internal capsule (CT). (C) Anterior cerebral artery infarct (pericallosal branch) (CT). (D) Posterior inferior cerebellar artery infarct (MRI). (Scans supplied by Frenchay Hospital, Bristol.)

state: grey matter can be distinguished from white matter; cortical surfaces are very distinct from surrounding CSF; a tumour, an infarct or an area of demyelination differs from normal adjacent tissues (*Fig.* 13.12).

Research: positron emission tomography

Positron emission tomography (PET) is a very specialized computerized radiographic scanning procedure which, unlike other methods, provides information about function. It differs from CT technically in that injected radio-labelled substances provide the source of radiation. In vivo biochemistry can be measured, using agents such as glucose, water, amino acids and oxygen. Positron emitting isotopes of carbon, oxygen, nitrogen and fluorine can be substituted chemically for non-radioactive in these natural substances: metabolic pathways and body functions can be studied qualitatively and quantitively. Thus blood flow studies use O-labelled water. A cyclotron produces the short-lived positron-rich radioactive isotopes which are used for labelling compounds to be injected intravenously.

A computer can reassemble radiographic 'slices' and demonstrate sagittal or coronal sections. It is even possible thereby to build up a three-dimensional picture of the whole brain, then remove an area and 'look inside'.

Neurochemical activity may be examined with labelled neurotransmitters or transmitter inhibitors. The tracer F–dopa images the dopamine-uptake capacity of nigrostriate neurons: in Parkinson's disease the decline of activity approaches 80% before symptoms become apparent; the putamen is demonstrably much more affected than the caudate nucleus. The activity of neural transplants into such patients can also be monitored. In epilepsy focal lesions can be identified. Functional changes in cerebral biochemistry may be revealed in psychiatric disorders. Types of dementia, including Alzheimer's disease can be differentiated. Cerebrovascular disorders can be investigated in detail.

Apart from investigation of pathological conditions, PET is an extremely sophisticated physiological research tool; new insights are being gained into functional anatomy such as cerebral blood flow during motor responses. One study provides detailed analysis of regional cortical activity during auditory and visual word processing (Petersen et al., 1988).

Chapter 14

Blood supply of the central nervous system

The brain requires active aerobic metabolism of glucose; if the arterial supply ceases for ten seconds, unconsciousness ensues, and after four minutes irreversible degeneration begins.

Arteries of the Brain

The brain is supplied by two pairs of arteries, the internal carotid and the vertebral; these anastomose on its inferior surface in the *circulus arteriosus* (of Willis) (*Fig.* 14.1); the communicating arteries forming this are usually too slender to compensate for major obstruction in supply. The cerebral and cerebellar arteries are in the subarachnoid space; their branches are either cortical or central, with little anastomosis between the superficial and deep areas supplied. Large *cortical branches* ramify in the pia mater; from them small rami enter the cortex and subcortical tissue. Surface anastomosis between the three major (anterior, middle and posterior) cerebral arteries is variable and usually limited; hence, if one is occluded, damage ensues. *Central branches* from the circulus arteriosus and adjacent parts of the three paired cerebral arteries supply the internal capsule, diencephalon and corpus striatum. These small but vital vessels form anteromedial, posteromedial, anterolateral and posterolateral groups (*Fig.* 14.1). The anterior and posterior choroidal arteries, respectively from the internal carotid and posterior cerebral, supply the choroid plexus and also provide central branches. Connexions between individual central arteries is very poor and most are 'end arteries'; hence their occlusion causes a 'stroke'. The cerebral arteries and their branches have thinner walls than other vessels of similar diameter.

Each *internal carotid artery*, traversing its canal in the petrous temporal bone and the upper part of foramen lacerum, enters the middle cranial fossa between the endosteum and the meningeal dura mater and turns forwards in the cavernous sinus. Its arched course thereafter is described as a 'carotid syphon' in angiograms (*see Fig.* 14.5). Turning up medial to the anterior clinoid process, it pierces the meningeal dura mater and arachnoid mater, enters the subarachnoid space, runs back below the optic nerve and then lateral to the optic chiasma; there, subjacent to the anterior perforated substance, it divides into the *anterior* and *middle cerebral arteries*. Its intrapetrosal part gives off a *caroticotympanic* branch to the tympanic cavity, the

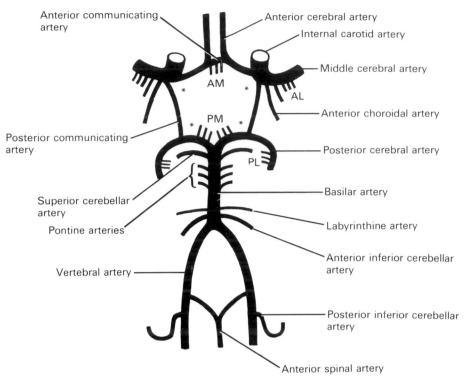

Fig. 14.1 Diagram of arteries at the base of the brain showing the circulus arteriosus. The groups of central branches are anteromedial (**AM**), anterolateral (**AL**), posteromedial (**PM**) and posterolateral (**PL**).

intracavernous part supplies *hypophyseal arteries* to the neurohypophysis and median hypothalamic eminence; from the latter a portal system extends to the adenohypophysis. Collateral branches within the subarachnoid space are the ophthalmic, posterior communicating and anterior choroidal arteries. The *ophthalmic artery* traverses the optic canal below the optic nerve, supplies orbital structures, the frontal and ethmoidal air sinuses, the frontal area of scalp and dorsum of nose. The *posterior communicating artery* arises near the terminal carotid bifurcation and runs posteriorly in the circulus arteriosus to join the posterior cerebral artery; usually slender, it may be large and give origin to the posterior cerebral artery. The *anterior choroidal artery* arises from the internal carotid just beyond the posterior communicating branch. Running posteriorly near the optic tract, it crosses the uncus to enter the choroid plexus in the inferior horn of lateral ventricle. It also supplies the optic tract, lateral geniculate nucleus, hippocampal formation, amygdaloid nucleus, globus pallidus, posterior limb and retrolentiform part of the internal capsule. Long and slender, it is prone to thrombosis.

Each *vertebral artery* ascends through the foramina transversaria of the upper six cervical vertebrae, curves behind the lateral mass of the atlas and

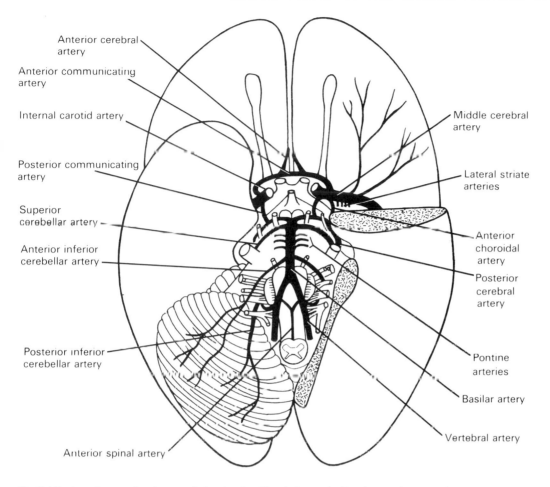

Anterior cerebral artery

Anterior communicating artery

Internal carotid artery

Posterior communicating artery

Superior cerebellar artery

Anterior inferior cerebellar artery

Posterior inferior cerebellar artery

Anterior spinal artery

Middle cerebral artery

Lateral striate arteries

Anterior choroidal artery

Posterior cerebral artery

Pontine arteries

Basilar artery

Vertebral artery

Fig. 14.2 Arteries at the base of the brain. The left cerebellar hemisphere and cerebral temporal lobe have been removed.

pierces the atlanto-occipital membrane, dura mater and arachnoid mater to enter the posterior cranial fossa via foramen magnum. The two vertebral arteries unite at the lower border of pons, forming the *basilar artery*, which ascends in the median pontine sulcus and bifurcates at upper border of pons into two *posterior cerebral arteries*.

Cerebral cortical blood supply *(Figs 14.2–14.5)*

Each *anterior cerebral artery*, the smaller terminal carotid branch, runs anteromedially above the optic nerve towards the longitudinal fissure, united there to its fellow by a short *anterior communicating artery*. It arches over the callosal genu, coursing posteriorly as the *pericallosal artery* on the corpus, giving off a *callosomarginal branch* which follows the sulcus cinguli. The

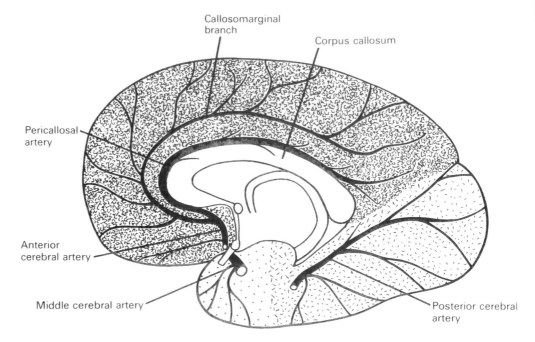

Fig. 14.3 The distribution of arteries on the medial surface of the right cerebral hemisphere.

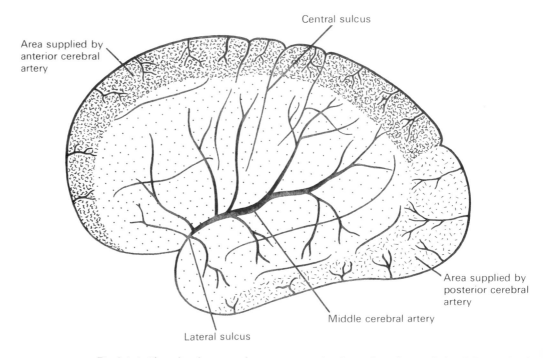

Fig. 14.4 The distribution of arteries on the lateral surface of the left cerebral hemisphere.

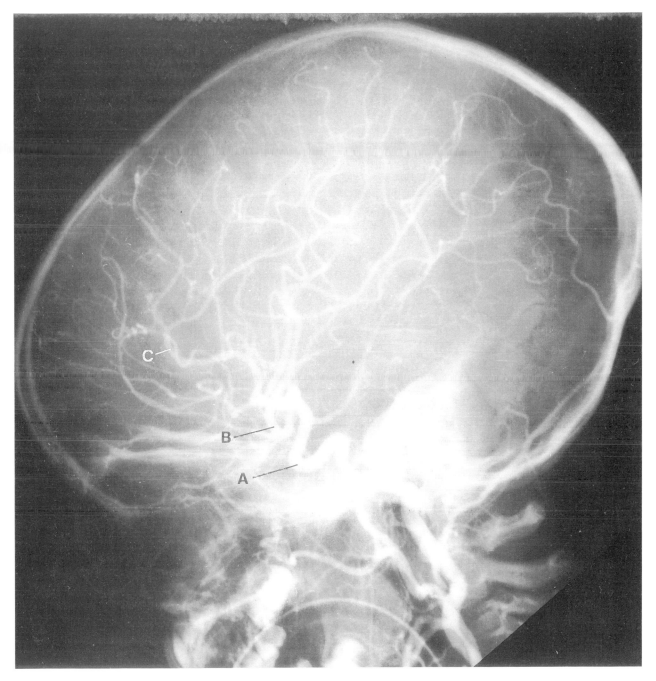

Fig. 14.5 Carotid angiogram. **A**, Carotid syphon; **B**, Middle cerebral artery; **C**,
Anterior cerebral artery.

cortical supply is to the orbital surface of the frontal lobe, to the medial hemispheric surface as far back as the parieto-occipital sulcus, and to an adjacent strip of the dorsolateral surface. This includes the 'leg area' of the motor cortex. Thrombosis of this vessel is uncommon.

Each *middle cerebral artery*, the larger branch and main continuation of the internal carotid artery, courses through the lateral fissure to the insula, supplying most of the dorsolateral surface (a narrow superior strip is supplied by the anterior cerebral artery, the occipital pole and inferior border by the posterior cerebral artery). This distribution includes the motor and sensory areas adjoining the central sulcus (except the 'leg area') and, in the dominant hemisphere, the speech and language areas. Cerebral thrombosis most commonly affects this artery, involving either the main trunk, cortical or central branches.

The two *posterior cerebral arteries* are the terminal branches of the basilar artery: both receive a posterior communicating artery from the internal carotid and then arch dorsally round the side of the midbrain to the tentorial surface of the cerebrum. Cortical branches supply the occipital lobe (medial, inferior and part of the lateral surface) and most of the inferior surface of the temporal lobe, including parahippocampal gyrus and uncus, but not the temporal pole. Vascular deprivation of the visual cortex causes blindness in the opposite visual field (contralateral homonymous hemianopia), often with 'macular sparing', the latter sometimes attributed to a branch of the middle cerebral artery reaching this area.

Central arteries

These small, deeply perforating branches are in four main groups (*Fig.* 14.1) but they occur elsewhere also.

1. The *anteromedial arteries*, arising from the anterior cerebral and anterior communicating arteries, enter via the anterior perforated substance to supply the anterior limb of internal capsule, head of caudate nucleus, putamen and anterior hypothalamus. They include the *medial striate artery*.

2. The *anterolateral (lateral striate) arteries*, arising from the proximal part of the middle cerebral artery, pierce the anterior perforated substance to supply the anterior and posterior limbs of the internal capsule and the caudate and lentiform nuclei. The largest branch, and the most susceptible to rupture, is termed the 'artery of cerebral haemorrhage'. It is appropriate to include in this group the *anterior choroidal artery*, arising from the internal carotid, previously described; its central branches supply the ventral region of the posterior limb and retrolentiform part of internal capsule.

3. The *posterolateral arteries*, arising from each posterior cerebral artery, supply the cerebral peduncle and the posterior part of thalamus, including the geniculate nuclei.

4. The *posteromedial arteries*, from the proximal part of the posterior cerebral and posterior communicating arteries, supply the cerebral peduncle and

enter the posterior perforated substance (between the peduncles), supplying the anterior part of thalamus, subthalamus and the central and
posterior regions of hypothalamus. The *posterior choroidal arteries*, two or
three on each side, arise from the posterior cerebral artery and enter the
third ventricle's choroid plexus via the transverse fissure, also supplying
the adjacent tectum and the superior part of thalamus.

Posterior cranial fossa

The brainstem and cerebellum are supplied by the vertebral and basilar
arteries.

Distribution of the vertebral artery

Small *meningeal branches* supply the dura mater. Two *posterior spinal arteries*,
arise from the vertebral artery or its posterior inferior cerebellar branches,
descend on each side behind the dorsal nerve roots, reinforced by intervertebral radicular arteries (*see* p. 262). They also supply the dorsal region of
the closed part of the medulla, including the gracile and cuneate nuclei.

A single *anterior spinal artery* is formed by two tributaries, one from each
vertebral artery, uniting in front of the medulla; as it descends in the cord's
ventral median fissure it is augmented by radicular arteries. Near its
commencement it supplies the paramedian medullary region, including the
pyramids, medial lemnisci and hypoglossal nerves (*see* p. 107).

Each *posterior inferior cerebellar artery*, the largest branch of the vertebral
artery, winds round the olive's caudal end, ascends behind vagal and
glossopharyngeal roots, then descends along the fourth ventricle's lateral
border and passes laterally into the cerebellum. This tortuosity may partly
explain its susceptibility to thrombosis, but this is sometimes secondary to
occlusion of the parent vertebral artery. The vertebral arteries are usually
unequal in size, sometimes markedly so. The cerebellar distribution is to the
inferior vermis, inferolateral surface of the hemisphere and to the fourth
ventricle's choroid plexus. En route the artery supplies the lateral medullary
region, dorsal to the olive and lateral to the hypoglossal nerve. This includes
the spinothalamic tracts, spinal trigeminal nucleus, nucleus ambiguus,
visceral efferent pathway, nucleus solitarius, dorsal vagal, vestibular and
cochlear nuclei, and the inferior cerebellar peduncle. Occlusion causes a
'lateral medullary syndrome' (*see* p. 107).

Distribution of the basilar artery

The basilar branches are bilateral and symmetrical (*Fig.* 14.2), and include
numerous small *pontine arteries*.

Paired *anterior inferior cerebellar arteries* supply the anterior and inferior
part of the cerebellum and also give off clinically important paramedian
pontine branches (*see Fig.* 5.18).

Each *labyrinthine artery*, arising directly from the basilar artery or from its anterior inferior cerebellar branch, accompanies the facial and vestibulocochlear nerves into the internal acoustic meatus, supplying the membranous labyrinth.

Each *superior cerebellar artery*, arising near the end of the basilar artery, is separated from the posterior cerebral artery by the oculomotor nerve. It curves round the cerebral peduncle with the trochlear nerve and ramifies over the superior cerebellar surface, supplying cortex and white matter, including the central nuclei. It gives branches to the superior cerebellar peduncle, inferior colliculus and pons.

Paired *posterior cerebral arteries*, form the terminal basilar bifurcation, their cortical, central and choroidal branches are described above.

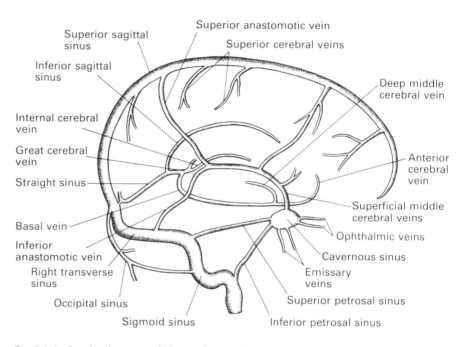

Fig. 14.6 Cerebral veins of the right cerebral hemisphere draining into venous sinuses.

Venous Drainage of the Brain (*Figs* 14.6 and 14.7)

Intracranial veins have no valves, their thin walls contain no muscle. All venous drainage passes to dural venous sinuses and must traverse the subdural space to reach these. Veins from the brainstem and cerebellum enter adjacent sinuses in the posterior cranial fossa. The cerebrum has external and internal veins. The external veins are in the subarachnoid space; the internal veins, draining deep structures and the choroid plexuses, emerge from the transverse fissure.

External cerebral veins

The *superior cerebral veins* drain the superolateral and medial surfaces of the cerebrum. They ascend, pierce the arachnoid mater, traverse the subdural space and enter the superior sagittal sinus or its lacunae. Traumatic anteroposterior displacement of the cerebral hemispheres may rupture these veins in the subdural cleavage plane, causing a subdural haemorrhage.

The *superficial middle cerebral vein* in each lateral fissure drains forwards to the cavernous sinus, is connected to the superior sagittal sinus by a *superior anastomotic vein* and to the transverse sinus by an *inferior anastomotic vein*.

The *deep middle cerebral vein* drains each insula, runs forward deep in the lateral fissure and is joined by an *anterior cerebral vein* to form the *basal vein*, which arches round the cerebral peduncle to enter the great cerebral vein.

Internal cerebral veins

A *thalamostriate vein* arises in the roof of each inferior ventricular horn, runs

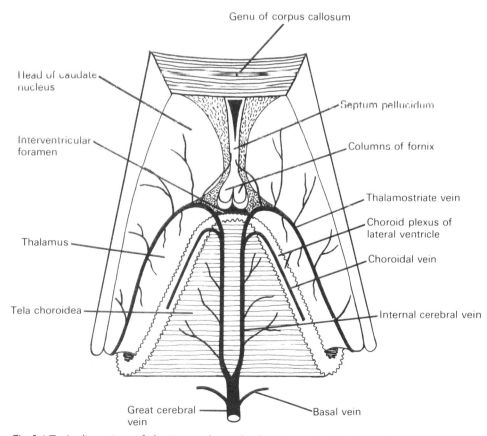

Fig. 14.7 A dissection of the internal cerebral veins and tela choroidea viewed from the posterosuperior aspect. The body and crura of the fornix have been removed.

along the medial side of the tail and body of the caudate nucleus and unites with the *choroidal vein* near the interventricular foramen, to form an *internal cerebral vein* (*Fig.* 14.7). The two internal cerebral veins run posteriorly in the tela choroidea to the transverse fissure, uniting beneath the splenium as the *great cerebral vein* (of Galen), which is joined by the basal veins before entering the commencement of the straight sinus.

Blood Vessels of the Spinal Cord

An *anterior spinal artery* and paired *posterior spinal arteries* descend throughout the cord in the pia mater, reinforced by multiple *radicular arteries* (from vertebral, deep cervical, posterior intercostal, lumbar and sacral vessels). The latter traverse all the intervertebral foramina and run medially to the cord along ventral and dorsal spinal roots to join the longitudinal spinal vessels. Very numerous, they are the major supply to the spinal cord below the cervical region. In the lower thoracic or upper lumbar region, usually on the left, one radicular artery, the *arteria radicularis magna (of Adamkiewicz)*, is particularly large and its occlusion may cause neural dysfunction. The posterior spinal arteries supply the dorsal grey and white columns; the rest of the cord is supplied by the anterior spinal artery.

The *veins of the spinal cord* follow the arterial pattern, draining by radicular veins to an epidural *internal vertebral venous plexus* which drains through the intervertebral foramina to vertebral, posterior intercostal, lumbar and sacral veins. This epidural plexus has no valves, and infection or malignant tumours may spread in it. It communicates with dural venous sinuses via the foramen magnum, hence prostatic or mammary tumours or a pleural abscess (empyema) may spread through it to the brain.

APPLIED ANATOMY

CEREBRAL ARTERIAL OCCLUSION

This commonly results from the embolism of a blood clot, usually secondary to arterial degeneration (atherosclerosis) in which a thrombus developing on damaged intima becomes detached. Atherosclerotic occlusion may occur in carotid or vertebral vessels in the neck or cranium. Occasionally embolism occurs in heart disease: in mitral stenosis a clot may form in the left atrium; in coronary ischaemia a 'mural thrombus' may develop on the endocardium; in bacterial endocarditis 'vegetations' on mitral or aortic valves may be detached. Rarely, in severe fractures, fat globules are swept into the circulation and may lodge in cerebral vessels.

The extent and pattern of nervous dysfunction, or 'stroke', depends on whether obstruction is in a main vascular trunk or confined to central or cortical branches.

As the main continuation of the internal carotid artery, the *middle cerebral artery* is most commonly invaded by emboli. Obstruction of its trunk produces such widespread cerebral ischaemia and oedema that death may result. Thrombosis in the *cortical branches* of the dominant hemisphere causes contralateral paralysis of the upper limb and lower facial muscles, with inability to speak or write and, if the language area (of Wernicke) is involved, difficulty in understanding words. Damage on the non-dominant side causes similar facial and upper limb paralysis but no sensory or motor aphasia. Obstruction of the *central supply* (lateral striate vessels) to internal capsule produces contralateral paralysis of upper and lower limbs (hemiplegia). Some cranial nerve nuclei such as the nucleus ambiguus, have a degree of bilateral cortical innervation and are either only partly affected or unaffected by a stroke. In 'pseudobulbar palsy', phonation, mastication and deglutition are seriously impaired because the corticonuclear fibres in the internal capsule of the other side had been previously affected by an asymptomatic vascular deprivation ('pseudobulbar' palsy means 'like a brainstem' lesion, as in bulbar poliomyelitis). For surveys on the incidence of residual dysarthria and dysphagia *see* Willoughby and Anderson (1984) and Gordon et al. (1987). The lower facial muscles have a contralateral cortical innervation, the upper facial muscles a bilateral one. The cortical innervation of trapezius is contralateral but of sternomastoid is ipsilateral.

Occlusion of *cortical branches* of the *posterior cerebral artery* results in contralateral visual field defects. The *central arteries*, including the posteromedial group and the posterior choroidal vessels, are clinically termed 'thalamogeniculate': damage to them causes hemianaesthesia and hemianopia; sensation is affected at thalamic level and recovery may be marred by severe intractable pain. Rarely, an obstructed central supply to the subthalamus produces hemiballismus, violent flailing movements in the contralateral limbs.

Thrombosis of the *anterior cerebral artery* is uncommon. Deprivation of the *cortical* supply results in paralysis and impaired sensation in the contralateral lower limb (paracentral lobule) and reduced awareness of it (superior parietal lobule). Occlusion of the *central branches* to the internal capsule is rare and produces contralateral weakness of the face and arm.

Since the *anterior choroidal artery* supplies the posterior limb of the internal capsule, retrolentiform area (optic radiation) and hippocampal formation, its obstruction may cause hemiparesis, hemianaesthesia, hemianopia and defective memory of recent events.

INTRACRANIAL HAEMORRHAGE

Extradural haemorrhage usually follows direct blows in the temporal region, with fracture of the squamous temporal bone and rupture of middle meningeal vessels. Typically there is transient unconsciousness due to concussion, then a lucid interval, followed by signs of progressively raised intracranial pressure, leading to coma as blood accumulates between the skull and dura mater. General signs of increased intracranial pressure include raised blood pressure, a slowing pulse rate and papilloedema. Untreated, this may be fatal within a few hours. As the brainstem and adjacent parts of the temporal lobes (parahippocampal gyrus and uncus) are displaced downwards through the tentorial hiatus, a 'tentorial pressure cone' develops: this causes traction on the oculomotor nerves, usually first on the side of the lesion, resulting in a *fixed dilated pupil* on that side. Later both pupils dilate and the limbs become spastic as the crura cerebri of midbrain are compressed.

Subdural haemorrhage follows sudden anteroposterior movement of the brain relative to the cranium. Rupture of a superior cerebral vein produces a subdural extravasation. If this is small the vein seals itself and a 'chronic subdural haematoma' then becomes surrounded by a fibrinous semipermeable membrane. Thus encapsulated, it slowly enlarges, producing headache, confusion and disturbance of memory — symptoms which may develop months after the original, often minor, incident.

Subarachnoid haemorrhage, usually due to rupture of a congenital aneurysm near the circulus arteriosus, causes sudden severe headache, nausea and vomiting, possibly followed by coma and death.

Cerebral haemorrhage, usually associated with hypertension, most frequently involves a lateral striate branch of a middle cerebral artery. If it is limited, there may be partial recovery with residual hemiplegia, due to a damaged internal capsule; extensive bleeding through the cortex or into the ventricles is fatal.

Chapter 15

Neurotransmitter pathways of the central nervous system

During the past twenty years advanced histochemical and neuroanatomical methods of investigation have been developed and applied to the nervous system. Initially the objective was to localize neurotransmitters at a cellular level through histochemical identification of either the neurotransmitter itself or one of its characteristic synthesizing enzymes. Techniques include fluorescence histochemical methods for monoamines, autoradiography for γ-aminobutyric acid (GABA) and, more recently, immunohistochemistry using antisera raised against neuroactive peptides, amino acids, amines or transmitter-synthesizing enzymes. In addition, histochemical methods have been combined with sophisticated tract-tracing techniques in order to define the projections of a neuron of known transmitter identity. Axon terminals take up injected horseradish peroxidase (HRP) or a fluorescent dye such as True Blue and transfer it by retrograde axonal transport to the soma, where it accumulates. Horseradish peroxidase can be demonstrated there by a simple enzyme histochemical technique, the fluorescent dyes by ultraviolet light. Both the histochemical and tract-tracing methods have been adapted for electron microscopy, resulting in greater resolution and accuracy of observation. Recent increased identification and location of neurotransmitters has resulted from advances in techniques of investigation.

Investigation has demonstrated neuron systems which utilize specific neurotransmitters. Pioneering work carried out on small rodents is now being confirmed by examination of human post-mortem nervous tissue. This rapidly developing branch of neuroanatomy has considerable pharmacological significance and is briefly surveyed here. The subject is dealt with comprehensively by Nieuwenhuys (1985) in his monograph *Chemoarchitecture of the Brain*.

Monoamine Systems

Neuron groups which synthesize monoamines are sited mainly in the brainstem and have diffuse projections. Included here are the catecholamines noradrenaline, dopamine and adrenaline and the indoleamine serotonin (5–HT). These were first located in reticular neurons by fluorescence techniques and more recently by using specific antisera. Transmitter-synthesizing *enzymes* peculiar to certain monoamine neuron systems can also be identified in this way. Thus tyrosine hydroxylase indicates the presence of noradrenaline or dopamine neurons. Identification of adrenaline neurons has resulted from immunohistochemical studies employing antisera raised against phenylethanolamine-N-methyl transferase (PNMT), the specific enzyme that methylates noradrenaline in adrenaline formation and is exclusive to adrenaline-containing neurons.

In the last decade there has been controversy about the nature of monoamine release from axon varicosities within the cerebral cortex since few of these appeared to have demonstrable synapses. It was thought that monoamines mostly pass via extracellular spaces to small regions of cortical neurons, a diffuse 'paracrine' effect. Improved techniques have recently shown that at least 90% of these axon varicosities have conventional synapses. Also against the concept of a diffuse non-synaptic effect is the discovery that the differential distribution of noradrenaline and 5–HT has regional cortical specificity and conforms to a fairly rigid intracortical laminar pattern (Parnavelas and Papadopoulos, 1989).

Noradrenaline neurons and pathways

There are several groups of noradrenaline neurons in the brainstem; they form two main systems, the locus ceruleus and the lateral tegmental. Their axons are long and branching, with profuse terminal networks and extend throughout the central nervous system.

The *locus ceruleus* is a pigmented nucleus, sited rostrally in the floor of the fourth ventricle, extending into the periaqueductal grey matter of midbrain, ventromedial to the trigeminal mesencephalic nucleus (*see Figs* 5.12 to 5.15). It consists entirely of noradrenaline-containing neurons and these comprise almost half the total number of such neurons in the central nervous system. The extensive projections of this nucleus are mostly ipsilateral. The major ascending pathway is termed the *dorsal noradrenergic bundle*. It traverses the midbrain tegmentum ventrolateral to the periaqueductal grey matter, enters the medial forebrain bundle, passing thence through the lateral hypothalamus to the septal area. As it ascends, the dorsal noradrenergic bundle gives branches to the superior and inferior colliculi, dorsal raphe nuclei, habenular nuclei and all the thalamic nuclei except for the dorsomedial and midline nuclei. Terminal branches innervate the septal area and join the cingulum to be distributed to the entire neocortex. Other branches pass to the amygdala, hippocampus and subiculum. There is also a small ascending projection to the hypothalamus in the dorsal longitudinal fasciculus.

The locus ceruleus projects to the cerebellar cortex and intracerebellar nuclei via the superior cerebellar peduncle. Noradrenaline released from cortical terminals has a powerful inhibitory effect on Purkinje neurons.

A descending pathway from the locus ceruleus in the central tegmental tract innervates the reticular formation throughout the pons and medulla, pontine nuclei and certain cranial nerve nuclei, including the dorsal vagal motor nucleus, the cochlear and trigeminal sensory nuclei. Thence it continues throughout the spinal cord, terminating in dorsal, lateral and ventral grey columns.

Through its extensive projections the locus ceruleus has roles in cortical activation, paradoxical sleep (*see* p. 232), facilitation and inhibition of sensory neurons and of preganglionic sympathetic neurons. Its action is not simply either excitation or inhibition but rather one of enhancing or diminishing the effects of other neurotransmitters. In general, in the waking state, it maintains a state of 'attention' and enables the individual to respond rapidly to emergency situations.

In Parkinson's disease and Alzheimer's disease there is a considerable loss of neurons in the locus ceruleus. This may partly explain the depression that commonly accompanies the former condition.

The *lateral tegmental system* comprises four groups of noradrenaline neurons, between caudal medulla and midbrain. Their axons ascend as a *ventral noradrenergic pathway* in the central tegmental tract, traversing the diencephalon in the medial forebrain bundle to reach the septal area. This system contributes a major innervation to most of the hypothalamus. In contrast to the locus ceruleus, distribution to the telencephalon is relatively limited and includes the olfactory cortex and amygdaloid nuclei. From the caudal medulla fibres descend to spinal grey matter.

The main functional significance of the lateral tegmental system is its noradrenaline innervation of the hypothalamus. Noradrenaline is apparently involved here in the regulation of the secretion of gonadotrophin, adrenocorticotrophic hormone and growth hormone. In the medulla there is innervation of the cardiovascular and respiratory control centres.

Dopamine neurons and pathways

Dopamine pathways are shorter than noradrenaline projections and have less extensive but very dense terminal fields of innervation. There are four main systems:

1. *Nigrostriate*. Dopamine neurons in the substantia nigra send axons to the caudate nucleus and putamen of the neostriatum. In Parkinson's disease degeneration of this system severely reduces the dopamine concentration in the neostriatum and substantia nigra.

2. *Mesolimbic*. The cells of origin of this system are located in the ventral tegmentum of the midbrain. Their axons ascend, enter the medial forebrain bundle and project to the limbic system. Excessive dopaminergic activity in this pathway simulates certain psychotic aspects of schizophrenia. Post-mortem examinations of brains from schizophrenics have reported gross asymmetry of dopamine concentrations in the amygdalae, that on the left being abnormally high (Reynolds, 1983; MacKay, 1984).

3. *Tubero-infundibular*. Axons from dopamine neurons in the infundibular nucleus of the hypothalamus enter this short tract which extends to the median eminence, infundibulum, supra-optic, paraventricular and dorsomedial hypothalamic nuclei. Dopamine probably inhibits release of pituitary prolactin and luteinizing hormone releasing hormone (LHRH) and also influences oxytocin and vasopressin secretion.

4. *Incertohypothalamic*. Axons from dopamine neurons in the zona incerta also project to the median eminence and influence endocrine secretion.

Adrenaline neurons and pathways

The concentration of adrenaline in the central nervous system is much lower than that of other catecholamines. In the rostral medulla two groups of adrenaline neurons are present bilaterally in dorsomedial and ventrolateral positions, the former adjacent to the nucleus solitarius. Axons of these adrenaline neurons terminate locally in the nucleus solitarius, dorsal nucleus of vagus and locus ceruleus; they ascend to the periaqueductal grey matter, hypothalamus (paraventricular and dorsomedial nuclei) and thalamus (midline nuclei); they descend to the intermediolateral cell column of the spinal cord. It is likely that they influence many visceral functions, including blood pressure, respiration, food intake, secretion of vasopressin and oxytocin.

Serotonin (5–HT) neurons and pathways

Serotonin neurons are chiefly located in the midline raphe nuclei of the midbrain, pons and medulla oblongata. They 'innervate virtually the entire central nervous system, thus comprising the most expansive central neuronal network yet described' (Nieuwenhuys, 1985).

Ascending pathways

Most of these originate from raphe nuclei in midbrain and rostral pons. They give branches to the substantia nigra and interpeduncular nucleus, join the medial forebrain bundle and supply many hypothalamic nuclei and the neostriatum. The most extensive distribution of these ascending fibres is via the fornix and cingulum to the limbic system.

There is widespread innervation of the neocortex, with regional and laminar specificity. Thus in the primary visual cortex serotonin is associated with sensory input (layer IV), noradrenaline with output (layers V, VI); there is more serotonin in area 17, more noradrenaline in area 18. These observations suggest that, in the visual cortex, serotonin is associated with initial signal processing, noradrenaline with higher order processing (Parnavelas and Papadopoulos, 1989).

Ascending fibres modulate behaviour. Destruction of serotonin neurons produces hypersensitivity to environmental stimuli, hyperactivity and insomnia. Serotonin is involved in 'slow wave sleep'. Lysergic acid diethylamide (LSD) depresses serotonin production and may produce hallucinations; hence *endogenous* inhibition of serotonin production might, in theory, result in mental disorder. Serotinergic fibres innervate small pial and intracerebral arteries and influence cerebral blood flow. A plexus of serotinergic fibres in ependyma extends through the ventricular system: this may release serotonin into cerebrospinal fluid; it may also regulate fluid production, flow and local neural uptake.

Migraine is a serotonin-related cerebrovascular disorder: the initial aura is accompanied by vasoconstriction, the subsequent headache by vasodilation. Migraine pain is attributable particularly to abnormal distension of meningeal vessels (served by the trigeminal nerve). The drug methysergide, a serotonin antagonist, is a potent migraine prophylactic but its use is limited by serious potential side effects, particularly retroperitoneal fibrosis. There are three main types of 5–HT receptors and several subtypes: recent research has led to the discovery of a previously unknown 5–HT_1-like receptor which mediates serotonin-induced vasoconstriction only in intracranial vessels. A drug named sumatriptan similar in structure to serotonin but acting only on these receptors has now been produced; trials indicate that it is highly effective in aborting an attack of migraine (Pramod, et al., 1989; Humphrey et al., 1990; Olesen and Edvinsson, 1991).

Brainstem and cerebellum

More caudal raphe nuclei innervate the reticular formation of pons and medulla. Serotinergic innervation of the locus ceruleus and substantia nigra has an inhibitory influence on the production of noradrenaline and dopamine respectively. Also supplied are the nucleus solitarius, dorsal vagal nucleus, nucleus ambiguus, trigeminal and facial nuclei. There is a projection to the cerebellar cortex and intracerebellar nuclei via the middle cerebellar peduncle.

Descending pathways

From raphe nuclei of the pons and medulla fibres descend in the dorsolateral spinal tract to synapse with enkephalin-containing neurons of the substantia gelatinosa. Enkephalin binds to opiate receptors of nociceptor afferent terminals, blocking impulse transmission to ascending pain pathways (*see Fig.* 4.11).

Cholinergic Systems

Acetylcholine is widely distributed throughout the central nervous system. Early attempts to localize cholinergic neurons employed, as a marker, the enzyme acetylcholinesterase (AChE), for which reliable enzyme histochemical methods were available. However, following the discovery that AChE is not confined to cholinergic neurons, it became urgent to develop a sensitive and reliable technique for the detection of choline acetyltransferase (ChAT) which is located only in cholinergic neurons. Only recently has an acceptable antiserum been raised against ChAT for use in immunohistological studies. The mapping of cholinergic systems in the central nervous system is still in progress.

ChAT-positive neuron somata have been identified, as expected, in ventral horn α and γ motor neurons and in preganglionic autonomic neurons of the brainstem and spinal cord.

Cholinergic pathways

1. *Habenulo-interpeduncular tract* (fasciculus retroflexus). This runs from the habenular nucleus of the epithalamus to the interpeduncular nucleus of the midbrain and is involved in autonomic control. The habenular nucleus receives a cholinergic innervation from the septum via the stria medullaris thalami.

2. *Septohippocampal pathway*. From the septal area cholinergic fibres project via the fornix to the hippocampus, a reciprocal pathway in the limbic system, necessary for memorization.

3. *Cholinergic projections from the basal forebrain*. In the human forebrain there is an anteroinferior aggregation of magnocellular nuclei which include the medial septal nucleus, nucleus of the diagonal stria, nucleus basalis (of Meynert) and substantia innominata. These vary in their arrangement and may be collectively termed a 'magnocellular basal nucleus'. Combined ChAT immunohistochemistry and retrograde tracing techniques have shown that these nuclei provide a cholinergic innervation to the entire neocortex, to the amygdala and hippocampus (affecting memory, affective response and behaviour), and to the olfactory bulb. These brain areas that receive a cholinergic innervation from the magnocellular basal nucleus have also been shown to synthesize nerve growth factor (NGF), suggesting a potential role in the treatment of local disorders such as Alzheimer's disease.

   In Alzheimer's disease, a form of senile dementia, there is gross reduction of acetylcholinesterase and choline acetyltransferase in all these areas, few neurons in the nucleus basalis and depressed cholinergic innervation. There is degeneration of the hippocampi and diffuse cortical atrophy. Affected brains are reported to have elevated aluminium concentrations (Crapper and McLachlan, 1987). Some cases of Parkinson's disease develop dementia and have depletion of neurons in the nucleus basalis. The pathological processes underlying the disorders of Alzheimer's and Parkinson's diseases may be related; occasionally the two conditions occur as a single complex. Recent clinical trials of an acetylcholinesterase inhibitor, Tacrine (THA), appear to provide amelioration of symptoms in Alzheimer's disease for a period of time, at least two years (Summers et al., 1986, 1989; Forsyth et al., 1989; Vida et al., 1989). However this form of therapy is ultimately flawed since it requires integrity of cholinergic neurons; moreover Alzheimer's disease is not simply a cholinergic deficit, other neurotransmitters are affected (Davis and Machs, 1986).

4. *Corpus striatum*. There are very high levels of acetylcholine in the neostriatum. Many intrinsic Golgi Type II neurons here are ChAT-positive. In addition, some nigrostriate fibres are cholinergic: anticholinergic drugs reduce the tremor of Parkinson's disease. In Huntington's chorea (*see* p. 195) there is a decrease of choline acetyltransferase in the neostriatum.

Amino Acid Systems

γ-aminobutyric acid (GABA)

This is the principal inhibitory neurotransmitter in the brain and its distribution is widespread; in the spinal cord its effect is mostly that of presynaptic inhibition. Of the many GABA neurons, most are local circuit interneurons in the cerebral cortex, cerebellar cortex (stellate, basket and Golgi cells), neostriatum and hippocampus. Examples of long-axoned GABA neurons are the Purkinje cells of the cerebellum, the striatonigral neurons (which degenerate in Huntington's chorea), pallidothalamic and nigrothalamic neurons.

Glycine

Neurons using glycine as a neurotransmitter appear to be restricted to local circuits in the spinal cord and medulla. These are always inhibitory in nature, e.g. the Renshaw interneurons of the ventral horn. Strychnine poisoning blocks glycine receptors and severe convulsions result. (For interrelated distributions of glycine and GABA in the spinal cord and their co-existence in some neurons *see* Todd and Sullivan, 1990.)

Glutamate

Glutamate neurons occur throughout the brain, probably as the major excitatory transmitter. Glutamate containing pyramidal cells provide fast point-to-point communication in corticostriate, corticopontine, corticorubral and corticotectal projections; also via corticospinal fibres from the *somatosensory cortex* to nucleus cuneatus and secondary sensory spinal neurons. In the cerebellar cortex, parallel fibres from granule cells release glutamate. The output of the hippocampus via the fornix to the septum uses glutamate. Glutamate interneurons are found in the hippocampus (Schaffer collaterals).

Peptide Systems

For many years peptides in the brain were only associated with hypothalamic hormones and releasing factors. Since 1970 over forty peptides, many of which were initially detected in the gut wall, have been found in neurons of the central and peripheral nervous systems. Peptides are widely distributed and detailed maps are available of enkephalin, substance P, somatostatin, neurotensin and cholecystokinin.

Neuroactive peptides differ from classical neurotransmitters in a number of respects. The latter may be synthesized at terminals but peptides can only be synthesized on ribosomes in the cell body. The effect of synaptic release lasts longer, since there are no rapid mechanisms for terminating this, and peptides are effective in low concentration. There is strong evidence that some peptides such as substance P act as neurotransmitters, but the function of others is less clear. Moreover, the so-called 'gut brain peptides' often co-exist with classical neurotransmitters in neurons. Their co-release usually modulates the action of these neurotransmitters rather than acting as independent transmitters. Neuromodulation works on a longer time scale than neurotransmission. Co-existence of peptides with neurotransmitters and even the presence of two neurotransmitters in one neuron is a complex subject, imperfectly understood (*see* Hökfelt et al., 1987).

The hypothalamus, amygdala, some brainstem nuclei and the dorsal grey column of the spinal cord are particularly rich in peptides; other areas such as the cerebellar cortex contain few. Peptides may occur both in Golgi Type I neurons, for example substance P in the habenulo-interpeduncular tract, and in Golgi Type II neurons, for example vasoactive intestinal polypeptide (VIP) in cortical interneurons. Substance P may be the neurotransmitter of certain primary sensory neurons mediating nociceptive sensations. Opioid peptides such as enkephalin modulate this input in endogenous analgesia (*see* p. 67).

Atrial natriuretic peptide (atriopeptin), recently located in myocytes of the cardiac atrial wall, is also present in the hypothalamus and brainstem where it is believed to be involved in cardiovascular regulation, fluid and electrolyte balance (Standaert et al., 1985). Peptide distribution and function form a rapidly expanding branch of neurobiological research.

Glossary: neuroanatomical and clinical terminology

Abducent. The sixth cranial nerve supplies the lateral rectus muscle, which abducts the eye, i.e. rotates it away from the midline. (L. *abduco* to lead away.)

Accessory. The eleventh cranial nerve is 'accessory' to the tenth (vagus); its cranial component joins the vagus and is distributed by it to the larynx and pharynx. The spinal component pursues a separate course, supplying sternomastoid and trapezius muscles.

Afferent. Conveying impulses from the periphery to the centre, centripetal, e.g. sensory fibres in peripheral nerves. (L. *afferre* to carry to.)

Agnosia. Inability to recognize and interpret sensory information, e.g. tactile, auditory, visual. (*a* neg.; Gr. *gnosis* knowledge.)

Allocortex. Phylogenetically old, three-layered cerebral cortex (archecortex and paleocortex). (Gr. *allos* other; L. *cortex* bark.)

Alveus. White matter on the ventricular surface of the hippocampus, mostly comprising fibres from hippocampus and subiculum passing to the fornix. (L. trough.)

Amygdala. Almond-shaped nuclear mass anterior to and above the tip of the inferior horn of the lateral ventricle. (Gr. *amygdale* almond.)

Aphasia. Language impairment following cortical damage: either inability to speak (motor aphasia) or failure of comprehension (sensory aphasia). (*a* neg.; Gr. *phasis* speech.)

Apraxia. Loss of acquired motor skills: inability to perform complex purposeful movements after cortical damage, although muscles are not paralysed. (*a* neg.; Gr. *praxis* action.)

Arachnoid. The delicate middle layer of the three meninges, attached to cerebral pia mater by a web of fine fibres; adheres to inner surface of dura mater in the vertebral canal. The subarachnoid space is 'under the arachnoid', between it and the pia. (Gr. *arachne* spider.)

Archecerebellum. Phylogenetically old part of the cerebellum, concerned with equilibration (flocculonodular lobe and lingula). (Gr. *arche* beginning.)

Archecortex. Phylogenetically old, three-layered cortex of the hippocampus and dentate gyrus. (Gr. *arche* beginning; L. *cortex* bark.)

Astereognosis. Inability to recognize familiar objects by feeling their shape. (*a* neg.; Gr. *stereos* solid; *gnosis* knowledge.)

Astrocyte. A star-shaped neuroglial cell with 'perivascular feet'. (Gr. *astron* star; *kytos* cell.)

Asynergy. Faulty synergy or cooperation between muscles. (*a* neg.; Gr. *synergia* cooperation.)

Ataxia. Loss of coordinated muscle action, resulting in unsteadiness of movement. (*a* neg.; Gr. *taxis* order.)

Athetosis. A condition resultant upon damage to the corpus striatum and characterized by involuntary slow writhing movements. (Gr. *athetos* without position; *osis* condition.)

Atrophy. A reduction in size of a previously normal organ or cell; severe atrophy is accompanied by some degree of degeneration. (Gr. *atrophia* a want of food.)

Autonomic. 'Self-governing': (visceral innervation). (Gr. *autos* self; *nomos* law.)

Autoradiography. A method for locating radioactive isotopes in tissue sections by prolonged exposure to a photographic emulsion. (Gr. *autos* self; L. *radius* ray; Gr. *graphein* to write.)

Axolemma. The delicate membrane surrounding an axon. (Gr. *axon* axis; *lemma* husk.)

Axon. The fibre which carries impulses away from a nerve cell body; (efferent process). (Gr. *axon* axis.)

Axon hillock. The region of a neuronal cell body, without Nissl granules, from which the axon arises.

Axonotmesis. The axons are crushed but endoneurial sheaths and other supporting connective tissue remain intact; followed by orderly axonal regeneration. (Gr. *axon* axis; *tmesis* a cutting.)

Axoplasm. Axonal cytoplasm. (Gr. *axon* axis; *plassein* to form.)

Baroreceptor. A vascular receptor responsive to blood pressure change, e.g. in carotid sinus. (Gr. *baros* weight.)

Basis pedunculi. (Crus cerebri). The ventral part of each cerebral peduncle, containing descending tracts. (Gr. *basis* base; L. *pedunculus* little foot.)

Brachium. In the brain this denotes a discrete short bundle of interconnecting fibres, e.g. inferior brachium from inferior colliculus to medial geniculate body. (L. arm.)

Brain. The intracranial part of the central nervous system, comprising cerebrum, brainstem and cerebellum.

Brainstem. Comprises midbrain, pons and medulla oblongata.

Bulbar. Refers to brainstem, e.g. corticobulbar fibres, bulbar palsy. Bulb is an old name for the medulla oblongata. (L. *bulbus* bulb.)

Calamus scriptorius. Caudal region of the rhomboid fossa, shaped like the tip of a pen. (L. *calamus* a reed, used to make writing pen.)

Calcar avis. An elevation on the medial wall of the lateral ventricle's posterior horn, produced by the deep calcarine sulcus. (L. *calcar* a spur; *avis* a bird.)

Cauda equina. The leash of lumbar, sacral and coccygeal nerve roots extending beyond the tip of the spinal cord. (L. a horse's tail.)

Caudal. (L. towards the tail.)

Caudate. (L. having a tail.)

Causalgia. A persistent burning pain which occasionally follows a peripheral nerve injury. (Gr. *kausos* heat; *algos* pain.)

Cerebellum. That part of the brain which occupies the posterior cranial fossa and is dorsal to the brainstem. (L. little brain, diminutive of *cerebrum*.)

Cerebrum. The major part of the brain, comprising the cerebral hemispheres and diencephalon. (L. brain.)

Chiasma. An evident x-shaped crossing, or decussation, of fibres, as in the optic chiasma. (Gr. *chiastos* to mark like a letter X.)

Chorea. Dysfunction of the corpus striatum, causing irregular involuntary movements of the limbs or face; formerly termed 'St.Vitus's dance'. (Gr. *choreia* dance.)

Choroid plexus. (Gr. *chorion* a membrane; *eidos* form; L. *plexus* a network.)

Chromatolysis. Disintegration and disappearance of Nissl bodies from nerve cells following axonal section. (Gr. *chroma* colour; *lysis* a loosing.)

Cinerea. e.g. tuber cinereum. (L. *cinereus* ash-coloured.)

Cingulum. A bundle of association fibres within the cingulate gyrus. (L. a girdle.)

Claustrum. A thin layer of grey matter between the insula and lentiform nucleus. (L. a barrier or wall.)

Colliculus. (L. a small eminence or hillock.)

Commissure. A bundle of nerve fibres uniting like structures on the two sides of the brain, e.g. corpus callosum; applied more generally in the spinal cord to describe fibres crossing the midline. (L. *commissura* a joining together.)

Contralateral. Situated in, or projecting to, the opposite side of the body. (L. *contra* opposite; *lateralis* from; *latus* side.)

Convolution. Synonymous with gyrus. (L. *convolutum* a fold.)

Corona radiata. Fibres which radiate out between internal capsule and cerebral cortex. (L. *corona* a crown.)

Corpus callosum. The great transverse commissure connecting the cerebral hemispheres. (L. *corpus* body; *callosus* hard.)

Corpus striatum. Grey matter situated within the cerebral hemispheres, comprising caudate and lentiform nuclei; myelinated fibres give sections a striped (striated) appearance. (L. *corpus* body; *striatus* striped.)

Corpus trapezoideum. A crossing of fibres of the auditory pathway, passing through or ventral to the medial lemniscus in the ventral part of the pontine tegmentum; of trapezoidal appearance in transverse section.

Cortex. External grey layer of cerebrum and cerebellum. (L. bark.)

Crus. (Crus cerebri: see basis pedunculi). (L. leg.)

Cytology. The study of cells. (Gr. *kytos* cell; *logos* word.)

Decussation. An X-shaped crossing of nerve fibres, uniting unlike structures on the two sides of brain or spinal cord, e.g. of pyramids; of superior cerebellar peduncles. (L. *decussare*, to divide crosswise, in the form of an X.)

Dendrite. The process of a neuron which conducts nerve impulses towards the cell body. (Gr. *dendron* a tree.)

Dentate. Like a tooth, toothed, e.g. dentate nucleus of cerebellum; dentate gyrus of hippocampal formation. (L. *dentatus* toothed.)

Denticulate. The denticulate ligament of the spinal cord's pia mater has small tooth-like lateral projections. (L. *denticulus* a small tooth.)

Diencephalon. That part of the brain between the telencephalon and mesencephalon; includes two thalami, the hypothalamus, subthalamus and epithalamus. (Gr. *dia* between; *enkephalos* brain.)

Diplopia. Double vision. (Gr. *diploos* double; *opsis* vision.)

Dura mater. The thick outer layer of the meninges, adjacent to hard parts, skull and vertebrae. (L. hard mother.)

Dys-. Greek prefix meaning difficult, hard, painful, etc.

Dysarthria. Difficulty in speaking. (Gr. *dys* difficult; *arthroun* to articulate.)

Dyskinesia. Disordered voluntary movement. (Gr. *dys* difficult; *kinesis* movement.)

Dyslexia. Impaired reading ability. (Gr. *dys* difficult; *lexis* speech.)

Dysmetria. Difficulty in accurately controlling (measuring) the range of movements. (Gr. *dys* difficult; *metron* a measure.)

Dysphagia. Difficulty in swallowing. (Gr. *dys* difficult; *phagein* to eat.)

Dysphasia. Difficulty in the understanding and expression of words. (Gr. *dys* difficult; *phasis* speech.)

Ectoderm. Outermost of the three primary embryonic layers, from which the epidermis and neural tube develop. (Gr. *ektos* outside; *derma* skin.)

Efferent. Conveying away from the centre, centrifugal, e.g. motor fibres in peripheral nerves. (L. *efferre* to carry away.)

Emboliform nucleus. A small plug-shaped intracerebellar nucleus. (Gr. *embolos* plug; L. *forma* form.)

Endoneurium. The delicate connective tissue sheath of a nerve fibre, within a peripheral nerve. (Gr. *endon* within; *neuron* nerve.)

Engram. A memory trace left on neurons by experience and learning, its nature as yet hypothetical. (Gr. *en* in; *gramma* mark.)

Entorhinal. The olfactory association cortex of the parahippocampal gyrus, posterior to the uncus (literally 'within the rhinencephalon'). (Gr. *entos* within; *rhis* the nose.)

Ependyma. Membrane lining the ventricles of brain and central canal of spinal cord. (Gr. *ependyma* upper garment.)

Epineurium. Connective tissue sheath surrounding a peripheral nerve. (Gr. *epi* upon; *neuron* nerve.)

Epithalamus. Part of the diencephalon dorsal to the thalamus: includes habenulae, pineal gland and posterior commissure. (Gr. *epi* upon; *thalamos* inner room.)

Falx cerebri. A sickle-shaped midline partition of dura mater between the cerebral hemispheres. (L. a sickle.)

Fasciculus. A small bundle of nerve fibres. (L. a small bundle.)

Fastigial nucleus. A small intracerebellar 'roof' nucleus on each side of the midline. (L. *fastigium* the apex of a gabled roof.)

Fimbria. Efferent fibres form a fringe along the medial side of the hippocampus, the fimbria of the fornix. (L. a fringe.)

Foramen. (L. an opening.)

Forceps. The frontal and occipital fibres of the corpus callosum form the U-shaped forceps minor and major. (L. a pair of tongs.)

Fornix. This comprises efferent fibres from the two hippocampi which arch over the thalami, below the corpus callosum, to reach the mamillary bodies.

(L. an arch.)

Fossa. e.g. the rhomboid fossa is the floor of fourth ventricle. (L. ditch.)

Fovea. e.g. the fovea centralis is a small central depression in the macula lutea. (L. a small pit.)

Funiculus. A column of white matter, dorsal, lateral or ventral in the spinal cord. (L. diminutive of *funis* cord.)

Ganglion. 1) A swelling comprising nerve cells located outside the central nervous system, e.g. dorsal root ganglion, autonomic ganglia. 2) As 'basal ganglia', applied collectively to certain areas of grey matter within the brain, having motor quality-control functions. (Gr. a swelling or knot.)

Geniculate. Abruptly bent, e.g. geniculate ganglion at the genu of the facial nerve; geniculate nuclei of thalamus. (L. *geniculare* to bend the knee.)

Genu. A knee-like structure, e.g. genu of corpus callosum. (L. knee.)

Glia. Interstitial, non-excitable, supporting cells of the central nervous system. (Gr. glue.)

Globose. Rounded, e.g. globose intracerebellar nucleus. (L. *globus* a ball.)

Globus pallidus. The inner and paler part of the lentiform nucleus; pallidum; paleostriatum. (L. *globus* a round mass; *pallidus* pale.)

Glomerulus. A small rounded synaptic configuration (in neuroanatomy), e.g. in the olfactory bulb; in the cerebellum around mossy fibre rosettes. (L. *glomero* to wind into a ball.)

Glossopharyngeal. The ninth cranial nerve is so-called because it supplies sensory fibres to tongue (posterior third) and pharynx. (Gr. *glossa* tongue; *pharynx* throat.)

Gyrus. Cerebral convolution. (L. from Gr. *gyros* a circle.)

Habenula. Part of epithalamus, comprising bilateral trigones and a commissure, between pineal gland and the thalami. (L. diminutive of *habena* a small strap.)

Hemi-. (Gr. half.)

Hemiballismus. Violent flinging movements of one side of the body due to a lesion in the opposite subthalamic nucleus. (Gr. *hemi* half; *ballismos* a jumping about.)

Herpes zoster. Viral infection of a sensory ganglion (spinal dorsal root, trigeminal, geniculate) causing pain and a vesicular rash in its cutaneous distribution, commonly intercostal or ophthalmic division of trigeminal. (Gr. *herpes* shingles; *zoster* a girdle.)

Hemiplegia. Paralysis of one side of the body. (Gr. *hemi* half; *plege* stroke.)

Heterotypical cortex. Primary motor or sensory areas of neocortex have their own characteristic structures: the six-layer pattern is obscured by blending of laminae II to V, with predominance here of either pyramidal or granular cells. (Gr. *heteros* different; *typos* pattern.)

Hippocampus. An elevation in the floor of the inferior horn of the lateral ventricle, part of the limbic system. (Gr. *hippokampos* a sea horse - from its appearance on coronal section.)

Homeostasis. The tendency of living organisms to maintain internal stability despite changing conditions. (Gr. *homoios* like; *stasis* position.)

Homotypical cortex. Association areas of neocortex all have a similar, six-layered structure. (Gr. *homos* the same as; *typos* pattern.)

Hydrocephalus. Increased volume of cerebrospinal fluid within the skull. (Gr. *hudro* water; *kephale* head.)

Hyper-. (Gr. above, over, excessive.)

Hyperacusis. Excessive perception of sound. (Gr. *akousis* hearing.)

Hyperaesthesia. Excessive sensitivity. (Gr. *aisthesis* sensation.)

Hypertrophy. Excessive growth, producing enlargement of an organ. (Gr. *trophe* nourishment.)

Hypo-. (Gr. under, below). May also be used to denote a deficiency.

Hypoglossal. The twelfth cranial nerve runs under the tongue, supplying its muscles. (Gr. *hypo* under; *glossa* tongue.)

Hypophysis cerebri. The pituitary gland. (Gr. *hypophysis* a growth below; L. *cerebrum* the brain.)

Hypothalamus. The region of the diencephalon below the thalamus, forming the floor and lower part of wall of third ventricle. (Gr. *hypo* under; *thalamos* inner room.)

Incisure. e.g. of Schmidt-Lanterman (in myelin sheath); tentorial (through which the brainstem passes). (L. *incisura* a slit or notch.)

Indusium griseum. A thin layer of grey matter clothing the upper surface of the corpus callosum. (L. a grey garment.)

Infarction. Vascular occlusion leading to death of tissue. (L. *in farcio* to stuff into.)

Infundibulum. Pituitary stalk; a funnel-shaped downgrowth of third ventricle which forms the neurohypophysis. (L. funnel.)

Insula. Cortex in depths of lateral cerebral fissure. (L. island.)

Internuncial neuron (interneuron). Small neuron interconnecting other neurons: e.g. Renshaw interneuron; flexor reflex arc; between corticospinal axons and ventral horn cells. (L. *inter* between; *nuncius* a messenger.)

Intra-. (L. within.)

Ipsilateral. Situated in, or projecting to, the same side of the body. (L. *ipse* self; *lateralis* from *latus* side.)

Kinaesthesia. The sense of perception of movement. (Gr. *kinesis* motion; *aisthesis* sensation.)

Lamina. e.g. lamina terminalis: the thin anterior wall of the third ventricle. (L. a thin plate or layer.)

Lemniscus. A ribbon-like bundle of nerve fibres ascending in the brainstem. Medial lemniscus: (continues dorsal column spinal pathway), formed after sensory decussation from nuclei gracilis and cuneatus, ascends to thalamus. Lateral lemniscus: auditory pathway betweeen superior olivary nucleus and inferior colliculus. Spinal lemniscus: spinothalamic and spinotectal tracts. (L. *lemniscus* from Gr. *lemniskos* a ribbon or fillet.)

Lentiform nucleus. A large lentil-shaped nucleus which, together with the caudate, comprises the corpus striatum. (L. *lens, forma* lentil shape.)

Leptomeninges. Arachnoid and pia mater. (Gr. *leptos* thin; *meninx* membrane.)

Limbic. (L. *limbus* a border.)

Limen insulae. Anterior part of insula. (L. *limen* threshold or boundary.)

Locus ceruleus. A pigmented nucleus of noradrenaline-containing neurons sited rostrally in the floor of fourth ventricle, extending into the periaqueductal grey matter. (L. *locus* a place; *caeruleus* dark blue.)

Macrosmatic. Keen sense of smell: for many animals this is a major component in perception of and response to the environment. (Gr. *macros* large; *osme* smell.)

Macula lutea. A slightly yellow spot in the retina at the posterior pole of the eye, in line with the visual axis, location of maximal visual acuity. (L. yellow spot.)

Mamillary bodies. A pair of small round swellings on the ventral surface of the hypothalamus. (L. diminutive of *mamma* little breast, nipple.)

Matter. e.g. grey matter. (L. *materia* substance.)

Medulla. Abbreviation for medulla oblongata, the caudal part of the brainstem. Note: medulla spinalis is an old term for spinal cord. (L. *modulla* marrow; *oblongus* more long than wide, oblong.)

Mesencephalon. Midbrain. (Gr. *mesos* middle; *enkephalos* brain.)

Meta-. (Gr. after.)

Metathalamus. Medial and lateral geniculate bodies. (Gr. *meta* after; *thalamos* inner room.)

Metencephalon. Pons and cerebellum. Rostral part of rhombencephalon. (Gr. *meta* after; *enkephalos* brain.)

Microglia. Small neuroglial cell. (Gr. *mikros* small; *glia* glue.)

Microsmatic. With a poorly developed sense of smell. (Gr. *mikros*; small; *osme* smell.)

Miosis. Constriction of pupil. (Gr. *meiosis* diminution.)

Mitral. Resembling a bishop's mitre. (Gr. *mitra* a headband or turban.)

Myasthenia. Muscular weakness. (Gr. *mys* muscle; *astheneia* weakness.)

Myelencephalon. Medulla oblongata. Caudal part of the rhombencephalon. (Gr. *myelos* marrow; *enkephalos* brain.)

Myelin sheath. White sheath around an axon, formed of concentric layers of lipid and protein. (Gr. *myelos* marrow.)

Myotome. That part of a somite which differentiates into striated muscle. (Gr. *mys* muscle; *tomos* cutting.)

Neo-. (Gr. *neos* new.)

Neocerebellum. Phylogenetically new part of the cerebellum, concerned with non-sterotyped, skilled and learned movements. (Gr. *neos* new; L. *cerebellum* small brain.)

Neocortex. Six-layered cerebral cortex, the most recently evolved, essential for motor skills and sensory programmes such as seeing, speaking, planning and all 'thought'. (Gr. *neos* new; *cortex* bark.)

Neostriatum. Caudate nucleus and putamen, the most recently evolved part of the corpus striatum. (Gr. *neos* new; L. *striare* striped.)

Neurapraxia. A temporary suspension of nerve conduction, a dysfunction commonly due to mild compression. (Gr. *neuron* nerve; *apraxia* no-action.)

Neurite. A neuronal process, either axon or dendrite. (Gr. *neurites* of a nerve.)

Neurobiotaxis. The tendency of nerve cells, during development, to migrate towards the principal source of stimuli: functionally associated centres in the brainstem may thereby become approximated. (Gr. *neuron* nerve; *bios* life; *taxis* arrangement.)

Neuroblast. An embryonic nerve cell. (Gr. *neuron* nerve; *blastos* germ.)

Neurofibril. Fine filaments in a nerve cell, usually extending from the processes and traversing the cell body. (Gr. *neuron* nerve; L. *fibrilla*, diminutive of *fibra* fibre.)

Neuroglia. Interstitial, non-excitable supporting cells of the central nervous system. (Gr. *neuron* nerve; *glia* glue.)

Neurolemma. The sheath surrounding a peripheral nerve fibre, comprising a longitudinal sequence of neurolemmal (Schwann) cells. (Gr. *neuron* nerve; *lemma* sheath.)

Neuron. A complete nerve cell, comprising cell body (soma), dendrites and an axon. (Gr. a nerve.)

Neurotmesis. Severance of nerve fibres. (Gr. *neuron* nerve; *tmesis* a cutting.)

Nociceptive. Responsive to injurious stimuli. (L. *noceo* to injure; *capio* to take.)

Nucleus. Can be used to describe either: (1) a microscopic cytological entity, the trophic centre of a cell or (2) a gross neuroanatomical feature, an aggregation of nerve cells in the central nervous system concerned with a particular function, e.g. nucleus proprius, nucleus gracilis. (L. a nut.)

Nystagmus. Rhythmic oscillatory movements of the eyes. (Gr. *nystagmos* nodding.)

Oculogyric. Refers to muscles which move the eyes, and their innervation. (L. *oculus* eye; *gyrare* to move in a circle.)

Oculomotor. The third cranial nerve innervates muscles which move the eyes. (L. *oculus;* eye; *motor* from *movere* to move.)

Oligodendrocyte. A neuroglial cell with few processes. An interfascicular oligodendrocyte forms myelin internodes on several axons in the central nervous system. Perineuronal oligodenrocytes are adjacent to cell bodies. (Gr. *oligos* few; *dendron* tree; *kytos* cell.)

Operculum. The convolutions of frontal, parietal and temporal lobes which cover the insula. (L. a lid or cover.)

Ophthalmoplegia. Paralysis of the extrinsic ocular muscles. (Gr. *ophthalmos* eye; *plege* a stroke.)

Pachymeninx. Dura mater. (Gr. *pachys* thick; *meninx* membrane.)

Paleo-. (Gr. *palaios* ancient.)

Paleocerebellum. Phylogenetically old part of the cerebellum; includes anterior lobe, uvula and pyramid; predominantly proprioceptive spinal input, serving stereotyped movements, posture, locomotion. (Gr. *palaios* ancient; L. *cerebellum* little brain.)

Paleocortex. Phylogenetically old, olfactory cortex. (Gr. *palaios* ancient; L. *cortex* bark.)

Paleostriatum. Globus pallidus, or pallidum, representing the corpus striatum of lower vertebrates. (Gr. *palaios* ancient; L. *striatus* striped.)

Pallidum. Paleostriatum, globus pallidus. (L. *pallidus* pale.)

Pallium. The cortex and superficial white matter of the cerebral hemispheres. (L. a cloak.)

Para-. e.g. paravertebral ganglia. (Gr. *para* beside, near, beyond.)

Paraesthesia. Distorted sensation, tingling, 'pins and needles'. (Gr. *para; aisthesis* perception.)

Paralysis. Loss of voluntary movement following neural injury, palsy. (Gr. *paralusis* to disable.)

Paraplegia. Paralysis of both lower limbs. (Gr. *paraplegie* paralysis.)

Paresis. Weakness, partial paralysis. (Gr. weakness.)

Peduncle. Stem or stalk. (L. *pedunculus* a little foot.)

Peri-. (Gr. around.)

Perikaryon. The cytoplasm around the nucleus. Sometimes loosely used as a synonym for neuronal cell body or soma; (Gr. *peri* around; *karyon* a nut.)

Perineurium. Connective tissue sheath around a bundle of nerve fibres. (Gr. *peri* around; *neuron* a nerve.)

Pes hippocampi. Paw-like anterior extremity of the hippocampus. (L. *pes* a foot.)

Pia mater. Vascular innermost meningeal layer investing the brain and spinal cord. (L. soft mother.)

Pineal. (L. *pinea* a pine cone.)

Plexus. A network of interlacing nerves or blood vessels. (L. *plecto* to interlace.)

Pneumoencephalography. Radiographic examination of the ventricular system following replacement of cerebrospinal fluid by air. (Gr. *pneuma* air; *enkephalos* brain; *graphein* to write.)

Pons. The portion of brainstem between midbrain and medulla; its ventral bridge-like appearance is due to transverse fibres passing into the two middle cerebellar peduncles. (L. bridge.)

Positron. This has the same mass and same charge as an electron but is positively charged. Positron-rich radioactive isotopes are used in positron emission tomography (PET). (L. *positivus* positive; Gr. *elektron* amber.)

Pre-. (L. *prae* before.)

Proprioception. Appreciation of the position, balance and movement of body parts, particularly during locomotion. (L. *proprius* one's own; *perceptio* perception.)

Prosencephalon. The forebrain: developmentally the most rostral brain vesicle; subdivides into diencephalon and telencephalon. (Gr. *pros* before; *enkephalos* brain.)

Prosopagnosia. Inability to recognise formerly familiar faces. (Gr. *prosopon* face; *agnosia* to know.)

Ptosis. Drooping of the upper eyelid. (Gr. a falling.)

Pulvinar. The posterior pole of the thalamus; it projects, overhanging the superior colliculus. (L. *pulvinar* a cushioned reclining seat used in Roman feasts.)

Putamen. Lateral portion of the lentiform nucleus. (L. a shell.)

Pyramidal tract. So-termed because the constituent corticospinal fibres traverse the medullary pyramids. The pyramidal system also includes corticobulbar tracts to cranial nerve motor nuclei.

Pyriform. Pear-shaped. (L. *pirum* pear; *forma* form.)

Quadrigemina. Corpora quadrigemina of the tectum: a group of four bodies, twinned. (L. *quattuor* four; *geminus* a twin.)

Quadriplegia. Paralysis affecting all four limbs. (L. *quattuor* four; *plege* a stroke.)

Raphe. A midline structure, e.g. nuclei of the raphe in the brainstem reticular formation. (Gr. *rhaphe* a seam.)

Receptor. This term is used in two quite different ways: 1) the sensory ending of a peripheral nerve, or an organ of special sense; 2) a protein in the cell membrane or cytoplasm which binds specifically to another molecule, e.g. neurotransmitter, hormone or drug: this binding initiates a modification of cell behaviour. (L. *receptum* from *recipere* to receive.)

Restiform body. The inferior cerebellar peduncle in its cord-like appearance on the dorsolateral surface of the medulla; excludes the (juxta-restiform) vestibular components which join it mesially. Sometimes used clinically as a synonym for the entire peduncle. (L. *restis* cord; *forma* form.)

Reticulum. A phylogenetically ancient network of nerve cells and fibres throughout the brainstem and spinal cord. (L. *reticulum* a little net.)

Rhinencephalon. The part of the cerebrum concerned with olfaction, large in lower vertebrates, small in humans. (Gr. *rhis* nose; *enkephalos* brain.)

Rhombencephalon. The hindbrain; the most caudal brain vesicle, subdivides into metencephalon (cerebellum) and myelencephalon (medulla oblongata). (Gr. *rhombos* rhomboidal; *enkephalos* brain.)

Rostrum. The rostrum of corpus callosum extends between the genu and lamina terminalis. (L. a beak or projection.)

Rubro-. (L. *ruber* red.)

Septal area. The area of cortex immediately anterior to the lamina terminalis and inferior to the rostrum of corpus callosum. (L. *saeptum* a partition.)

Septum pellucidum. The midline partition between the anterior horns of the lateral ventricles; extends between corpus callosum and fornix. (L. *saeptum* partition; *pellucidus* transparent.)

Somatic. Pertaining to the body framework as distinct from viscera; neural efferents to skeletal muscle, afferents from skin, muscle, joints, etc. (Gr. *somatikos* of the body.)

Splenium. The rounded posterior end of the corpus callosum. (Gr. *splenion* a bandage or pad.)

Stria terminalis. Efferents from the amygdaloid nucleus to septal area and hypothalamus form an elongated narrow bundle medial to the tail of the caudate nucleus in the inferior horn, and in the boundary between caudate nucleus and thalamus in the body of the lateral ventricle. (L. *stria* a narrow band; *terminalis* of a boundary.)

Striatum. The caudate nucleus and putamen; neostriatum. (L. *striatum* striped.)

Sub-. (L. under.)

Subiculum. Transitional zone between three-layered hippocampal cortex and six-layered parahippocampal gyrus. (L. a little layer.)

Substantia gelatinosa. Grey matter of gelatinous appearance forming the apex of the dorsal grey columns of the spinal cord.

Substantia nigra. A broad plate of neurons, some containing melanin pigment, between the basis pedunculi and tegmentum of midbrain.

Subthalamus. Region of the diencephalon beneath the posterior part of thalamus, behind hypothalamus.

Sulcus. (L. groove, furrow.)

Sympathetic. A division of the autonomic nervous system. (Gr. *sympathein* feeling with, i.e self responsive.)

Synapse. The site of unidirectional communication between the axon of one neuron and the cell surface of another. (Gr. *synapsis* contact.)

Syndrome. A group of symptoms and signs which characterize a disease. (Gr. *syndromos* a running together.)

Syringomyelia. A chronic disease involving cavitation and gliosis of the central canal of the spinal cord, sometimes extending to the medulla. (Gr. *syrinx* a tube; *myelos* marrow.)

Tanycyte. A specialized type of neuroglial cell in the ependymal floor of the third ventricle. (Gr. *tanyein* to stretch; *kytos* a cell.)

Tapetum. Fibres from corpus callosum forming the roof and lateral wall of posterior horn and the lateral wall of inferior horn of the lateral ventricle. (L. *tapete* a carpet.)

Tectum. Roof of midbrain. (L. roof.)

Tegmentum. The midbrain tegmentum, between substantia nigra and tectum is continuous with the pontine tegmentum, the dorsal region of pons. (L. a covering.)

Tela choroidea. A membrane developed from pia and ependyma, including choroid plexuses: forms roof of third ventricle and medial part of floor of body of lateral ventricles; roofs fourth ventricle. (L. *tela* a web; Gr. *chorion* membrane; *eidos* form.)

Telencephalon. The cerebral hemispheres; a subdivision of the prosencephalon. (Gr. *telos* end; *enkephalos* brain.)

Tentorium cerebelli. The horizontal dural fold between the cerebellum and cerebral hemispheres. (L. *tentorium* a tent.)

Thalamus. Part of the diencephalon, on each side of the third ventricle. (Gr. *thalamos* an inner room.)

Tomography. Sectional radiography of the body. (Gr. *tomos* cutting; *graphein* to write.)

Trigeminal. The fifth cranial nerve has three major divisions. (L. *trigeminus* threefold, triplets.)

Trochlear. The fourth cranial nerve supplies the superior oblique eye muscle, whose tendon angles through a ligamentous sling. (L. *trochlea* a pulley.)

Trophic. Pertains to functions concerned with nutrition and hence to growth: e.g. trophic influence of nerve growth factor, atrophy, hypertrophy. (Gr. *trophe* nourishment.)

Uncinate. Uncinate fasciculi: 1) a bundle connecting orbital surface of frontal lobe with cortex of temporal pole; 2) aberrant fibres from fastigial nucleus hook over opposite superior cerebellar peduncle. (L. *uncinus* hook-shaped.)

Uncus. A hook-shaped medial protrusion at the rostral end of the parahippocampal gyrus: olfactory cortex. (L. a hook.)

Uvula. Part of the inferior vermis of cerebellum. (L. a little grape.)

Vagus. The tenth cranial nerve is the longest, with an extensive distribution. (L. wandering.)

Vallecula cerebelli. The deep midline ventral fossa of the cerebellum, floored by the inferior vermis. (L. a little valley.)

Velum. The superior and inferior medullary vela are slender membranes roofing the fourth ventricle. (L. a curtain or veil.)

Ventricle. (L. *ventriculus* a little belly.)

Vermis. The median portion of the cerebellum. (L. a worm.)

Vertigo. Dizziness. (L. movement.)

Zona incerta. A rostral extension of the midbrain reticular formation into the subthalamus.

Bibliography

Barlow H.B. and Mollon J.D. (eds) (1982) *The Senses* Cambridge, Cambridge University Press.

Basmajian J.V. (1978) *Muscles Alive*. Baltimore, Williams & Wilkins.

Berg D.K. (1984) New neuronal growth factors. *Annu. Rev. Neurosci.* 7, 149–170.

Björklund A., Lindvall O., Isacson O., Brudin P., Wictorin K., Strecker R.E., Clarke D.J. and Dunnett S.B. (1987) Mechanisms of action of intracerebral neural implants: studies on nigral and striatal grafts to the lesioned striatum. *Trends Neurosci.* **10**, 509–516.

Bloedel J.R., Dichgans J. and Precht W. (eds) (1985) *Cerebellar Functions*. New York, Springer-Verlag.

Braitenberg V. (1967) Is the cerebellar cortex a biological clock in the millisecond range ? *Prog. Brain Res.* 25, 334–346.

Brazier M.A.B. and Petsche H. (eds) (1977) *Architectonics of the Cerebral Cortex*. New York, Raven Press.

Brodal A. (1981) *Neurological Anatomy in Relation to Clinical Medicine*. Oxford, Oxford University Press.

Brodal A. and Pompeiano O. (1957) The vestibular nuclei in the cat. *J. Anat. (Lond.)*, **91**, 438–454.

Brodmann K. (1909) *Vergleichende Lokalisationslehre der Grosshirnrinde in ihren Prinzipien dargestellt auf Grund des Zellenbaues*. Leipzig, Barth.

Brooks V.B. (1986) *The Neural Basis of Motor Control*. New York, Oxford University Press.

Carpenter M.B. and Sutin J. (1983) *Human Neuroanatomy*. Baltimore, Williams & Wilkins.

Cheney D.L. (ed.) (1990) Nerve growth factor: an update. *Neurosci. Facts, Fidia Res. Found.* **1**, 4

Choudhury B.R., Whitteridge D. and Wilson M.E. (1965) The function of the callosal connections of the visual cortex. *Quart. J. Exp. Physiol.* **50**, 214–219.

Cotman C.W. (1978) *Neuronal Plasticity*. New York, Raven Press.

Cowan W.M. and Cuénod M. (1975) *The use of Axonal Transport for Studies of Neuronal Connectivity*. Amsterdam, Elsevier.

Crapper D.R. and McLachlan P.H. (1987) *Memory, Aluminium and Alzheimer's Disease*, *see* Milgram et al. (1987), pp. 45–59.

Crosby E.C., Humphrey T. and Lauer E.W. (1962) *Correlative Anatomy of the Nervous System*. New York, Macmillan.

Davies A.M. and Lumsden A. (1990) Ontogeny of the somatosensory system: origins and early development of primary sensory neurons. *Annu. Rev. Neurosci.* **13**, 61–73.

Davis K.L. and Mohs R.C. (1986) Cholinergic drugs in Alzheimer's disease. *New. Engl. J. Med.* **13**, 1286–1287.

Davson H. (1980) *Physiology of the Eye.* London, Churchill Livingstone.

Daw N.W., Jensen, R.J. and Brunken W.J. (1990) Rod pathways in mammalian retinae. *Trends in Neuroscience.* **13**, 3, 110–115.

De Robertis E. (1967) Ultrastructure and cytochemistry of the synaptic region. *Science* **156**, 907–914.

del Río-Hortega P. (1920) La microglía y su transformación en células en basoncito y cuerpos gránulo-adiposos. *Trab. Lab. Invest. Biol.* Madrid. **18**, 37–82.

Eccles J.C. (1977) An instruction—selection theory of learning in the cerebellar cortex. *Brain Res.* **127**, 327–352.

Eccles J.C., Llinás R. and Sasaki K. (1966) The excitatory synaptic action of climbing fibres on the Purkinje cells of the cerebellum. *J. Physiol. (Lond).* **182**, 268–296.

Emson P.C. (1983) *Chemical Neuroanatomy.* New York, Raven Press.

Fisken R.A., Garey L.J. and Powell T.P.S. (1975) The intrinsic, association and commissural connections of area 17 of the visual cortex. *Phil. Trans. R. Soc. Lond.* **B, 272**, 487–536.

FitzGerald M.J.T. (1985) *Neuroanatomy Basic and Applied.* London, Baillière Tindall.

Forsyth D.R., Surmon D.J., Morgan R.A. and Wilcock G.K. (1989) Clinical experience with and side effects of Tacrine Hydrochloride in Alzheimer's disease: a pilot study. *Age and Ageing.* **18**, 223–229.

Garey L.J., Jones E.G. and Powell T.P.S. (1968) Interrelationships of striate and extrastriate cortex with the primary relay sites of the visual pathway. *J. Neurol. Neurosurg., Psychiat.* **31**, 137–157.

Gordon C., Hewer R.L., and Wade D.L. (1987) Dysphagia in acute stroke. *Brit. Med. J.* **295**, 411–414.

Grant, J.C.B. (1949) *Atlas of Anatomy.* London, Baillière Tindall

Graybiel A.M. (1977) Direct and indirect preoculomotor pathways of the brainstem: an autoradiographic study of the pontine reticular formation in the cat. *J. Comp. Neurol.* **175**, 37–78.

Grossman A. and Besser G.M. (1985) Prolactinomas. *Br. Med. J.,* **290**, 182–184.

Hökfelt T., Millhorn D., Seroogy K. et al. (1987) Coexistence of peptides with classical neurotransmitters. *Experientia.* **43**, 768–780.

Hubel D.H. and Wiesel T.N. (1974) Sequence regularity and geometry of orientation columns in the monkey striate cortex. *J. Comp. Neurol.* **158**, 267–294.

Hubel T.H., Wiesel T.N. and Le Vay S. (1977) Plasticity of ocular dominance columns in monkey striate cortex. *Phil. Trans. R. Soc. Lond. (Biol)* **278**, 377–409.

Humphrey P.P.A., Feniuk W. and Perren M.J. (1990) Anti-migraine drugs in development: advances in serotonin receptor pharmacology. *Headache,*

30 (suppl. 1), 12–16.

Hutchings M. and Weller R.O. (1986) Anatomical relationships of the pia mater to cerebral blood vessels in man. *J. Neurosurg.* **65**, 316–325

International Nomenclature Committee (1980) *Nomina Anatomica.* 5th edn. Baltimore, Williams & Wilkins.

Ito Masao (1984) *The Cerebellum and Neural Control.* New York, Raven Press.

Jeanmonod D., Rice F.L. and Van der Loos H. (1981) Mouse somatosensory cortex: alterations in the barrelfield following receptor injury at different early postnatal ages. *Neurosci.* **6**, 1503–1535.

Johansson H. and Silfvenius H. (1977) Axon-collateral activation by dorsal spinocerebellar tract fibres of group 1 relay cells of nucleus Z in the cat medulla oblongata. *J. Physiol. (Lond).* **265**, 341–369.

Jones D.G. (1975) *Synapses and Synaptosomes.* New York, Wiley.

Jones D.G. (1988) Synaptic trends and synaptic remodelling in the developing and mature neocortex, *see* Petit and Ivy (1988), pp. 21–42.

Kandel E.R. and Schwartz J.H. (1983) *Principles of Neural Science.* New York, Elsevier.

Kitai S.T. and Weinberg J. (1968) Tactile discrimination study of the dorsal column system in the cat. *Exp. Brain Res.* **6**, 234–246.

Kretschmann H.J. (1988) Localisation of the corticospinal fibres in the internal capsule in man. *J. Anat. (Lond.).* **160**, 219–225.

Kuffler S.W. (1973) The single-cell approach in the visual system and the study of receptive fields. *Invest. Ophthalmol.* **12**, 794–813.

Langley J.N. (1921) *The Autonomic Nervous System.* Cambridge, Heffer.

Levi-Montalcini R. and Hamburger V. (1951) Selective growth-stimulating effects of mouse sarcoma on the sensory and sympathetic nervous system of the chick embryo. *J. Exp. Zool.* **116**, 321–361.

Levick W.R. and Dvorak D.R. (eds) (1986) The retina – from molecules to networks. *Trends Neurosci.* **9**, 5.

MacFadyen, D.J. (1984) Posterior column dysfunction in cervical spondylotic myelopathy. *Can J. Neurol. Sci.* **11**, 365–370.

MacKay A.P.V. (1984) High dopamine in the left amygdala. *Trends Neurosci.* **7**, 107–108.

Madrazo I. (1990) Cell implantation in Parkinson's disease. *Br. Med. J.* **301**, 874.

Marsden C.D. (1982) Basal ganglia disease. *Lancet,* ii, 1141–1147.

Melzack R. and Wall P.D. (1965) Pain mechanisms: a new theory. *Science* **150**, 971–979.

Milgram N.W., MacLeod, C.W. and Petit T.L. (1987) *Neuroplasticity, Learning and Memory.* New York, Alan R. Liss.

Nieuwenhuys, R. (1985) *Chemoarchitecture of the Brain.* New York, Springer-Verlag.

Olesen J. and Edvinsson L. (1991) Migraine: a research field matured for the basic neurosciences. *Trends Neurosci.* **14**, 3–5.

Ottoson, D. (1983) *Physiology of the Nervous System.* London, Macmillan.

Papez J.W. (1937) A proposed mechanism of emotion. *Arch. Neurol. Psychiatry.* **38**, 725–743.

Parnavelas J.G. and Papadopoulos G.C. (1989) The monoaminergic inner-vation of the cerebral cortex is not diffuse and nonspecific. *Trends Neurosci.* **2**, 315–319.

Patten J. (1977) *Neurological Differential Diagnosis*. London, Starke.

Panfield W. and Rasmussen T. (1950) *The Cerebral Cortex of Man*. New York, Macmillan.

Pert C.B., Snowman A.M. and Snyder S.H. (1974) Localization of opiate receptor binding in synaptic vesicles of the rat brain. *Brain Res.* **70**, 184–188.

Petersen S.E., Fox P.T., Posner M.I., Mintum, M. and Raichle M.E. (1988) Positron emission tomographic studies of the cortical anatomy of single word processing. *Nature.* **331**, 585–589.

Petit T.L. and Ivy G.O. (eds) (1988) *Neural Plasticity, A Lifespan Approach*. New York, Alan R. Liss.

Petrie K., Conaglen J.V., Thompson L. and Chamberlain K. (1989) Effect of melatonin on jet lag after long haul flights. *Br. Med. J.* **298**, 705–707.

Pramod R., Saxena P.R. and Ferrari M.D. (1989) 5-HT$_1$-like receptor agonists and the pathophysiology of migraine. *Trends Pharmacol. Sci.* **10**, 200–204.

Press G.A., Amaral D.G. and Squire L.R. (1989) Hippocampal abnormali-ties in amnesic patients revealed by high-resolution magnetic resonance imaging. *Nature.* **341**, 54–57.

Purves D. and Lichtman J.W. (1985) *Principles of Neural Development*. Massachusetts, Sinauer Associates.

Ramón y Cajal S. (1900) *Textura del Sistema Nervioso del Hombre y de los Vertebrados*. Madrid, Moya.

Ramón y Cajal S. (1908) Structure et connexion des neurons. In *Les Prixs Nobel en 1906*, pp. 1–25. Stockholm, Norstedt and Söner.

Ramón y Cajal S. (1911) *Histologie du système nerveux de l'homme et des vertébrés*. Paris, Maloine.

Rexed B. (1954) A cytoarchitectonic atlas of the spinal cord in the cat. *J. Comp. Neurol.* **100**, 297–379.

Reynolds D.V. (1969) Surgery in the rat during electrical analgesia induced by focal brain stimulation. *Science.* **164**, 444–445.

Reynolds G.P. (1983) Increased concentrations and lateral asymmetry of amygdala dopamine in schizophrenia. *Nature.* **305**, 527–529.

Sarnat H.B. and Netsky M.G. (1974) *Evolution of the Nervous System*. Oxford, Oxford University Press.

Shepherd G.M. (1990) *The Synaptic Organization of the Brain*. Oxford, Oxford University Press.

Sigal R., Doyon D., Halimi P.H. and Atlan H. (1988) *Magnetic Resonance Imaging*. New York, Springer-Verlag.

Sinclair D.C. (1967) *Cutaneous Sensation*. Oxford, Oxford University Press.

Snyder S.H. (1986) *Drugs and the Brain*. New York, Scientific American Books.

Springer S.P. and Deutsch G. (1981) *Left Brain, Right Brain*. San Francisco, Freeman.

Standaert D.G., Saper, C.B. and Needleman P. (1985) Atriopeptin: potent hormone and potential neuromediator. *Trends Neurosci.* **8**, 509–511.

Stein D.G., Rosen J.J. and Butters N. (1974) *Plasticity and Recovery of Function in the Central Nervous System.* New York, Academic Press.

Strata P. (ed.) (1989) *The Olivocerebellar System in Motor Control.* New York, Springer-Verlag.

Summers W.K., Majovski L.V., Marsh G.M., Tachiki, K. and Kling A. (1986) Oral tetrahydroaminoacridine in long-term treatment of senile dementia, Alzheimer type. *N. Engl. J. Med.* **315**, 1241–1245.

Summers W.K., Tachiki, K.H. and Kling A. (1989) Tacrine in the treatment of Alzheimer's disease. *Eur. Neurol.* **29** (suppl. 3), 28–32.

Sunderland S. (1945) Intraneural topography of the radial, median and ulnar nerves. *Brain.* **68**, 243.

Sunderland S. (1978) *Nerves and Nerve Injuries*, 2nd edn. London, Churchill Livingstone.

Szentágothai J. (1985) The neuronal architectonic principle of the neocortex. *Ann. Acad. Bras. Cienc.* **57**, 249–258.

Szentágothai J. (1987) The architecture of neural centres and understanding neural organization. In: McLennan H., Ledsome J.R., McIntosh C.H.S., Jones D.R. (eds), *Advances in Physiological Research.* New York, Plenum Press.

Thompson R.F. (1987) Identification of an essential trace circuit in the mammalian brain, *see* Milgram et al. (1987), pp 151–172.

Todd A.J. and Sullivan A.C. (1990) Light microscope study of the coexistence of GABA-like and glycine-like immunoreactivities in the spinal cord of the rat. *J. Comp. Neurol.* **296**, 496–505.

Vallbo Ä.B. (1971) Muscle spindle response at the onset of isometric voluntary contractions in man. Time difference between fusimotor and skeletomotor effects. *J. Physiol. (Lond.)* **218**, 405–431.

Vida S., Gauthier L. and Gauthier S. (1989) Canadian collaborative study of tetrahydroaminoacridine (THA) and lecithin treatment of Alzheimer's disease: effect on mood. *Can. J. Psychiatry.* **34**, 165–170.

Vierck C.J. (1974) Tactile movement detection and discrimination following dorsal column lesions in monkeys. *Exp. Brain Res.* **20**, 331–346.

Von Voss Hermann (1971) Tabelle der absoluten und relativen muskelspindelzahlen der menschlichen skelettmuskulatur. *Anat. Anz.* **129**, 562–572.

Wall P.D. (1970) The sensory and motor role of impulses travelling in the dorsal columns towards cerebral cortex. *Brain.* **93**, 505–524.

Wall P.D. (1978) The gate control theory of pain mechanisms. A re-examination and re-statement. *Brain.* **101**, 1–18.

Wall P.D. and Noordenbos W. (1977) Sensory functions which remain in man after complete transection of dorsal columns. *Brain.* **100**, 641–653.

Walton J. (1987) *Introduction to Clinical Neuroscience*, 2nd edn. London, Baillière Tindall.

Warwick R. (1953) Representation of the extraocular muscles in the oculomotor nuclei of the monkey. *J. Comp. Neurol.* **98**, 449–504.

Weller R.O. (1990) Personal communication.

Williams A. (1990) Cell implantation in Parkinson's disease. *Br. Med. J.* **301**, 301–302.

Williams P.L., Warwick R., Dyson M. and Bannister L.H. (1989) *Gray's Anatomy*. Edinburgh, Churchill Livingstone.

Willoughby E.W. and Anderson N.E. (1984) Lower cranial nerve motor function in unilateral vascular lesions of the cerebral hemisphere. *Br. Med. J.* **289**, 791–794.

Wysocki C.J. (1979) Neurobehavioral evidence for the involvement of the vomeronasal system in mammalian reproduction. *Neurosci. Biobehav. Rev.* **3**, 301–341.

Young J.Z. (1978) *Programs of the Brain*. Oxford, Oxford University Press.

Zaimis E. and Knight J. (eds.) (1972) *Nerve Growth Factor and its Antiserum*. London, Athlone Press.

Zeki S.M. (1970) Interhemispheric connections of prestriate cortex in monkey. *Brain Res.* **19**, 63–75.

Zhang E.T., Inman C.B.E. and Weller R.O. (1990) Interrelationships of the pia mater and the perivascular (Virchow-Robin) spaces of the human cerebrum. *J. Anat.* **170**, 111–123.

Index

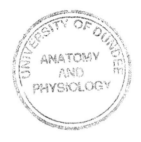